PREVENTING BOUNDARY VIOLATIONS IN CLINICAL PRACTICE

Preventing Boundary Violations in Clinical Practice

THOMAS G. GUTHEIL
ARCHIE BRODSKY

THE GUILFORD PRESS
New York   London

© 2008 Thomas G. Gutheil and Archie Brodsky
Published by The Guilford Press
A Division of Guilford Publications, Inc.
72 Spring Street, New York, NY 10012
www.guilford.com

Paperback edition 2011

Printed in the United States of America

This book is printed on acid-free paper.

Last digit is print number: 9 8 7 6 5 4 3 2

Library of Congress Cataloging-in-Publication Data

Gutheil, Thomas G.
  Preventing boundary violations in clinical practice / Thomas G. Gutheil,
Archie Brodsky.
      p. ; cm.
  Includes bibliographical references and index.
  ISBN 978-1-59385-691-5 (hardcover : alk. paper)
  ISBN 978-1-4625-0443-5 (paperback : alk. paper)
  1. Psychotherapist and patient—Moral and ethical aspects.   2. Psychotherapists—
Professional ethics.   3. Boundaries—Psychological aspects.   4. Interpersonal relations.
I. Brodsky, Archie.   II. Title.
  [DNLM: 1. Professional–Patient Relations—ethics.   2. Psychotherapy—ethics.
3. Counseling—ethics.   4. Ethics, Professional.   5. Transfer (Psychology)
WM 62 G984p 2008]
  RC480.8.G88 2008
  616.89′14—dc22

                                                                2008002942

To the clinicians, patients, victims, and attorneys
who over the decades
have taught us all about boundaries

About the Authors

Thomas G. Gutheil, MD, is Professor of Psychiatry, Department of Psychiatry, Beth Israel Deaconess Medical Center, Harvard Medical School, where he is Assistant Director of Medical Student Training and Co-Founder of the Program in Psychiatry and the Law. One of the world's leading forensic psychiatrists, he is a past president of the American Academy of Psychiatry and the Law and current president of the International Academy of Law and Mental Health. Dr. Gutheil is coauthor of the widely used *Clinical Handbook of Psychiatry and the Law,* which won the American Psychiatric Association's Manfred S. Guttmacher Award for outstanding contribution to the forensic psychiatric literature (an award Dr. Gutheil has shared three times). Among his numerous other awards and honors are the American Psychiatric Association's 2000 Isaac Ray Award for outstanding contributions to forensic psychiatry and several awards for teaching, including a Lifetime Achievement in Mentoring Award at Harvard Medical School. Among Dr. Gutheil's more than 250 scholarly journal articles and book chapters are publications recognized as foundational in the description and analysis of boundary issues in clinical practice. Dr. Gutheil lectures worldwide and is regularly consulted by attorneys, licensing boards, and institutions on boundary questions, risk management, and malpractice prevention.

Archie Brodsky is Research Associate in the Department of Psychiatry, Beth Israel Deaconess Medical Center, Harvard Medical School, where he is Co-Founder of the Program in Psychiatry and the Law. He is coauthor of *Sexual Dilemmas for the Helping Professional,* a pioneering work on clinical and ethical boundaries in mental health treatment. Among the 15 trade and professional books he has coauthored in the mental health field are *Love and Addiction; The Truth about Addiction and Recovery; Medical Choices, Medical Chances;* and *Clinical Supervision in Alcohol and Drug Abuse Counseling.* A co-winner (with Dr. Gutheil) of the Guttmacher Award, Mr. Brodsky is a member and former chair of the Human Rights Committee at Massachusetts Mental Health Center.

Acknowledgments

Much of the thinking in this book derives from years of discussions with members of the Program in Psychiatry and the Law, Beth Israel Deaconess Medical Center, Harvard Medical School. The Program was co-founded and co-led (together with the authors) for a quarter-century at Massachusetts Mental Health Center by Harold Bursztajn, MD, with whom we have enjoyed (and we do mean enjoyed) a stimulating dialogue throughout that time. Robert Simon, MD, Kenneth Pope, PhD, Glen Gabbard, MD, Gary Schoener, PhD, Larry Strasburger, MD, and Paul Appelbaum, MD, provided extensive conceptual contributions over those decades, as well as encouragement and coauthorship of related work.

We are indebted to several anonymous reviewers for appreciating the general applicability of the clinical and ethical principles presented here, transcending differences in theory and practice. The insights of these reviewers have guided us in speaking ecumenically to a broad readership of clinicians. Not at all anonymous was the contribution of Robert Goisman, MD, who showed with concrete examples how the same principles can be understood and applied in cognitive-behavioral as well as psychodynamic terms. The book is richer for his input and that of Frank Dattilio, PhD, on the practical challenges faced by clinicians in maintaining boundaries in today's institutional, regulatory, and legal environments. Linda Jorgenson, JD, Michael Commons, PhD, Patrice Miller, PhD, Eric Drogin, JD, PhD, and Patricia Illingworth, JD, PhD, also contributed useful ideas and information.

This book could not have evolved and ripened as it did without the steadiness of purpose (and personnel) shown by an independently owned publisher, The Guilford Press. We are deeply grateful for Guilford's sustained interest and faith in this project, which has benefited immeasurably from the insight, judgment, patience, and tact of our editor, Jim Nageotte, ably assisted by Jane Keislar. Barbara Watkins's editorial intervention, as skillful as it was timely, enabled us to communicate our ideas more efficiently and inclusively. Ellen Dubie, Tom Gutheil's office assistant at Massachusetts Mental Health Center, provided valuable administrative assistance.

Finally, Tom thanks Shannon, Janine, Alexa, Tia, and Dylan for love without boundaries and support in countless ways. Archie thanks Ed Bauman as well as various friends for keeping him on track, and most of all Vicki for her understanding, steady support, and many sacrifices on the home front.

Contents

PART III. Implications

Introduction

Dilemmas concerning the boundaries of the therapist–patient relationship arise commonly, and well-intentioned clinicians at all levels of training and experience struggle with them daily. When you are driving to work and you see one of your patients jogging at the side of the road, do you wave to each other? What do you do when you are at a party, cocktail in hand, only to see a patient of yours walk in the door? How (and how quickly) do you respond when a patient suddenly hugs you at the end of a session? Do you accept a gift that a patient brings to make up for causing you some inconvenience?

Questions like these have serious clinical, ethical, and legal implications. How they are resolved can have both an immediate and long-term impact on a patient's well-being and progress in treatment. For the clinician, the potential consequences extend to termination of employment and loss of license. Dual relationships (including sexual boundary violations) were the most frequent cause of disciplinary actions against psychologists in the United States in the period from 1983 to 2005 and the second leading cause among Canadian psychologists between 1983 and 2006 (Pope & Vasquez, 2007). Alleged boundary violations are also a leading cause of malpractice suits against mental health professionals.

There are clear cases of boundary violation, most often cases of sexual or financial exploitation. However, the great majority of boundary questions that arise in clinical practice are outgrowths of what T. S. Eliot called "a hundred indecisions, . . . a hundred visions and revisions" that occur in the normal course of therapy. Subtle determinations must be made day by day, moment by moment, requiring understanding and

1

judgment on the part of the clinician and (if possible) the patient. Subsequent inquiries may involve a supervisor, administrator, forensic evaluator, professional society ethics committee, licensing board, attorney, judge, or jury. All of these actors may bring different perspectives to the inquiry, perspectives that ought to be informed by current knowledge and scrupulous case-by-case analysis. Still, it is the clinician—any clinician—who is on the front line, making immediate decisions in the interest of the patient.

Inexperience and inadequate training do get clinicians in trouble, but not even the most experienced therapist is home free. On the contrary, as is made clear in Chapter 10 of this book, age and status bring special vulnerabilities. A therapist dealing with illness, divorce, sexual dysfunction, unfulfilled ambitions, retirement, and mortality may feel driven to cross previously sacrosanct lines. There is also the pitfall of feeling "above the law," that is, above professional review and sanctions. No one is so eminent that he or she cannot benefit from learning, reflection, supervision, consultation, and documentation. The vulnerability to crossing boundaries in nontherapeutic ways comes from elemental needs and feelings, together with a misdirection of the clinician's desire to help and a misapplication of the assumption of mutuality and reciprocity in human relationships (Genova, 2001).

Whether you are a psychiatrist, a clinical psychologist, a substance abuse counselor, or a community mental health worker, you will experience the relational pushes and pulls of the clinician–patient dyad. These relational currents and the ethical issues that flow from them play a part in cognitive-behavioral therapy (CBT), dialectical behavior therapy (DBT), reality therapy, family systems therapy, psychodynamic therapy, and any other type of "helping" relationship (Wachtel, 2007). To be sure, if you provide exposure therapy for phobias or panic disorder, or applied behavior analysis for autism or developmental disability, you will work within different boundaries from those of an insight-oriented therapist in private office practice. Likewise, if you live among residents you supervise in a group home, you will be exposed and accessible to your clients in ways for which there is no parallel in one-to-one psychotherapy. Such contextual variables necessarily figure in boundary determinations.

Nonetheless, when you dispense something—whether pills or words—that a patient may experience as a magic potion that can make him or her well, the patient may develop an emotional attachment and make personal attributions about you. Whether or not you think in terms of the unconscious and of transference and countertransference, you still offer, in some form, the promise of life, hope, or improved health to a person in pain and fear. Thus, it is not just a therapist's lapses and weaknesses that lead to boundary problems. Rather, it is the interaction of two separate and unique individuals. The pressure to lose perspective can come from the therapist, the patient, or both, and each patient brings a new set of challenges.

In managing the constantly shifting boundaries of the patient–therapist dyad, then, there is no substitute for clinical understanding, whether that understanding is expressed in terms of "transference" and "countertransference" or what some CBT practitioners refer to as "therapy-interfering behaviors" (Linehan, 1993). For a proper understanding and resolution of boundary questions in daily practice, we need to shift the focus from the surface to the depth of a patient–therapist interchange—that is, from a given act to its therapeutic (or countertherapeutic) purpose, meaning, impact, and—above all—context.

AN EVOLVING UNDERSTANDING

It is difficult to identify one precise point at which the notion of boundaries in relation to therapeutic work first entered the field. Freud captured one dimension of boundary theory when he likened the dispassion and objectivity of the psychoanalyst to that of a surgeon. He also cautioned against misreading transference love as a real experience and against personal involvement with the analysand. Most important, he made clear that it would be a disaster for the patient and the treatment if the analyst acted on the patient's sexual overtures (Freud, 1915/1958c). Yet, Freud himself conducted an analysis while walking with an analysand on the banks of the Danube. Freud also

> sent patients postcards, lent them books, gave them gifts, corrected them when they spoke in a misinformed manner about his family members, provided them with extensive financial support in some cases, and on at least one occasion gave a patient a meal. (Gutheil & Gabbard, 1993, p. 189, citing Lipton, 1977)

Much of this activity might be explained as "other times, other customs."

Similar boundary excursions, and worse, occurred regularly in the early decades of psychoanalysis and psychotherapy. A famous instance was the alleged affair between Carl Jung, an early follower who broke with Freud, and Sabina Spielrein, his first analysand and, later, research assistant (Gabbard, 1995a; Person, 2003). Another follower of Freud, Sandor Ferenczi, analyzed his mistress and then her daughter, with whom Ferenczi fell in love. The three—mother, daughter, and Ferenczi—lived together for a while (Gabbard, 1995a; Hoffer, 1991). Donald Winnicott, an important figure in the early development of child psychology, analyzed a close friend, socialized with patients, and took a child patient into his house as a boarder (Little, 1990; Winnicott, 1949). Masud Khan, a protégé of Winnicott and a striking, charismatic, and perhaps even psychopathic figure in early British analysis,

> gossiped freely about his A-list social life . . . and his other patients, going so far as to arrange a liaison between [his analysand] and a female patient. . . . The three of them—the two patients and their analyst—even played poker together. (Khan cheated.) (Boynton, 2002, p. C2)

By modern reckoning—perhaps by any reckoning—these extremes clearly deviated from basic therapeutic principles and probably caused harm to the patients involved. Strikingly, in these early incidents, little harm accrued to the therapists, and the latter were not uncommonly supported by colleagues, including Freud (Gabbard, 1995a).

By mid-century the recommended "surgeon-like" detachment of Freud and his followers (whether or not actually adhered to) generated a reaction in the form of "humanistic" therapies that permitted greater warmth and self-disclosure on the part of the therapist (see Farber, 2006). In the 1960s intense feeling and meaningful experience were sought through freewheeling therapeutic approaches, from therapeutic use of lysergic acid (LSD) to nude marathons in hot tubs. Various "communal" therapies (sometimes led by self-aggrandizing gurus) promoted a virtually complete relaxation of boundaries, in some cases extending to outright promotion of therapist–patient sex (e.g., Shepard, 1971).

The first significant awareness of problematic boundary issues in the form of sexual misconduct emerged from the clinical research of Masters and Johnson (1970), who observed numerous cases of sexual dysfunction resulting from sexual relations with psychotherapists. They went so far as to recommend that therapist sexual misconduct be prosecuted as a form of rape (Masters & Johnson, 1976). At around the same time, the famous case of *Roy v. Hartogs* (1975) set a precedent for large civil damage awards for victims of such misconduct (Freeman & Roy, 1976). Other highly publicized cases followed, along with national survey research on the extent of reported or self-reported sexual misconduct by mental health professionals as well as physicians (Gartrell, Herman, Olarte, Feldstein, & Localio, 1986, 1987; Gartrell, Herman, Olarte, Localio, & Feldstein, 1988; Gartrell, Milliken, Goodson, Thiemann, & Lo, 1992; Gechtman, 1989;

Holroyd & Brodsky, 1977; Kardener, Fuller, & Mensh, 1973, 1976; Perry, 1976; Pope, Keith-Spiegel, & Tabachnick, 1986; Pope, Tabachnick, & Keith-Spiegel, 1987; Searight & Campbell, 1993). Reviewing the major incidence surveys of the 1970s and 1980s (while acknowledging the uncertain reliability of self-reports), Pope (1988) found aggregate averages of 8.3% of male therapists and 1.7% of female therapists who reported sexual involvement with patients or clients. (For other reviews of incidence data, see Gabbard & Nadelson, 1995; Hankins, Vera, Barnard, & Herkov, 1994; Pope, 1990b, 2001; Schoener, 1989b; Williams, 1992.) Among more than 1,000 cases of sexual misconduct of all kinds seen up to that time by the Walk-In Counseling Center of Minneapolis, Gonsiorek (1989) found that approximately 80% of the cases involved male therapist–female client, 5% male therapist–male client, 2% female therapist–male client, and 13% female therapist–female client. These estimates have not changed substantially since then, although incidence rates undoubtedly have fluctuated with variations in training practices, disciplinary sanctions, and publicity.

The articles that began to appear in the literature about this formerly taboo area in the 1970s and 1980s generally used the term "boundary violation" simply to describe sexual relations between therapist and patient (e.g., Stone, 1976). Early books on the subject were similarly selective in focus (Burgess & Hartman, 1986; Gabbard, 1989; Pope & Bouhoutsos, 1986; Smith & Bisbing, 1988). Some of these books focused on the personal experiences of patients (Bates & Brodsky, 1989; Freeman & Roy, 1976; Plasil, 1985; Walker & Young, 1986) or of therapists (Rutter, 1989a). A compendium of clinical, research, teaching, administrative, and policy perspectives on the subject came out of the pioneering work of the Walk-In Counseling Center of Minneapolis (Schoener, Milgrom, Gonsiorek, Luepker, & Conroe, 1989).

Two sensational cases crystallized public awareness of therapist sexual misconduct and therapeutic boundaries, for good and for ill. One was a 1989 Colorado case dramatized in the PBS *Frontline* documentary "My Doctor, My Lover," in which psychiatrist Jason Richter was held liable for having a sexual relationship with a woman who had recently been his patient (Storring, 1991). This case was complicated by the defense's aggressive attempts to discredit the plaintiff's subsequent therapist, who had made the well-intentioned error of involving herself in her patient's legal action (Edelwich & Brodsky, 1991, pp. 228–229; Thompson, 1989). The other was the Massachusetts case of Margaret Bean-Bayog, MD, a Harvard-trained, Harvard-affiliated psychiatrist (in which Dr. Gutheil was retained as an expert by Dr. Bean-Bayog's attorneys). Arguably, this was not a case of boundary violation at all, but was simply made to appear that way by weeks of lurid headlines. Dr. Bean-Bayog had treated Paul Lozano, a medical student with a history of severe depression, suicidal feelings, and sadomasochistic preoccupations, as well as significant substance abuse. Mr. Lozano died of an overdose of cocaine months after leaving treatment. His family sued after the discovery of concrete objects—flash cards, children's books, and stuffed animals—which Dr. Bean-Bayog had used early in therapy to help the patient cope with his intense neediness and dependency while she took a long vacation (he subsequently "outgrew" his need for such toys). Even more damaging was the discovery of private notes in which Dr. Bean-Bayog had unwisely recorded the fantasies she had in response to the patient's sadistic fantasies. These notes, which Mr. Lozano apparently had stolen from her home, were disclosed to the media by the plaintiff's attorney and portrayed as real-life communications. The public was given the impression that Dr. Bean-Bayog had totally lost objectivity and become emotionally enmeshed and possibly sexually involved with Mr. Lozano. To avoid further distortions, humiliations, and the risk of financial ruin, Dr. Bean-Bayog voluntarily gave up her medical license, and she and her insurer agreed to settle the civil case. As a result, the case was essentially tried in the media instead of in the proper forums (Maltsberger, 1995).

At about the same time, two larger social and professional movements appear to have combined to broaden the concept of boundaries in psychotherapy beyond the single issue of sexual relations between therapist and patient. The first was the growing awareness of child sexual abuse; clinicians observed the resultant sensitivity in survivors to suggestions of potential abuse that might occur when therapy began to feel personal or eroticized. The second development was observation of boundary problems experienced by patients with certain personality disorders such as borderline personality disorder, both in their families of origin and subsequently in the therapy; patients would sometimes reenact their childhood boundary confusions with the therapist (Averill et al., 1989; Gabbard, 1993; Gabbard & Wilkinson, 1994; Gutheil, 1985, 1989, 1991; Herman, Perry, & Van der Kolk, 1989).

From these two trends emerged a paradigm of multiple forms of boundary phenomena that became the focus of both theoretical and practical discussion (Borys & Pope, 1989; Epstein & Simon, 1990; Gutheil & Gabbard, 1993; Simon, 1992). Book-length examinations of this broader conception of boundary maintenance were addressed to psychoanalytically oriented therapists (Gabbard & Lester, 2002), frontline counselors and staff members in human services agencies (Edelwich & Brodsky,

1991; Reamer, 2001), and psychotherapists and helping professionals generally (Epstein, 1994; Peterson, 1992). Other books have dealt with areas such as clinical and forensic issues in the treatment of victims of sexual exploitation by therapists (Pope, 1994), assessment and rehabilitation of offending therapists (Irons & Schneider, 1999; Strean, 1993), and boundaries in supervisory and academic contexts (Celenza, 2007).

One benefit of the heightened interest in boundary violations and sexual misconduct in the 1980s and early 1990s was to stimulate quantitative research on a range of interconnected subjects. In addition to the incidence data summarized earlier, researchers investigated therapists' feelings of attraction to patients (Bernsen, Tabachnick, & Pope, 1994; Pope et al., 1986; Pope & Tabachnick, 1993; Rodolfa et al., 1994), therapists' attitudes and behavior with respect to various forms of physical contact and other boundary incursions (Borys & Pope, 1989; Herman, Gartrell, Olarte, Feldstein, & Localio, 1987; Lamb & Catanzaro, 1998; Pope, 2001; Pope et al., 1987; Stake & Oliver, 1991; for cross-cultural comparison, see Miller, Commons, & Gutheil, 2006), sexual and nonsexual relationships with former clients (Akamatsu, 1988; Anderson & Kitchener, 1996; Conte et al., 1989; Herman et al., 1987; Lamb et al., 1994; Pope et al., 1987), therapists' reports of patients' sexual involvements with previous therapists (Gartrell et al., 1987; Pope & Vetter, 1991), and sexual involvement between students or trainees and their teachers or supervisors (Bartell & Rubin, 1990; Clayton, Weeks, & Vieweg, 1991; Gartrell et al., 1988; Glaser & Thorpe, 1986; Heru, Strong, Price, & Recupero, 2004; Lamb & Catanzaro, 1998; Pope, Levenson, & Schover, 1979). Epstein, Simon, and Kay (1992) surveyed psychiatrists to test the usefulness of Epstein & Simon's (1990) "Exploitation Index" (described in Chapter 13). Some 43% of the respondents reported that the warning signs compiled in the index alerted them to at least one potentially counterproductive behavior in their practice. Some 29% made changes in future treatment practice as a result.

Predictably, the intense (some might say obsessive) preoccupation with boundaries in therapy that had taken hold by the 1990s led to a swing of the pendulum in the opposite direction. Some commentators have expressed concern that professional associations and leading figures in the field are giving practitioners and trainees an overly restrictive, liability-driven message that emphasizes "don'ts" at the expense of "dos" (Coale, 1998; Kroll, 2001; Lazarus, 1994; Martinez, 2000). Such training, these critics argue, does not allow for legitimate variations in treatment methods. As a result, it may inhibit therapists from exercising appropriate flexibility and creativity in the patient's best interest. Indeed, a therapist who is too fixated on avoiding boundary violations may be risking liability for other forms of substandard or unethical practice, such as failing to maintain an effective treatment alliance or showing disrespect for a patient.

This serious concern is addressed in Chapter 11 of this book. In fact, pertinent areas of therapeutic technique and ethics are being reassessed—for example, the question of appropriate self-disclosures by therapists (Barrett & Berman, 2001; Farber, 2006; Knox & Hill, 2003; Maroda, 1994; Psychopathology Committee of the Group for the Advancement of Psychiatry, 2001; Renik, 1995; Stricker & Fisher, 1990; see Chapter 5). However, in most cases it is not the American Psychiatric Association, the American Psychological Association, or the National Association of Social Workers that applies ethical guidelines in a sweeping, formulaic manner. Rather, it is state boards of registration and the courts that sometimes lose sight of the individualized, context-dependent clinical perspective that should inform the assessment of alleged boundary violations. The insensitivity of some regulatory boards and the susceptibility of juries to inflammatory testimony and arguments are realities for which clinicians must be prepared.

Nonetheless, it is not risk management that properly drives clinical decisions. Good therapeutic technique is practiced in the interest of the patient's well-being and development. As a bonus, good therapy is also good risk management. This book is informed, therefore, by the fundamental principle that boundary issues are clinical issues first, ethical issues second, and legal issues third. An ethically and legally defensible negotiation of boundaries between patient and therapist is grounded in an understanding of the patient and the clinical process.

THERAPEUTIC BOUNDARIES IN THE POPULAR IMAGINATION

Fictional and dramatic representations hold up a mirror to the explorations and debates taking place in the professions. F. Scott Fitzgerald's *Tender Is the Night*, as novel and film, centers on a psychiatrist who falls in love with and marries a patient. Interestingly, in light of what has since been learned about risk factors that make patients vulnerable to sexual involvement with therapists, the patient, Nicole Diver, had had an incestuous relationship with her father (see Chapter 10). In this novel, published in 1934, the psychiatrist, Dick Diver (like the early psychoanalysts discussed above), did not have to face ethics hearings and professional sanctions for his involvement with a patient, although the marriage as well as Dr. Diver's professional relationship with his partner in practice did break up for reasons directly or indirectly related to Nicole's mental illness.

Immediately after World War II, Alfred Hitchcock's movie *Spellbound* dramatized a romantic relationship between therapist and patient that included many boundary excursions—for example, flight from the hospital resembling a "field trip," a picnic together, and other "nontraditional" activities. In the decades that followed, boundary excursions were portrayed in Brian DePalma's *Dressed to Kill* and *Lovesick*; the former includes a homicidal psychiatrist. Interesting twists on the above can be found in the films *Prince of Tides* and *Final Analysis*. Both involve a sexual and romantic relationship between the psychiatrist and the *sibling* of a patient, a brother in *Prince of Tides* and a sister in *Final Analysis*. A remarkable detail in *Final Analysis* is the psychiatrist's assertion that he has obtained an ethics consultation from the American Medical Association (AMA) as to the appropriateness of his liaison with the designated patient's sister. The psychiatrist claims that he has found no bar to this practice. Whether or not the AMA's ethics code contained an explicit prohibition against this practice at the time, such a relationship would be precluded on grounds of general inappropriateness and loss of objectivity, especially for the duration of the treatment.

No such nuanced analysis need be applied to *Basic Instinct II*, in which a forensic psychiatrist blunders into a series of boundary violations, beginning by treating as a patient a person he has examined in a legal context (see Chapter 12 for reasons to avoid this dual role). At one point, in a kind of scenario discussed in Chapter 6, he goes to a party only to find his examinee/patient, a murderous borderline personality, among the guests. When he tries to leave unobtrusively, she pursues him to the door. Walking disasters such as this fictional therapist do appear in a few case examples in this book; fortunately, they are relatively rare.

More recently, the television show *The Sopranos* played a significant role in public perceptions of therapy and in stimulating professional and lay discussion of boundary issues. The program includes therapy sessions between a Mafioso leader, Tony Soprano, and his therapist, Dr. Jennifer Melfi. (For a detailed analysis of the dynamics of the Soprano–Melfi relationship, see Siegel, 2004.) Some of the more memorable incidents include: Soprano's attack on Dr. Melfi when he is enraged by her ill-advised diagnostic summary of his mother; her having to do therapy sessions in a motel room because her life has been threatened by gangsters fearful she may have been told dangerous secrets; and a highly charged moment when—after Dr. Melfi has been brutally raped by a known assailant—she visibly weighs revealing this to Soprano (a revelation that would surely bring fatal vengeance down on the perpetrator), yet holds her tongue. This would be about the most extreme boundary violation imaginable–to use a patient to exact murderous revenge.

ETHICS CODES AND CLINICAL JUDGMENT

The ethics codes of the major mental health professional organizations all prohibit sexual relations with patients and require clinicians to avoid dual or multiple relationships that have the potential to compromise therapy or harm the patient (see, e.g., American Association for Marriage and Family Therapy, 2001; American Psychiatric Association, 2006; American Psychological Association, 2002; National Association of Social Workers, 1999).

Although there are variations in some areas, such as personal relationships with *former* patients (see Chapter 9), the codes all emphasize the underlying principles of respect for patients' human rights and dignity and acting in the patient's interest rather than one's own.

Knowledge of your professional ethics code, applicable laws and regulations, and agency policies and procedures is a foundation of good practice. Then it is up to you to build on that foundation. As Pope and Vasquez (1998) caution:

> Ethics codes cannot do our questioning, thinking, feeling, and responding for us. Such codes can never be a substitute for the active process by which the individual therapist or counselor struggles with the sometimes bewildering, always unique constellation of questions, responsibilities, contexts, and competing demands of helping another person. . . . Ethics must be practical. Clinicians confront an almost unimaginable diversity of situations, each with its own shifting questions, demands, and responsibilities. Every clinician is unique in important ways. Every client is unique in important ways. Ethics that are out of touch with the practical realities of clinical work, with the diversity and constantly changing nature of the therapeutic venture, are useless. (pp. xiii–xiv)

We cannot hope to address all the different forms and guises in which boundary problems arise, especially given the current proliferation of treatment methods and settings. In addition, any guidelines for practice may need to be applied differently in the case of children, the elderly, patients with a chronic disease or disability, patients who lack basic life skills, a depressed versus a psychotic patient, or a patient with a specific phobia as opposed to a personality disorder. By modeling the application of clinical understanding to a range of situations as they arise, we aim to help readers educate their clinical judgment in preparation for the innumerable real-life variations that no book or training program can anticipate. The case examples in the chapters that follow are intended as stimuli to reflection and discussion. Instead of simply listing the locations of icebergs to avoid, they help develop navigational skills for spotting and steering clear of such obstacles. A map or chart will take you only so far when the waters are constantly shifting; you need to navigate in real time.

You can think of this book as a "supervisor on a bookshelf." Still, only a real, living supervisor knows the local terrain and the standards and protocols that apply to the case at hand. As discussed in Chapter 13, consultation with experienced colleagues can best illuminate the salient factors to be considered and the judgments to be made in a given clinical context. Such consultation can be supplemented as needed by a review of relevant literature.

This is not to say that maintaining clinical and ethical boundaries is as easy as it may sound on paper, even in a book that acknowledges uncertainty and controversy as thoroughly as this one does. Patients can be forceful, insistent, and quite manipulative about bestowing a hug or a kiss. You may decline to accept a patient's gift only to find that it has been left with your office assistant. Confronting such intrusions can be challenging and stressful. Legal and professional constraints, too, may set practical limits on individualized clinical judgment. As noted above, regulatory boards, judges, and juries do sometimes decide cases on the basis of the superficial appearance rather than the deeper ramifications of a clinician's conduct.

Nonetheless, therapists who use informed clinical judgment to support reasonable, patient-centered responses to boundary dilemmas are well armed to defend unorthodox practices to their peers and, secondarily (if needed), in court. In the end, the gold standard for evaluation is that any therapeutic intervention be *for the patient*. In deference to this bedrock principle, this book is at least as much about therapeutic technique as it is about risk management. We will not object too strenuously if readers take the subjects addressed here as entry points to a consideration of broader clinical questions. That is as it should be. Good clinical practice—treating the patient effectively as well as ethically—is what boundary maintenance is about.

CONTENT AND ORGANIZATION OF THIS BOOK

This book is divided into three parts. Part I, "Foundations," lays out definitions and principles underlying the establishment and maintenance of boundaries in the therapeutic interchange. Challenges to the maintenance of a secure therapeutic frame are shown to arise out of the intimacy and mutual vulnerability inherent (to a greater or lesser degree) in the therapist–patient dyad. Part II, "Explorations," applies this understanding to the patient-centered, context-sensitive recognition, management, and assessment of a wide range of specific boundary issues. Beginning with a discussion of the therapist's role and the pitfalls of role reversal, boundary dilemmas in the areas of time, place, money, services, gifts, self-disclosure, communication, out-of-office contacts, clothing, physical contact, and sexual misconduct are explored through analysis of numerous case examples.

Part III, "Implications," generalizes from these analyses and reviews literature pertinent to questions of broad significance in the field. Before the fact, there is prevention of boundary violations through education and training, alliance-based interaction and intervention, self-monitoring and self-reflection, and consultation with colleagues, supervisors, and consultants. After the fact, there is forensic evaluation—including assessment of the merits of claims of misconduct—in civil litigation as well as in state licensing board and professional ethics committee hearings. Also discussed in Part III are foreseeable (although not universal) harms that can result from sexual misconduct and other serious boundary violations, risk factors in both therapists and patients for involvement in boundary violations, maintenance of boundaries with former patients, and obstacles to understanding the interactive character of therapist–patient boundary issues. In addition, we reinterpret the commonly observed "slippery slope," or progression of boundary violations from mild to severe, as something over which the clinician can exercise knowledgeable choice rather than accept fatalistically.

Much of the burden of this investigation of boundaries in psychotherapy, especially in Part II, is carried by analysis of case examples adapted from the authors' consultative experience (both clinical and forensic) as well as from published legal and clinical reports. Some of these vignettes are fictional, while those drawn from life are disguised or made into composites. The extensive use of such vignettes exemplifies our method of working toward deep understanding through critical examination of cases that probe the limits of theory.

PART I

Foundations

CHAPTER 1

Definitions and Dilemmas

"What does all this have to do with me?" you might ask. "Why do I need a book about understanding and maintaining therapeutic boundaries?" After all, you might think, "This couldn't happen to me. I'm not one of those 'bad apples' who give the profession a bad name by exploiting patients. I'm an ethical practitioner, and I've been doing this work for too long to be susceptible to that kind of thing."

In fact, the pitfalls of boundary maintenance do not just confront manipulative predators or the very inexperienced. The vast majority of practitioners who encounter perplexing boundary questions are not 'bad apples,' but mainstream professionals from a range of fields and orientations who find themselves up against the exigencies of daily practice. Unprepared by training, overwhelmed by personal vulnerability, ambushed by circumstance, lulled into complacency by high professional attainment—in one way or another they are "in over their heads." Boundary violations do not necessarily arise from bad character, as Gutheil and Gabbard (1993) point out: "Bad training, sloppy practice, lapses of judgment, idiosyncratic treatment philosophies, regional variations, and social and cultural conditioning may all be reflected in behavior that violates boundaries" (p. 189). In this real, messy world where boundaries may be less clear than they seem, many unsuspecting clinicians may regret having thought *"This couldn't happen to me"* (Norris, Gutheil, & Strasburger, 2003).

> A patient told her therapist, "We'll have to stop our sessions because my husband is being transferred to Los Angeles." From the informa-

15

tion revealed by the patient, the therapist concluded that her husband's company's stock would rise in value. The therapist then bought a large amount of the stock. In addition to facing professional sanctions, he was prosecuted for insider trading.

At a summer barbecue a therapist noticed that one of his patients had arrived with his family. The therapist wondered whether it would be most appropriate to leave immediately. Then again, he was tempted to stay and gather data about the patient that could be useful for the therapy. "This is a new perspective from which to look at this patient," he thought, "and I don't know much about his family. I can talk to his wife and kids and find out what this is really all about."

A therapist was caught by surprise when a patient suddenly hugged her on her way out at the end of a session. By the time she thought about what she might say, the patient had left the office. The therapist had had enough exposure to boundary issues to feel uncomfortable about what had happened but not enough to know what to do about it, either at the time or thereafter. So she left the issue undocumented, unexamined, and unresolved. Some weeks later she received a letter from the patient's attorney.

Some therapists commit clear improprieties, and some are predatory individuals who should not be practicing. Far more common, however, are conscientious professionals caught in clinical dilemmas that turn into ethical and even legal problems. In many cases a clinician is genuinely uncertain about what is the right thing to do. Often, too, unrealistic expectations or irrational inferences lead a patient to misconstrue normal professional behavior as intrusive or disrespectful.

Boundaries are often subtle and difficult to discern, and the answers to clinicians' dilemmas are not cut-and-dried (see Glass, 2003). Indeed, these answers can vary greatly with circumstances. Some of the cases heard by the courts or boards of registration have come about because of inexperience, inadequate training, or life crises on the part of clinicians. Others are rooted in the clinical dynamics of patients whose suggestibility is touched off by the media or for whom accusation becomes a shortcut to resolution. Often there is an interaction between the two: patients can provoke or misinterpret, but therapists are not always equipped to deal with such problems in the most professional manner. In this uncertain atmosphere, clinicians struggle to maintain a professional demeanor, to do their best on behalf of their patients, and to avoid having questions raised about their conduct even when they have acted in an entirely proper manner.

The following perceived boundary violations represent a spectrum of formal complaints brought before the American Psychiatric Association ethics committee (J. Lazarus, 1993):

- Therapist accepting gifts from patient
- Therapist taking patient to lunch
- Therapist giving patient a ride home
- Therapist using insider information obtained from patient
- Therapist accepting a party invitation from patient
- Therapist asking patient for advice
- Therapist giving patient gifts in return for referrals of other patients
- Therapist hugging patient
- Therapist making personal revelations to patient
- Therapist writing introduction to patient's book lauding the therapy
- Therapist introducing own children to patient
- Therapist joining patient's book discussion group

The authors' forensic experience and reports in legal publications indicate that other mental health professionals face similar accusations. Questions and conflicts surrounding these and other therapeutic boundary crossings can be stressful for both patient and therapist. They can have serious consequences for the therapy and for the patient's well-being as well as legal and professional consequences for the therapist (extending to loss of license and livelihood). How can the practicing clinician prepare to cope with such questions?

DOING THE LAUNDRY:
THE IMPORTANCE OF CONTEXT

When, if ever, is it appropriate for a patient to do a clinician's laundry? This question can serve as a *gedanken* ("thought") experiment to introduce the subject of clinical boundaries. The idea of a patient's being given dirty clothing to handle will strike most people as inappropriate, a clear boundary violation. That is a reasonable reaction, provided that the contract for therapy is to explore the patient's way of living and any symptoms of psychiatric disorders the patient may have. Within this contract, it is difficult to see how the patient's performing personal services for the therapist serves a therapeutic purpose. Indeed, such an arrangement is likely to contaminate the therapy and exploit the patient for the therapist's benefit (Hundert & Appelbaum, 1995).

Now, put the laundry question into some different contexts. First, handling dirty laundry might be part of an exposure exercise in exposure and response-prevention treatment for obsessive–compulsive disorder. Next, suppose the patient is living in a residential rehabilitation program where the goal is not simply personal growth and development but learning to survive through cooperation with others in a communal setting. The house leader performs some therapeutic functions but also structures and participates in the daily life of the community. Chores are allocated equitably for the benefit of all. Here the patient has made an informed choice, in the form of a contract, to live and share domestic responsibilities with fellow residents, including the clinician. Therefore, doing the clinician's laundry, along with everyone else's, is not automatically a departure from the therapeutic contract.

Finally, consider a patient who is being treated by a cognitive-behavioral therapist for intense fear in public settings. In keeping with the plan outlined at the beginning of treatment, the patient is to complete the therapy by going through a fear-inducing real-life situation in the presence of the therapist. If going to the laundromat has been a difficult task for the patient, the therapist might propose, "I'll walk you through going to the laundry, negotiating the various steps in the process." To accomplish this, the patient may bring in a bag of laundry, or the therapist may provide a dirty sweatshirt as a training tool. Either way, *the purpose is to benefit the patient*, not to promote personal intimacy between patient and therapist or to secure unpaid labor for the therapist. Doing laundry together in this structured way is within the boundaries of the treatment for which the patient has contracted.

BOUNDARY CROSSINGS

A *boundary* is the edge of appropriate behavior at a given moment in the relationship between a patient and therapist, as governed by the therapeutic context and contract. It may be defined by the physical, psychological, and/or social space occupied by the patient in the clinical relationship. Where the boundary line actually falls, or is perceived to fall, depends on the type and stage of therapy and may be subject to judgment and interpretation. Therapeutic boundaries are not hard-and-fast. Rather, they are movable and context-dependent, and their placement depends on a number of factors in the clinical situation. Both the flexibility of therapeutic boundaries and the limits of that flexibility can be understood by exploring the nature and significance of boundary *crossings*, as distinct from boundary *violations* (Glass, 2003; Gutheil & Gabbard, 1993, 1998).

A boundary *crossing* is a departure from the usual norms of therapy, that is, the verbal and physical distances normally maintained in a therapeutic interaction. It frequently happens that, intentionally or not, a clinician interacts with a patient in a way that is unusual or uncharacteristic of standard psychotherapy. We will use the term "boundary crossings" to refer to benign deviations from standard practice, those that are harmless, are nonexploitative, and may even support or advance the therapy. Examples include extending a hand to help a patient who has stumbled and fallen, giving a ride to a patient who is stranded in a blizzard, and giving a patient (based on need) a number for reaching the therapist in an emergency. If a patient comes into the office sobbing because she has just been informed of a sudden death in her family, withholding the human gesture of accepting the patient's embrace would likely be hurtful and might endanger the therapy. As Karl Menninger is reputed to have taught, "When in doubt, be human."

A RIDE IN A BLIZZARD: MANAGING A BOUNDARY CROSSING

A patient is left stranded after a therapy session by a severe, unanticipated blizzard that has shut down public transportation and made walking hazardous. As the therapist begins to drive home, she sees the patient struggling in the snow. Should the therapist offer the patient a ride?

As a rule (with exceptions such as exposure exercises in CBT), interactions between patient and therapist take place only in the office and are limited to the content of therapy. At the same time, effective therapy presupposes having a live patient. Humanitarian concern and common sense call for coming to the patient's rescue in an emergency. However, this entails crossing a well-established clinical boundary of meeting only in the office. The therapist can manage this excursion in an above-board, professional manner by observing the following guidelines:

1. Behave professionally while in the car together. Do not engage in personal revelations or exchanges that would be inappropriate in the office.
2. Do not attempt to conduct therapy outside the office. The drive home should not be a continuation of the office hour.
3. Document the boundary crossing as relevant data. Have it on re-

cord that the therapist exercised clinical judgment and considered the possible impact of the incident on the patient and the therapy.

4. At the next office session, debrief the patient and open up the incident for exploration.
5. Make note of the boundary crossing in supervision. A therapist who is not in regular supervision should obtain a consultation if anything about the incident appears to present special problems for the patient or for the therapist. This step is especially important if the therapist becomes aware of a reluctance on his or her part to document the incident.

If an interaction with a patient feels like something that cannot be written down as part of the therapeutic record, it is a potential problem. If it cannot be brought back to therapy and discussed with the patient, it is a potential problem. The same is true if it cannot be submitted to the informed judgment of a colleague or supervisor. These principles of good clinical practice would apply even if there were no legal or professional sanctions to fear. In addition, if these precautions are not taken, a subsequent review may conclude that the therapist tried to cover up a misjudgment or impropriety. This clearcut example of professionalism does not resolve all the complexities presented by therapeutic boundaries, but it points the way to coping with those complexities ethically and effectively.

Psychoanalytically trained therapists view boundary crossings as an inevitable manifestation of the shifting distance between therapist and patient in the course of the therapeutic encounter. By processing these crossings with the therapist, the patient learns to question habitual assumptions and behavior patterns. Cognitive-behavioral therapists address boundary crossings (referred to by Linehan, 1993, as "in-session behaviors") in an analogous way. Practitioners need to be alert to the occurrence of boundary crossings that may raise clinical, ethical, or legal questions and be prepared to process them therapeutically, both for the patient's benefit and to minimize the risk that a boundary crossing may turn into a boundary violation.

BOUNDARY VIOLATIONS

Some boundary *crossings* are inadvisable because of their intent (i.e., they are not done in the service of the patient's well-being and growth and involve extratherapeutic gratifications for the therapist) and/or their effect (i.e., they are not likely to benefit the patient and entail a significant risk of harming the patient). Such unwarranted and dangerous crossings, which essentially exploit the patient, are called boundary *violations*. A boundary *violation* is a boundary crossing that takes the therapist out of the professional role. Violations are typically exploitative or done for the therapist's rather than the patient's benefit, and they have a potential to harm the patient. Indeed, good intentions will count for little in subsequent forensic evaluations if the therapist's actions are found to have had a foreseeably harmful impact (especially on a previously traumatized patient).

As will be shown in Part II, boundary violations can range from seeing the patient at an inappropriate time or place to having a social, financial, or sexual relationship with the patient. Whereas either the patient or therapist can initiate a boundary crossing, the word "violation" implies the transgression of an ethical standard, a judgment that is made only about the therapist. A patient may initiate behavior that presents a serious threat of a boundary violation, such as disrobing in the office or impulsively kissing the therapist. However, since the therapist retains responsibility for maintaining boundaries, whether this provocative behavior leads to a boundary violation actually depends on the therapist's response.

Unfortunately for the well-meaning clinician, it is not always possible to avoid boundary crossings simply to avoid any chance of committing a boundary violation. Psychoanalytically oriented therapy, for instance, is conceived theoretically in terms of how the patient and therapist approach and retreat from boundaries and how they negotiate the boundary crossings that inevitably occur in this process. Such crossings and negotiations occur, and are appropriately recognized, in other types of therapy as well (see Kohlenberg & Tsai, 2007; Leahy, 2001, 2003b; Linehan, 1993; Safran & Segal, 1996).

Whether a given act constitutes a boundary violation can rarely be assessed outside of the therapeutic context in which the act takes place. The exceptions are egregious instances such as sex with a patient and insider stock trading based on a patient's revelations. Rather, clinical boundaries are set by the therapeutic contract, which limits the types of interactions the patient and therapist will have in the service of a stated therapeutic goal. (The therapeutic contract is discussed in greater detail in Chapter 3.) It is in this context-driven framework that boundaries either are or are not crossed or violated. A key question to ask in considering possible boundary violations, before or after the fact, is *"Cui bono?"* (For whose benefit?). If it is demonstrably *for the patient*—that is, for the health or benefit of the patient—it is at least presumptively within the boundaries of therapy.

BOUNDARY VIOLATIONS
AND RESPONSIBILITY: THREE AXIOMS

The word "violation" necessarily raises questions of accountability. Who is responsible for transgressing the permissible limits of therapeutic exchange? If the patient initiates the transgression, is the patient at fault? These questions are especially urgent in a political atmosphere in which any acknowledgment of the patient's contribution to and participation in an extratherapeutic interaction with a clinician has been referred to as "blaming the victim." This critical issue will be discussed more fully in Chapter 11. Here, we present three axioms developed by the authors as ground rules for discussion and analysis (Gutheil & Gabbard, 1992, 1993). These fundamental principles make clear that seeking to understand the etiology of boundary violations is not the same as condoning or excusing them.

> **Axiom I:** *The responsibility for setting and maintaining boundaries always belongs to the clinician. The patient is not blamed or stigmatized for violating therapeutic boundaries.*

Only the clinician has a professional code to violate; the patient has no such code. Therefore, only the clinician can be culpable, blameworthy, or subject to civil or (in some states) criminal liability. This is true even if (as is often the case) the patient initiates the boundary challenge. Does the patient have any boundaries to maintain? Although the patient does in fact join the therapist in establishing the therapeutic frame (Spruiell, 1983), the patient's boundaries are more flexible and forgiving (Gutheil & Gabbard, 1993). As one senior clinician puts it: "There are three rules of therapy. You come on time. You pay your money. And we treat each other with respect. Everything else is negotiable" (C. Gates, personal communication, 1968). Indeed, one might question whether the patient even needs to come on time. The therapist should not be late, but if the patient is willing to pay the full fee for less than a full hour, the meaning this behavior has for the patient can be explored.

Of course, the patient cannot be allowed to assault the therapist physically. Indeed, the immediate need to restrain the patient may necessitate physical contact that would otherwise be a boundary violation. With that major exception, enactments, or actions, that would be unethical on the part of a therapist become, on the patient's part, material for therapy. Subject to no code, the patient is free to request, demand, pout, or vent. The patient can call the therapist "Shrinkie," make flirtatious gestures, or threaten to discontinue therapy or commit suicide.

A patient who asks a therapist to have sex is not violating any ethical code and is not punished. Rather, the therapist sets limits ("that's not therapy") and explores the meaning of the patient's wish for sex with the therapist. If the patient persists in propositioning the therapist over a long period of time, as with any other unproductive behavior, questions can be raised about the progress and effectiveness of the therapy. Such questions are to be resolved (usually with a consultant) by the usual criteria for re-directing or terminating therapy.

Axiom II: *In any interaction between two people, the actions of both play a contributing role. However, by Axiom I, the fact that the thera-pist and patient are in that sense responsible for their actions cannot be translated into blaming the patient/victim.*

Any interaction does have two sides. A competent adult patient is accountable for his or her actions (even if, in a psychoanalytic model, driven by unconscious forces) in the very general sense that we are all responsible for everything we do. But the moral equality, or role sym-metry, between patient and clinician ends there. Entering into the ther-apeutic relationship for different purposes, the two parties have un-equal power and responsibility within that relationship. The clinician has a fiduciary responsibility to safeguard and promote the well-being of a vulnerable patient. Therefore, to analyze boundary violations as complex interactions between two people that reflect a variety of dy-namics on both sides in no way blames the patient or relieves the clini-cian of responsibility.

Humbert Humbert's plea for understanding in *Lolita*—"She seduced me!"—is no defense for a therapist who has sex with a patient, even if she *did* seduce him. Part of a clinician's job is not to be seduced; the patient has no such job description. It is only to be expected, not condemned, that patients will initiate a good many boundary crossings. These crossings are predictable expressions of the problems for which patients seek treat-ment, and patients often rationalize them as such. But therapists must not meet patients' rationalizations with their own (e.g., "I'm giving this pa-tient the relationship she needs"). Rather, they need to keep in mind that the processes begun by patients' boundary crossings are a normal and—if skillfully handled—beneficial part of therapy.

Axiom III: *Careful, candid, clinically informed exploration of profes-sional misconduct, with attention to actual cause-and-effect relation-ships, will, in the long run, be beneficial to patients, illuminating to the mental health professions, and valuable to society.*

Various factors appear to have contributed to the current disinclination to study the therapeutic dyad as the fertile ground from which boundary violations grow. On one side, there is the insistence on political correctness that sees any examination of the patient's contributing role in the situation as an attack on the patient, inflicting added trauma on an already devastated victim (Gutheil & Gabbard, 1992). On the other side, at least within psychiatry, there has been less effort to understand the interaction between therapist and patient during a time when a more straightforward medical model of treatment has gained ascendancy (Schultz-Ross et al., 1992). The result has been the common division of labor in which the psychiatrist dispenses medication while other practitioners assume responsibility for the patient's psychotherapy, with its inevitable relational features (outlined in, e.g., Norcross, 2002; Safran & Muran, 1998, 2003; Wachtel, 2007).

Rigorous empirical study will offer the most reliable route to effective preventive strategies (see, e.g., Twemlow, 1995a, 1995b, 1997). Such exploration will not necessarily be pleasant, comfortable, reassuring, or politically palatable. Nonetheless, we must face what really is before us if we are to have any hope of reducing the incidence of serious boundary violations without extinguishing the creativity and spontaneity of therapy.

Following these axioms, the case vignettes in this book are presented with full attention to the relevant dynamics of the dyad but with a clear emphasis on the clinician's ethical responsibility. The following case is illustrative.

> A woman in her late 20s who complained of depression and troubled relationships had been seeing a male therapist for several months. During one session she asked the therapist if she could take off her clothes to relax. In the complaint she later filed with the licensing board, she stated that the therapist had simply replied, "It's your session." In his version of the story, the therapist claimed that he had said nothing. Paralyzed by helplessness, dismay, and dread in a situation he had never before faced, he watched helplessly as the patient stripped to the waist. He then ran into the adjoining office and searched desperately for the applicable code in a book of regulations.
>
> This patient had already crossed boundaries with the therapist by appearing at public events in which he was involved. She was simultaneously seeing a female therapist, whom she accompanied on shopping trips as well as to the therapist's medical appointments. The second therapist was prescribing medications for her. Neither therapist knew about the other.

Patients do initiate or provoke boundary violations. This patient drew two therapists into a web of manipulation and enmeshment. She sought to reassure herself that she had the upper hand in knowledge and power. A highly publicized "crackdown" on boundary violators gave her a way to exert further control by embroiling one of the therapists in a complaint process. Although this was, on the surface, what she wanted, it was not what she (or her insurer) was paying for. Therapeutically, her behavior might have opened a window on the way she dealt with people outside of therapy, but she needed a therapist to open that window for her. Both therapists, by their failure to set limits, served her ill. By allowing her to act out in her habitual ways, they did not help her confront the sources of her behavior and learn to deal differently with her feelings. That clinical failure is their responsibility, not hers.

Preventive and remedial strategies for this kind of situation, including how the therapist might better have reacted to the unanticipated emergency, will be considered in Chapter 7. The therapist did not intend or initiate misconduct, but in his understandable discomfort he was unprepared to respond to the challenge in a professional manner. In the stress of the moment he took refuge in a book of regulations. Concerned first to protect himself from possible sanctions, he neglected to attend to the patient clinically. His ill-considered reaction exemplifies the harm done by a messianic crusade against boundary violations that ignores critical contextual factors as well as essential distinctions as to the type and severity of boundary crossings.

REALITY VERSUS PERCEPTION OF MISCONDUCT: THE "SLIPPERY SLOPE"

An important concept in boundary theory is the so-called slippery slope that leads incrementally from minor boundary crossings to more serious violations, often culminating in sexual misconduct. This metaphoric image has been under attack as too alarmist and as unnecessarily stigmatizing (by association with sexual misconduct) with respect to small, innocent, and sometimes beneficial deviations from standard practice. The criticism will be discussed and the "slippery slope" reinterpreted in less rigid, more reasonable, terms in Chapter 11. It is useful at the outset, however, to establish some guidelines for understanding.

First, sexual misconduct on the part of a clinician usually is preceded by relatively minor boundary excursions. It is a common pattern, and it does get people in trouble. There can be little doubt that a therapist who allows—let alone asks—a patient to disrobe during a session is at increased risk for progressing to sexual misconduct. However, not all boundary crossings or even boundary violations lead to sexual misconduct (in fact, most do not), and by themselves they do not constitute evidence of sexual misconduct. Rather, the "slippery slope"—as a legal term applied to a clinical situation—more often describes the law's *perception* of the progression of boundary violations than it does the reality. However unfairly, juries, judges, ethics committees of professional organizations, and state licensing boards often believe that the occurrence of boundary violations, or even crossings, is presumptive evidence of, or corroborates allegations of, sexual misconduct (Gutheil & Gabbard, 1993).

Where therapists do proceed down the "slippery slope," it is often through a combination of rationalization, blackmail, and fatalism. Initially, the boundary transgressions may be sufficiently small that the therapist can rationalize that nothing out of the ordinary or potentially harmful is happening. Then the patient drops the other shoe: "OK, you've been hugging me. Now it's time to take the next step." "Now, I can't possibly refuse," thinks the flustered, intimidated therapist, "because then the patient will get angry and file a complaint about the hugging." (See Chapters 8 and 11 for further discussion of such situations.)

It is prudent, therefore, to pay attention to the flow of actual and potential boundary crossings in your practice. If there is any ambiguity about the appropriateness of your treatment, a blurring of boundaries may be taken as a sign of substandard treatment in the event of a lawsuit resulting from a bad outcome. And if you are accused of sexual misconduct, the fact finder may take the position that a lesser boundary violation lends credence to the allegation.

For clinical, ethical, and legal reasons, clinicians of all disciplines should be alert to the dynamics of any therapeutic encounter and any ongoing relationship with a patient, and keep their eyes and minds open to possible motivators and precipitants of boundary crossings in the patient, in the clinician, or in the interaction. Ideology and good intentions can subvert good practice if they prevent one from attending to the turbulent complexity of a patient's psyche or the demons and temptations that beset one's own.

WHEN DOES A BOUNDARY CROSSING BECOME A VIOLATION?

How can you tell when a boundary crossing becomes or risks becoming a boundary violation? Sometimes a crossing takes on the character of a violation when it is part of a repetitive pattern or is followed by more overt boundary violations. When an individual act is looked at in isolation, the judgment depends on clinical considerations. Was the act in question undertaken in the interest of the patient? What effects might it have on this particular patient? Did the therapist deal with the crossing in an ethical, professional manner?

Answering these questions requires posing more questions. What, in a particular exchange between two particular individuals, does it mean to act in the patient's interest, to anticipate possible effects on the patient, or to respond in a professional manner? One useful guideline is that a boundary crossing is more likely to be benign if it is discussible and is in fact discussed with the patient (and, if called for, with a supervisor or consultant). A therapist who, instead of acting in an oblivious or self-protective manner, works through such an incident with the patient is acting to restore the professional role and repair the relationship. Moreover, clinical exploration of a potential or inadvertent boundary violation often defuses its potential for harm and may benefit the patient and advance the therapy.

The character and significance of a boundary crossing are highly context-dependent (Gutheil & Gabbard, 1998). One context that needs to be taken into consideration is professional discipline. A CBT practitioner who accompanies a patient out of the office for the purpose of encountering a feared situation and a case manager who makes home visits to give a patient practical assistance are acting within their defined, theoretically based professional roles, which are not the same as that of a psychoanalyst when it comes to out-of-office contacts. Boundaries can also shift with changing treatment practices and settings. For example, in the era of extended inpatient treatment, therapists commonly conversed with their patients during leisurely walks on the hospital grounds; this gave many patients a feeling of comfort, safety, and peace. In today's more impersonal hospital settings, patients and clinicians often are not together long enough to get to know each other and so taking a walk outside the hospital with a patient is more likely to be seen as problematic. Other relevant contexts include the therapeutic task at hand, the therapist's style and approach, the patient's needs, the stage of treatment, and the options and constraints presented by the geographic and community setting (Simon & Williams, 1999).

A critical context is that created by cultural differences. To take a historical example, an Austrian psychoanalyst who immigrated to the United States found that he needed to stop helping female patients put on and take off their overcoats. In his native Vienna he would have been considered rude had he neglected this routine courtesy. In the United States, however, a vulnerable patient might develop erotic feelings toward the analyst on the basis of this minimal physical contact, and a gesture taken for granted in other cultures (or in previous eras) might be misconstrued as a boundary violation not only by the patient but also by a jury or regulatory board. To take a contemporary example, a Brazilian immigrant patient for whom incidental physical contact would seem customary and normal might find a therapist's display of diplomas on the office wall (taken for granted in the United States) pretentious and off-putting (Miller et al., 2006).

As this example illustrates, the significance of a boundary crossing is to be found in "the psychological meaning of the event to the patient and the therapist" (Waldinger, 1994, p. 225). For the Austrian analyst, helping patients on and off with their coats had no special psychological meaning; he was not acting out of neediness, wish for contact, or self-aggrandizement. It was, however, his professional responsibility to discern the psychological meaning that this "innocent" act might have for American women and to change his behavior accordingly. It is a distressing fact of life that patients experiencing the insecurity, anguish, grief, and grievance often associated with psychiatric disorders may interpret the most proper, unobjectionable behavior on a therapist's part as exploitative and harmful. No clinician can anticipate all such delusions that may arise. Nonetheless, it helps to be aware of some common ways in which patients whose own boundary maintenance is weak—such as paranoid patients, those with borderline personality disorder (Gutheil, 1989, 2005b, 2005c), and those who have been abused—can show a hypersensitivity to boundary crossings (see Chapter 10).

Two contrasting cases, described in greater detail by Waldinger (1994), show the importance of personal history and context in how patients react to boundary crossings. In the first case, a 25-year-old woman came to an outpatient clinic complaining of dissociative episodes during a severe economic crisis in her life. Her male psychotherapist agreed to see her without charge, a deviation from standard practice at the clinic that seemed justified by the patient's circumstances. Several weeks later the patient began to express the fear that the therapist was trying to take advantage of her. After a suicide attempt was narrowly averted, the therapist sought consultation. The patient told the consultant that when she was an adolescent her brother had given her gifts in exchange for sex. She feared that her therapist would similarly demand anything he wanted from her in return for free treatment. The consultant then recommended that the therapist discuss the patient's fears in treatment and that he negotiate a small fee with the patient to establish a clearer boundary.

In the second case, a 46-year-old man had been in therapy with a female therapist for 5 years. His main concerns were his troubled marriage and his overly close relationship with his mother. His mother's unexpected death precipitated a suicidal crisis, hospitalization, and divorce. Now living alone, the patient was more dependent on his therapist for support than he previously had been. As he began to reconstitute, he acknowledged how alone he felt and expressed gratitude toward the therapist for her stable presence in his life. At the end of that session, he asked her if he could give her a hug. Caught off guard, the therapist made an on-the-spot judgment that it would harm the patient if she refused. She explored this incident at her next session with the patient, who said the hug had reassured him that "someone could still stand me." Still worried that her maternal feelings toward the patient had drawn her into a boundary violation, the therapist sought consultation. The consultant not only found no evidence that the patient had been harmed, but agreed that it might have hurt the patient to refuse his hug at that pivotal point in his recovery. The consultant expressed confidence that henceforth the patient would be strong enough to discuss rather than enact his yearnings for connection.

In the first of these cases, the patient experienced what the therapist intended as a helpful boundary crossing as though it were a boundary violation. In the second, the patient experienced what would normally be called a potential boundary violation as life-saving support. Thus, the very same act (such as calling a patient by his first name or agreeing to schedule more frequent sessions with a patient) may turn out to be either a boundary crossing or a boundary violation, depending on the contexts in which it occurs. Waldinger (1994) summarizes the practical significance of the two cases as follows:

> Both therapists had departed from their standard practices with patients—a clear indication for self-examination and consultation. If these examples had occurred in psychopharmacological treatment or cognitive therapy, the need for consultation would have been just as great. (p. 227)

Both therapists saw the need for self-examination and consultation. Not coincidentally, although both patients had been suicidal, neither case resulted in lasting harm to the patient, and neither led to a lawsuit or an ethics complaint. Indeed, the great majority of therapists' deviations from their usual practice do not result in boundary violations, let alone malpractice suits or complaints to licensing boards. Nonetheless, any deviation from standard practice warrants reflection as to the clinical rationale for the action being taken and any warning signs of a boundary violation (see Chapter 13).

Boundary questions arise in a number of areas, including gifts and services, modes of personal address, various forms of self-disclosure, times and places for therapeutic interactions, accidental and deliberate contacts outside the office, billing practices, and physical contact. Which professional responsibilities carry over to a clinician's personal time outside the office, and which do not? A therapist needs to be attentive to various boundary issues that emerge, as these may facilitate or block the patient's autonomous strivings—in other words, as they present opportunities or pitfalls for therapy. How does one steer clear of inadvisable and dangerous boundary crossings without losing the flexibility needed to support the patient's growth? How can one plan and manage boundary crossings that might help the patient? Finally, how can one best recover from inadvertent or ill-considered boundary crossings, thus preventing the so-called slippery slope of escalating boundary violations that is truly inevitable only when it is presumed to be so?

As the chapters that follow will show, there are basic clinical principles that can guide the clinician through these thickets, even while any given situation may demand its own individualized resolution. Such resolution can be as simple as *"Cui bono?"* and as complex as an unprecedented set of contingencies for which no rulebook, no algorithm, exists. Much of the time, the clinician can go far toward a solution by asking, "Who is this for, anyway? What goals, whose goals, are being served? Is it in the service of the therapy, of the therapeutic contract, and of the patient's autonomy and growth? Am I getting something out of it beyond the satisfaction of a job well done and the experience and wisdom gained from practice?" Protecting the patient from harm and enhancing the patient's welfare are the primary goals, but they must be achieved in a highly charged clinico-legal environment in which the therapist's safety also is salient. Reconciling these sometimes divergent needs and priorities is a challenge to be met through deep understanding and well-developed therapeutic technique.

In the discussion thus far, we have tried to show that clinical boundary questions are characterized by neither rote simplicity nor unmanageable complexity. In many cases it is by no means obvious what is appropriate professional behavior, but there are ways to think about such situations so as to resolve one's doubts reasonably and responsibly. We turn to that in the next chapter.

CHAPTER 2

Therapy and Its Limits

"I see patients only for short-term counseling," you might say. "How can they develop any feelings toward me?" The answer to this question lies in the distinction between the special characteristics of particular therapies and the common features of all therapies. These can be called, respectively, pragmatic and relational factors.

Pragmatic factors are the distinguishing features of different schools, theories, approaches, concepts, and techniques of therapy. In these terms, for example, free association is different from directive therapy under hypnosis. Jungian therapists, rational-emotive therapists, reality therapists, client-centered therapists, cognitive-behavioral therapists, family therapists, group therapists, and addiction counselors all say and do different things—but always for the purpose of helping the patient. That is where the relational factors come in.

Relational factors are the universal, generic characteristics of any helping relationship—the bedrock of all therapy and counseling (for detailed analysis, see Norcross, 2002; Safran & Muran, 1998, 2003; Wachtel, 2007). Whatever else you do as a mental health clinician, you are charged with the responsibility of helping a patient by forming a relationship that enables you to exert a benign, constructive influence on his or her feelings, thoughts, and actions. This characterization holds true even when the relationship is structured as purely pharmacological and limited to 10 minutes of contact, 2 minutes of which are spent writing prescriptions; even that is not just a one-dimensional interaction. Once the patient makes the effort to come to your office with the aim of improving his or her condition, a relationship is formed. Trust is extended and hopes are aroused.

31

In "talk" therapies, the subtleties of verbal interaction take on an importance that they do not have in less purely verbal modalities. What the therapist says to the patient, as well as when and how, may vary greatly according to the therapist's treatment philosophy and personal style. The common factor that cuts across all these differences is a fundamental ethical principle: *primum non nocere* (first, do no harm). As was emphasized in Chapter 1, everything said and done in treatment must be for the benefit of the patient. The clinician's job is always to act in the service of the patient's well-being.

Short-term therapy, personal counseling in various life settings (college, military, employment, prison, residential treatment), couple counseling, psychopharmacology, cognitive and behavioral therapies, psychiatric nursing, medical treatment, social work, and pastoral counseling all have relational dimensions that can give rise to boundary crossings and violations. In this book we concentrate on the relational factors that underlie all forms of therapy. The clear and simple ethical imperative of boundary maintenance—always act in the patient's interest—follows from an understanding of these relational factors.

We do not prescribe rules for maintaining boundaries in different therapies. In the unpredictable give-and-take between patient and therapist, most rules eventually break down or prove inadequate. Our approach, therefore, is to present numerous case examples of how basic clinical and ethical principles apply to a variety of situations. These principles and illustrative examples constitute the most practical preparation a clinician can have when unfamiliar, unanticipated situations arise in the heat of practice.

THE THERAPEUTIC DYAD

We have all observed, and felt, how physical proximity and ongoing contact with others regularly create emotional closeness. Consider the bond that forms when people work together at close quarters over an extended period of time—for example, in college dormitories and military units where people are thrown together 24 hours a day. These bonds are not necessarily sexual, but they are certainly emotional, and they can lead to sexual involvements.

Sitting in a room alone with someone and listening and responding to their most intimate revelations is bonding in a special way. This bonding may seem most intense in the analytic setting, but it is not absent from any therapy situation. If you see a patient in 15-minute sessions for 10 weeks, those structural limits do not necessarily constrain the patient's capacity to idealize, to imagine, to wish, or to long for closeness. Your 15 minutes of listening may be 15 minutes more than the patient's husband listens to her. Likewise, for a man who grew up without loving parents, a little nurturance can be a powerful stimulant. A patient may build you up into an all-knowing "expert" who can dispense miracle cures and solve all of his or her problems. This wish to have the therapist satisfy all of the patient's needs, not just therapeutic needs, has been termed the *golden fantasy* (Gutheil, 1989; Smith, 1977). A needy, dependent patient's expressions (explicit or implicit) of this wish can put tremendous pressure on the therapist to assume other, nontherapeutic roles in the patient's life.

Clinicians may miss these patterns and their ethical implications in the sincere belief that "I just prescribe"; "I'm just doing a procedure"; "We're not having a full therapeutic relationship"; or "This is not really my patient—I'm just covering for someone." On the contrary, any clinical interaction is subject to the relational features described here, and any clinician can benefit from an elementary understanding of them. In particular, the seemingly impersonal act of prescribing medication is a form of concrete exchange between clinician and patient that reverberates with unspoken symbolism (Gutheil, 1982b).

If you are dispensing a magic potion, something that carries with it a promise of healing or relief from suffering, then you may become, for the patient, a giver of life, of health. In the patient's fantasy life, you may become the equivalent of a parent feeding a child. (Of course, a therapist need not concretely hand a patient a pill in order to be perceived and internalized as a benign, nurturing figure.) As one unsophisticated patient told his therapist, "Taking the medication is like eating a little piece of you." A character in John Updike's novel *Couples* remarks that she has learned in psychotherapy that when she takes a pill she is symbolically being impregnated by her pharmacist father. Patients who commit suicide with an overdose of a prescribed medication may be expressing feelings of dependency, betrayal, or blame; indeed, attorneys, judges, and juries have been known to echo this "magical thinking" by holding clinicians liable for malpractice just because they provided, for a legitimate therapeutic purpose, the chosen means of suicide (Bursztajn, Gutheil, Brodsky, & Swagerty, 1988).

Therapists have their own feelings and fantasies. (The word "fantasy" is used here in its everyday meaning, not as a technical psychoanalytic term.) In the case of prescribing, for example, a psychiatrist may medicate a patient to support the patient's well-being and growth, to make the patient more malleable and receptive to treatment recommendations, to gratify one's own need for power by making the patient dependent on the medication, or—as a worst case—to drug the patient into having sex. Decades ago, when psychodynamic therapy was the dominant modality, an overreliance on medication was commonly attributed to an intolerance of the patient's feelings, which the therapist was trying to banish or suppress instead of helping the patient work through them. Today, routine prescribing as a form of avoidance is difficult to explore since it has become the norm in psychiatry.

More generally, just as a patient may want you to be an ideal parent, an ideal mate, an ideal provider, you may want to believe that you can be everything to the patient. This wish is not necessarily pathological in origin. It can arise, instead, from normal feelings, desires, and vulnerabilities. When all your efforts to help the patient are to no avail, it is natural to look beyond the usual therapeutic modalities for ways to break the stalemate. You may be frustrated by the limits set by managed care, by institutional policies and procedures, by the patient's resistance, or by the limits of therapy itself. The urge to reach out to someone in a more fully "human" way can seem irresistible, especially when you have experienced suffering similar to the patient's in your own life, making your empathy and affinity with the patient especially keen. That's why you're in the helping professions (Eber & Kunz, 1984; Groesbeck & Taylor, 1977; Miller, 1981; Sussman, 1992). Ironically, the very motives that make you want to help others—a responsiveness to suffering and a desire to ameliorate it—can draw you into emotional entanglements with patients (Edelwich & Brodsky, 1991). These aims, broadly therapeutic in origin, have led even experienced therapists, who would be expected to know better, to cross over the line from representing and modeling people in the patient's life, while empathically exploring the conflicts this process reveals, to *becoming* one of those people (Dewald & Clark, 2001; Gabbard & Lester, 2002).

It can be a strain to stay within the limits of the therapist's role when to do so runs counter to our ordinary experience of mutuality, that of giving fully when we feel strongly and *getting something back for it*. When we expend so much energy empathizing with someone else's feelings, we want to get back some "fellow feeling" from the other person, just as with our families and friends. As clinicians, however, we are not permitted such gratification. This seemingly unnatural lack of reciprocity, a sense that we are always putting out and never taking in, can leave us feeling frustrated and deprived. As a result, we may be susceptible to overinvolvement with patients at a personal level, looking to them to replenish our depleted emotional reserves, even as we risk becoming clinically inattentive and detached (Genova, 2001).

Overidentifying with the outcomes of therapy, taking a patient's progress or lack of it personally, can lead to overt boundary violations if we insert ourselves into patients' lives to bring about desired outcomes instead of limiting ourselves to appropriate professional interventions. At the extreme, even a therapist who is not by nature sexually exploitative but who identifies strongly with a patient's yearning for a satisfying sexual relationship might (in the absence of clear professional boundaries) start thinking about gallantly stepping into the breach. There are indeed predators who take advantage of their position of power to exploit vulnerable people. Yet, there are also cases of sexual misconduct by therapists that result from "a profoundly failed treatment alliance" (Schultz-Ross, Goldman, & Gutheil, 1992, p. 506).

This understanding of the interaction between therapist and patient is described, in the analytic tradition, in terms of *transference and countertransference*. Transference means that the patient reacts to the therapist as a surrogate for significant people in the patient's life. In countertransference the therapist reacts to the patient in terms of similar associations. For example, a patient's sexual feelings toward a therapist may reflect a desire to achieve equality of power with an authority figure such as a parent (Person, 2003). Analytically oriented therapists regard transference and countertransference as parts of the process of therapy, to be understood for what they reveal about the patient's conflicts and the reactions the patient provokes in others. Person (2003) explains how sexual feelings in therapy (if not acted out) can serve a therapeutic purpose:

> [The erotic transference] may confer on the patient a new appreciation of the possibilities inherent in relationships (sometimes through an identification with a therapist's empathy and kindness). The therapeutic usefulness of the erotic transference is twofold: the wealth of psychological material it yields in understanding both erotic and power issues and the strength of the emotional charge that initially sustains the patient through some hard work. However, to the degree that it persists, it becomes a limitation in the analysis. (p. 31)

Transference and countertransference are not, however, part of the vocabulary and repertoire of many clinicians today. Nor is it necessary to use this terminology to understand the emotional currents from which boundary violations arise. From a CBT perspective, transference can be understood in terms of stimulus generalization, whereby the patient reacts to a situation according to its perceived degree of similarity to other situations. Slovenko (1991) puts the question of transference in perspective:

Transference feelings are particularly intense in the psychoanalytic situation. However, . . . [a]ll human relationships are tinged with transference. Every relationship is a mixture of a real relationship and transference phenomenon. (p. 603)

In everyday terms, the patient and therapist are thrown into a tinder-box of emotions. The patient is vulnerable by virtue of the very problems that brought him or her to therapy. The therapist is made vulnerable by the nature of the situation as well as perhaps his or her own personal problems. Chapter 10 lists specific vulnerabilities, or risk factors, in both clinicians and patients (some of which are illustrated in the intervening chapters) that can exacerbate the inherent, universal pitfalls of the therapeutic dyad.

THE THERAPEUTIC FRAME

Psychotherapists from Freud onward have recognized the need to turn the highly charged atmosphere of the dyad into a safe space for the patient's intimate explorations (Havens, 1989; Winnicott, 1965). The concept of *the therapeutic frame* developed out of this effort to take advantage of the benefits while minimizing the risks of the emotional dynamics of the dyad (Bleger, 1966; Epstein, 1994; Gabbard & Lester, 2002; Langs, 1976, 1982; Spruiell, 1983). The therapeutic frame can be visualized as "an envelope or membrane around the therapeutic role that defines the characteristics of the therapeutic relationship" (Gutheil & Gabbard, 1993, p. 190). Its primary purpose is to "define a fluctuating, reasonably neutral, safe space that enables the dynamic, psychological interaction between therapist and patient to unfold" (Simon, 1992, p. 272). Elements of the frame include the office setting, the scheduling and duration of appointments, fee arrangements, and the treatment contract, which covers the purpose, goals, methods, and process of treatment. Thus, the frame structures where, when, and how the therapist and patient will interact.

The therapeutic frame consists of boundaries that block off intrusive, threatening, or misleading behaviors without blocking off human contact. Maintenance of this stable, flexible frame allows the therapist's empathy and identification with the patient to move across the interpersonal space without confusing the patient about the therapist's motives. It provides continual reassurance that the therapist cares about—and is not trying to take advantage of—the patient. The patient can then think, "This is a place where I might be able to expose and explore the irrational stuff inside me" (Epstein, 1994, p. 120).

Within these general guidelines, the therapeutic frame is created by the therapist and patient in a way that reflects the unique characteristics of those two individuals and of the dyad they form. The frame may expand and contract spontaneously in the normal process of therapeutic interaction. Moreover, the therapist and patient may agree to extend the frame by a deliberate revision of the therapeutic contract. Sometimes, however, instead of extending the frame at the patient's request, the therapist holds to the existing limits, for it is the therapist's responsibility to maintain an appropriate frame in the interest of the patient.

SETTING LIMITS

In maintaining the frame, the therapist not only protects ethical boundaries but often advances the therapy as well. Most therapists, whether analytic or cognitive-behavioral, believe that it is an essential developmental experience for a child to be told "No." The frustration of the child's primitive wishes contributes to building self-control and a mature personality structure. Children who do not experience reasonable adult restraint may, as adults, still operate out of primitive wishes. This deficiency of learning begins to be corrected when a therapist says, "No, you can't sit on my lap." Thwarting this infantile wish gives the patient the opportunity to reflect on his or her frustration. The patient can then ask, "What does this mean? How is it different from the way my father violated me when I was a child? How does one person differ from another? How does the present differ from the past?"

By contrast, if the therapist accedes to the patient's wish, not only is an ethical boundary violated, but a clinical opportunity is missed. The therapist is simply allowing the patient to relive dysfunctional childhood experiences by repeating behaviors learned in a very threatening environment. The therapy goes slack from a loss of the creative tension that fuels a patient's progress. Maroda (1994) explains this essential feature of analytic therapy:

> *The objective of an analytic treatment is to go beyond the establishment of a good working relationship or positive transference to a stage of dynamic conflict.* A successful treatment is predicated on the notion of the relationship developing to a point at which the patient's conflicts and deficits are expressed within the context of the therapeutic relationship. (pp. 67–68; italics in original)

In analytic and nonanalytic therapies alike, limit setting can serve a useful clinical function. Moreover, it can have a significant clinical impact even when granting the patient's request would not constitute a boundary violation, as in the following case:

> A woman who had had several years of analysis (her analyst had since died) moved to another city, where she began weekly therapy with a male psychiatrist. The patient, who presented as a healthy woman with conflicts that were normal for a person in her life situation, said that she would like to see the therapist twice a week. The therapist replied, "We'll have to talk a bit, at least for a few sessions, to see whether twice-weekly sessions are warranted." Under the strain of what would seem a small deprivation, the patient unexpectedly regressed to attention-seeking behavior, calling the therapist frequently on slight pretexts. In the office she played hide-and-seek with the therapist by sitting on the floor out of his field of vision. The therapist realized that the patient's apparent competence and ordinary neurotic complaints masked intermittent regressed states that reflected her unmet longings and still-active childhood impulses.
>
> After 6 months of intensive therapy, the patient asked the therapist, "These things you've been listening to me tell you—should I be listening to myself, too?" The question marked the beginning of therapy for this patient. Until then she had said anything to keep a peaceful rapport going with the therapist. From this vantage point, her therapist could understand, and help her understand, that her campaign to have him see her twice a week had been part of a power struggle, an attempted seduction (in nonsexual terms) of, and wish for seduction by, the therapist. The patient had imagined that if she behaved herself, she would be rewarded with the gratification of more frequent sessions, that is, more of the therapist's time and attention.
>
> Indeed, part of what brought her to this pivotal point of awareness was the therapist's refusal to play his part in the seduction. After he had turned down her request several times, she told him, "If you hadn't held up that brick wall, I wouldn't have discovered how much I was beating my head against it." Once she realized, "Gosh, I'm going crazy over not being able to see my therapist twice a week," she could ask, "I wonder what that means and why that should happen."

Had the therapist granted without exploration this patient's "innocent" request, he would not have been subject to an ethics review, since it was within his professional discretion to see this patient twice a week (as opposed to, say, seeing her at the end of the day and going out for coffee with her afterward). Yet, his firmness in setting limits led to a clinical breakthrough in which the patient learned something important about herself. Once she could ask "Why is that?," therapy had begun for her. For the therapist, this case was a lesson in the need to be alert to boundary questions even when they are not anticipated and not evident.

For many patients, therapy is, among other things, about setting, adjusting, or extending limits. People whose lives are constricted by fear, guilt, prolonged grief, low self-esteem, lack of assertiveness, phobias, abnormal inhibitions, or obsessive rituals generally need to extend their limits. At the same time, they may need to set limits on their indulgence in dysfunctional behavior patterns on which they have relied for familiarity and reassurance. Conversely, destructive boundary-breaking behavior may stem from a sense of severe limits imposed by one's circumstances or inadequacies. Substance abuse, for example, can be seen in this dual light as a form of antisocial acting out typically motivated by objective or subjective deprivation and limited opportunity (Peele, 1998; Peele & Brodsky, 1975; Peele, Brodsky, & Arnold, 1991).

When people who have drawn narrow boundaries around themselves, or have had those boundaries imposed on them by an abusive environment, begin to learn to cope more effectively with life, they may initially assert themselves in inappropriate ways simply because they do not know any better. In therapy they can experience what it is like to be encouraged, not punished, for taking appropriate risks, as well as to be restrained when they make false starts. This corrective experience takes different forms in different kinds of therapy; for example, in dialectical behavior therapy (DBT) a therapist may refrain from visiting a patient who has been hospitalized for self-injury, in order not to reinforce parasuicidal behavior (Linehan, 1993). Nonetheless, there is an underlying developmental process that most forms of therapy are designed to support. *So, while the testing of limits can lead to boundary violations in therapy, it is part of the very process of growth and development that therapy is intended to facilitate.*

ETHICAL PRINCIPLES FOR MAINTAINING THERAPEUTIC BOUNDARIES

The job of a therapist—of whatever school—is to guide and support the patient through a delicate growth process, full of both opportunity and risk. As the patient "pushes the envelope" of life's constraints to discover where his or her true boundaries lie, the therapist must respect the boundaries of the dyad, perhaps "pushing the envelope" of standard practice, but only in a professional capacity and only for the patient's benefit. In the emotional intensity and close bond that may develop between clinician and patient lie inequalities of power and responsibility that require the clinician to set aside self-interest in the service of the patient's vital interests: health and illness, well-being and suffering, even life and death (Perlin, 1996).

In the face of the controversy (discussed in Chapter 11) over whether therapeutic boundaries have become overly strict and legalistic, it should be emphasized that these boundaries are derived from long-established ethical principles that inform all clinical work. These principles, as summarized by Gutheil and Simon (2002), are as follows.

Respect for the Dignity of the Patient

This fundamental principle can be said to underlie all the others. To respect the human dignity of the patient is to avoid depersonalizing or taking advantage of the patient.

Respect for the Patient's Authentic Goals or Choices

The therapist and patient work together to achieve the patient's health-directed goals as agreed to in the therapeutic contract. These goals might include fostering health, freedom from symptoms, increased responsibility, and the ability to make free choices. The therapist does not interpose his or her own personal needs, such as dominance, dependency, or sexual gratification.

Respect for the patient's goals means respect for the patient's *autonomy* and *self-determination*. Autonomy is the patient's independence and separateness as a self-directing person (Simon, 1992). Supporting the patient's autonomy can be contrasted with exerting *undue influence* by taking advantage of a position of power and trust—for example, by sexually exploiting the patient. Therapy can be thought of as a form of "due influence," in which the therapist seeks to persuade the patient to move toward the goals of treatment. Such persuasion, in which the therapist engages the patient's capacity to reason, is to be distinguished from coercion, in which the therapist aims to manipulate the patient by undermining the patient's reasoning capacity (Malcolm, 1992).

The therapist fosters self-determination by helping the patient reach the point where therapy is no longer necessary, as opposed to inducing prolonged dependence on the therapist. This principle is important because it is normal for patients to transfer their dependence on others to the therapist. This immature attachment becomes the last obstacle for the patient, duly influenced by the therapist, to overcome.

Respect for Fiduciary Relationship

Mental health and other health professionals have a fiduciary relationship with their patients—that is, a relationship based on trust and good faith (Jorgenson, 1995d; Jorgenson, Hirsch, & Wahl, 1997). Attorneys, accountants, stockbrokers, and executors act as fiduciaries when they manage a person's financial affairs. A clinician assumes a parallel responsibility. Instead of money, however, the patient places his or her intimate revelations, emotional vulnerability, and hopes and prospects for a better life in trust with the clinician. The clinician must manage these "assets" in the patient's best interest and not for personal gain, material or otherwise.

Many clinicians honor the fiduciary relationship through practice in keeping with two clinical and ethical principles long maintained by analytic therapists: *neutrality* and *abstinence*. According to the principle of neutrality, the therapist, while forming an alliance with the patient's healthy aspirations, remains dispassionate about the patient's choices and outcomes (Hoffer, 1985). By not becoming personally invested in the patient's success or failure, the therapist is better able to support the patient's autonomy and avoid undue influence. Although this principle of neutrality might appear to be violated when, for instance, a CBT practitioner "weighs in" in favor of certain choices a patient makes (such as doing therapy homework), the therapist's investment in what the patient chooses to do is tactical, for the patient's benefit, not personal and emotional on the part of the therapist. As this example illustrates, judgment and flexibility are needed in applying ethical principles to different types of therapy and contexts of practice. One therapist may laugh openly at a patient's jokes, while another may not—so long as both are acting in the patient's interest.

Freud's (1915/1958c) principle of abstinence is especially helpful in understanding and preventing boundary violations, even if one does not practice strictly in accord with this principle. The principle "holds that the therapist abstains from seeking personal gratification from the therapeutic relationship, beyond receiving a fee and taking satisfaction from the work itself" (Gutheil & Simon, 2002, p. 590; cf. Novey, 1991). The work, of course, is to care for others, and the main satisfaction comes from engaging with this challenge and contributing one's best professional skills to serve the patient and the goals of therapy. It is also natural to feel gratified by seeing someone benefit and progress in life, as long as one refrains from burdening the patient, and the therapy, with one's own expectations and interventions. Abstinence includes not acceding to the patient's or therapist's wish for immediate gratifications in therapy, such as that of easy, time-filling communication that enables the patient to avoid confronting inner conflicts. (Such diversion is to be distinguished from conversation that sets the patient at ease and establishes trust and rapport.) This clinical principle takes on ethical dimensions with respect to self-seeking behavior such as seeking the patient's praise or admiration or using the patient as a personal confidant.

The idea that a clinician has a fiduciary responsibility to act in the patient's best interest is consistent with four other established ethical principles: *altruism* (doing for others, even at cost to oneself), *beneficence* (doing good), *nonmaleficence* (doing no harm), and *compassion* (acting out of a feeling for the suffering of others). Together, these and the other ethical tenets outlined here constitute universal norms for clinical practice that cut across professional lines, applying (for example) to clergy and primary care physicians as well as to psychotherapists. They are benchmarks against which to measure the deviations described in Part II of this book.

PART II

Explorations

CHAPTER 3

Role, Time, Place

This chapter addresses three basic areas where boundary violations often begin and, with timely intervention, can end. The
concept of role is part of the foundation of therapeutic boundary maintenance, since most boundary violations constitute some form of role conflict,
role deviation, or role reversal. Time and place are elementary structural
components of the therapeutic frame, literal boundaries that, by limiting
and containing the interchange, help keep it safe and productive.

ROLE

When a patient says to a therapist, "I can't trust you unless you let me sit
on your lap," or "I need you to write a letter to my boss telling him to go
easy on me," the therapist may answer, "That's not what therapy is." In
establishing such a boundary, the therapist defines the limits of the role
he or she can play in the patient's life. All of the boundary violations discussed in this and the next five chapters represent, in some form, a stepping out of role on the part of the clinician. Therefore, an understanding
of the clinician's role underlies any effective strategy for preventing
boundary violations.

A great many boundary violations could be prevented if clinicians
simply asked themselves, "Is this something a therapist does?" One overzealous resident in a psychiatric hospital, acting on the mistaken belief
that a patient was being sought by police, fingerprinted the patient. Out
of anxiety and a beginner's naiveté, the resident took on a law enforcement role. That is not what a therapist does. Likewise, sweeping the office

floor or keeping the therapist's books is not what a patient can be permitted to do, although just such events have actually occurred.

What Is a Therapist's Role?

Psychotherapy has been defined as "the intentional use of verbal techniques to explore or alter the patient's emotional life in order to effect symptom reduction or behavior change" (Hundert & Appelbaum, 1995, p. 347). Opinions may differ as to whether this definition needs to be expanded to include cognitive-behavioral techniques such as behavioral activation, but there is no underlying difference when it comes to ethical (as opposed to practical) limits on the therapist's role. An analytic therapist's job might be described as that of a *hired co-investigator*. "Hired" implies a contractual relationship with monetary compensation. "Co-" suggests an alliance, a collaborative relationship. "Investigator" focuses the therapist's role on exploration and discovery. There is a close parallel here with Beck's (1991) concept of "collaborative empiricism" as the foundation of the treatment alliance in CBT. If you find yourself doing something other than "investigating" (in this broader sense that accommodates different therapeutic approaches) collaboratively with the patient, you may be straying from the therapist's role and task.

The role of a therapist is indeed a special one in the patient's life. Typically, a patient comes to therapy with expectations that include close and careful attention, empathy, and understanding in a comfortable, supportive environment. These demands, which may represent a sharp break with the patient's previous relationships with important people in his or her life, are appropriately met by the therapist. This does not mean, however, that the therapist goes to the extreme of becoming the ideal, totally accepting or nurturing, parent—let alone lover—of the patient's fantasies. Such perfect gratification, bypassing the tension and conflict from which the patient needs to learn and grow, would raise unrealistic expectations both of the therapist and of life outside therapy (Gutheil & Gabbard, 1993). Renouncing those aspirations by staying within the limits of the therapist's role entails losses for both patient and therapist, as Stark (1995) notes:

> For therapists who are at the receiving end of the patient's relentless entitlement, it means an ability to confront the reality that we will never be the perfect mother both we and the patient would have wanted. We must grieve the reality of our own very real limitations. We will then be able to tolerate being in the position of saying no. But our ability to say no in the face of the patient's unremitting insistence that we say yes will give her

the opportunity to come to terms with the reality that things are not always as she would have wanted them to be. (p. 199)

At the other extreme, the abstinence required of an analytic therapist does not extend to total frustration of the patient's wishes (Viederman, 1991). Rather, the therapist needs to distinguish between patient demands that perpetuate preexisting psychological dynamics and "growth needs" that require some gratification in the service of breaking those patterns (Casement, 1990). A therapist who projects care and concern, together with appropriate limit setting, is serving the patient's growth needs. In this sense, the difference between an analytic therapist and a CBT practitioner who reinforces positive accomplishments is at most one of degree.

Although the ethical boundaries of the therapist's role do not preclude empathy, positive regard, and a supportive attitude toward the patient, that role stops short of identifying *personally* with the patient's success. Such overidentification can burden the patient by interfering with the patient's autonomous growth. To facilitate genuine growth, the therapist must be able to "let go." In any case, as Gabbard and Wilkinson (1994) note, the therapist cannot impose a cure:

> Therapists must also reconcile themselves to the notion that certain patients may not be interested in giving up lifelong modes of adaptation such as chronic suicidality or sadomasochistic relatedness. . . . Two thousand years ago Seneca the Younger noted, "It is part of the cure to wish to be cured." It is not too late to heed his advice. (p. 66)

A therapist with a narcissistic need to have a patient get better may be tempted to go beyond the normal repertoire of therapeutic techniques in a misguided attempt to "save" or "rescue" the patient. When therapy is driven by the therapist's need to feel competent, worthy, powerful, or all-knowing by virtue of his or her influence on the patient's life, there can be as much a conflict of interest (albeit an intangible one) as when a therapist exploits a patient sexually or financially (Epstein & Simon, 1990). Again, we emphasize that this narcissistic investment on the therapist's part is not to be confused with supportive encouragement, such as the "cheerleading" by which a dialectical behavior therapist reinforces constructive behavior and skill development (Dimeff & Koerner, 2007; Linehan, 1993).

Informed Consent and the Therapeutic Contract

The therapeutic frame, as described in the preceding chapter, is established by a treatment contract (oral or written, but always documented), which defines the purpose and methods of therapy (see Caudill, 1997b, pp. 275–279; Epstein, 1994, pp. 120–121). The contract is a working agreement by which the therapist and patient set out their goals and specify how, where, when, and for how long they will interact. The contract helps both therapist and patient by creating shared expectations as to what may and may not happen in therapy (Gutheil, 1982a).

Although the term "contract" sounds legalistic, the treatment contract can best be thought of as a shared understanding about how therapy will proceed and how progress can be assessed. This agreement may be expressed orally in an early session or may be co-created during the course of therapy. Written contracts are, however, commonly used by clinicians who work with multiple clients in high-conflict situations (e.g., some family mediators, family systems counselors, and parenting coordinators). In such cases a detailed contract specifies the limits of the clinician's responsibility to each individual and to the family as a whole.

The content of the contract will, of course, reflect the type of therapy the patient agrees to undertake. Psychoanalytic, cognitive-behavioral, client-focused, existential, narrative, or community-oriented therapists can use the contract to establish and communicate norms and expectations consistent with their respective methods. For example, feminist and relational therapists, as well as some contemporary analytic therapists, emphasize active interchange and the co-creation of interpersonal reality (sometimes referred to as "intersubjectivity") rather than strict interpersonal boundaries (see, e.g., Combs & Freedman, 2002; Jordan, 1995; Renik, 1995).

Within the broad limits of acceptable practice, the contract may allow for therapeutic innovations in the interest of the patient. If modalities are to be employed that are not customarily associated with the type of therapy being practiced, these should be discussed and incorporated into the contract. This would be the case, for example, if a psychodynamic therapist anticipated using modalities normally employed by cognitive-behavioral therapists, such as home visits, outings to confront feared situations, or active instruction in life skills. If such departures are not anticipated at the outset, the contract may be changed by mutual agreement to include them during the course of therapy. In this way, the contract can help determine whether a given event is a boundary crossing (either planned or occurring inadvertently while following an agreed-upon plan and process) or a boundary violation.

The contract is created by informed consent. Informed consent is a fundamental ethical and legal principle that underlies all clinical practice (Berg, Appelbaum, Lidz, & Parker, 2001; Croarkin, Berg, & Spira, 2003; Pope & Vasquez, 2007). To obtain the patient's informed consent to a recommended treatment, the therapist explains what the treatment involves, its risks and benefits, and the risks and benefits of alternative treatments, including no treatment at all. The patient can then choose freely whether to undertake the proposed treatment or any other (see Epstein, 1994, pp. 147–150). This essential process safeguards the patient's autonomy and fosters the therapeutic alliance (Gutheil, 1982a; Simon, 1992).

Likewise, as therapy proceeds, the therapist honors the ethical principles of respect for the patient's dignity, autonomy, and self-determination by adhering to the contract (Gutheil & Simon, 2002). Not to give the patient the treatment he or she contracted for, even if the patient at times demands or wishes for something else, is not only disrespectful but also unethical and countertherapeutic, and may give rise to legal or disciplinary action. The contract gives the therapist a basis for setting limits when the patient asks, pleads, or insists that the therapist step out of role. Citing the contract if necessary, the therapist responds to boundary challenges by exploring the meaning of the patient's behavior rather than acceding to the patient's request. In this way, the patient's attention can be redirected to the wishes, fears, and needs that motivate the patient's demands. If therapy becomes stalled in exploring the patient's repeated attempts to induce the therapist to act in some other role, the therapist again reminds the patient of what the two of them contracted to do. For example, a therapist might say, "We can't spend every session on your asking me whether you can sit on my lap when we agreed to work on your depression (anxiety, etc.)."

By Axiom I (presented in Chapter 1), it is the therapist's responsibility to maintain boundaries in a therapeutic manner. A reality therapist can say, "That's not how you meet your needs." A psychoanalyst can ask, "What comes to mind when you ask that question?" If the patient appears to react to the therapist's firmness with discomfort or shame, the therapist can attempt to alleviate such feelings with reminders of the goals of therapy or with reassuring remarks such as "We're not here to judge; we're here to understand."

Role Conflicts and Multiple Relationships

In a cartoon in *The New Yorker*, a woman is lying on the analytic couch as a male therapist sits behind her taking notes. The therapist asks, "Are you uncomfortable discussing this because I'm a man or because I'm your husband?" (Gregory, 2001, p. 98). This is an absurdly obvious example of the kinds of role conflicts that clinicians must avoid. Clearly, one does not accept family members or other close associates as patients; conversely, one does not associate personally with family members of, or other intimates of, patients (Hundert & Appelbaum, 1995).

In individual (as opposed to family or couple) therapy, a therapist must maintain confidentiality by refraining from discussing the patient's condition and treatment with family members without the patient's explicit permission. The therapist may step outside the confidential relationship in an emergency—for example, if it becomes necessary to call the patient's spouse and say, "I'm very concerned about your husband, who appears suicidal. Please tell me if you know where he is." The therapist and patient may also involve the spouse or other family member in the therapy in an adjunctive role. In this vein, the therapist might say, "Let's get your wife in here, and let's talk." With the patient's agreement, and after a discussion of the purpose, the spouse may be involved in the treatment in specified ways—for example, by facilitating the patient's plan to stop drinking or to lose weight. In such cases it is essential to clarify this adjunctive role to both patient and spouse: the therapist is not treating the spouse, and the treatment is for the patient's benefit (see Epstein, 1994, pp. 123–124).

Many of the boundary questions discussed throughout this book involve some form of dual relationship, such as a financial, social, or sexual relationship coexisting with the therapeutic relationship. The ways in which such conflicts of interest can compromise therapy and exploit and harm patients have been thoroughly discussed and documented (e.g., Kitchener, 1988; Pope, 1991). Since the focus of this book is on boundary issues that arise in the therapist–patient dyad, we will not deal specifically with multiple relationships in areas such as referrals, solicitation of business, and advertising (Epstein, 1994, pp. 127–143; Reamer, 2001, pp. 143–147). However, multiple relationships are also manifested in contexts such as monetary transactions, gifts, and services (Chapter 4), unintended personal encounters outside the office (Chapter 6), and the conflict between therapeutic and institutional or forensic roles (Chapter 12). The ethics codes of the major professional associations call for avoidance of multiple relationships that have the potential to compromise therapy and harm the patient. At the same time, clinicians must be prepared to make ethical and practical choices when circumstances create the prospect of a multiple relationship with a patient (Pope & Wedding, 2008; see Chapter 13).

Role Deviation: "Helping" Outside of Therapy

"What should I do about . . . ?" "I need you to write a letter to my boss saying he shouldn't be so hard on me because I have a mental disorder." "Would you please help me balance my checkbook?" Such "innocent" requests by patients can lead to the pitfall of *role deviation*, wherein a therapist assumes nontherapeutic roles in a patient's life. When you become a patient's personal or financial adviser, or "run interference" for the patient out in the world, you are not doing therapy—except when such services have been contracted for. The following situations represent commonly occurring dilemmas, all the more insidious because they typically involve no intent on the therapist's part to exploit the patient for personal gain.

Gratuitous Advice

When a therapist dispenses offhand personal advice (e.g., "Two out of three women you'll meet are no good"), therapeutic exploration can be disrupted. (This cautionary statement does not apply either to therapeutic limit setting or to the focused directiveness characteristic of approaches such as reality therapy and life-skills training.) Like other boundaries, this one was not rigorously respected in the early days of psychotherapy. Freud, for example, is reported to have advised one of his patients, a fellow analyst, to divorce his wife and marry a patient (Gay, 1988). Today, the risks of domination and dependency resulting from a therapist's expression of judgmental attitudes and directive advice are better recognized. Special care should be taken in the transition zone "between the chair and the door," where the therapist, having stayed in role throughout the session, may throw off unguarded remarks as the patient is leaving. A permissible (and necessary) exception is to warn the patient about logistical risks specific to the therapy setting, such as "Watch your step; the parking lot is icy" (Gutheil & Simon, 1995).

The discriminations that need to be made in this area are sometimes delicate ones. Coaching can be a dimension of therapy, but that dimension needs to be made explicit in the contract. Otherwise, although the impulse to correct a patient's naive expectations and cushion the adjustment to painful realities may be strong, the therapist's role is not to lecture but to facilitate the patient's self-exploration and learning through experience. The same words may be appropriate or inappropriate, depending on the context. For example, it is usually not therapeutic to volunteer the sentiment "It's a cold world out there," whether as factual information or as personal opinion. These same words, however, might be used to mirror the pain and frustration the patient has expressed after experiencing a series of rebuffs. Such a reflective statement invites the patient to acknowledge and confront his or her feelings. Again, the patient's needs and the therapeutic contract determine the appropriateness of the intervention.

Extratherapeutic Interventions

What if a patient asked, "Can't you call my boss and tell him to lay off me?" (This kind of "favor" requested by a patient is to be distinguished from situations such as insurance or Medicaid forms, parole reports, work-disability forms, or return-to-work plans, in which a clinician performs a mandated or prescribed extratherapeutic function. Nor is it to be equated with staged desensitization to anxiety-producing work situations.) Rather than agree to such a request, there are numerous therapeutic responses directed toward helping the patient cope with a stressful work environment. These include "How does that make you feel?" and "Let's talk about ways you can communicate with your boss." The therapist might suggest role playing: "Let's go through the kind of exchange you might have; I'll play your boss." But when the therapist gets on the phone or writes a letter to the employer, the therapist has stepped out of role and become a diplomat, a negotiator. At the extreme, this active "helping" can lead to the role conflict involved in attempting to conduct an objective evaluation of the patient (Strasburger, Gutheil, & Brodsky, 1997) or to the ethical compromise of "special pleading" through false diagnoses or dishonest reports. As a rule, a therapist refrains from intervening in a patient's life to do what the patient needs to do for him- or herself. Rather, the therapist provides an environment in which the patient can work through conflicts and develop strength for living.

Balancing the Checkbook

If there is one surprisingly common case of role deviation, it is probably the therapist's offer to balance a patient's checkbook, a simple act with complex implications. This is not, ipso facto, impermissible, but it is not what a therapist is there to do, and it can create, maintain, or exploit an artificial dependency. A request for such assistance can be an early sign that a patient is seeking to blur therapeutic boundaries. Likewise, when the therapist offers to balance the patient's checkbook, boundaries become blurred.

The authors' clinical and forensic experience suggests that the seemingly benign act of balancing a patient's checkbook is a fairly common early precursor to sexual misconduct. This may be because of the signal importance of money in our society. A checkbook is more than the routine, cut-and-dried thing it appears to be. If I open my checkbook to you, I am giving you a private look at what may be very personal and conflicted issues in my life. Moreover, money is itself a major area of serious boundary violations (see Chapter 4). A therapist who gets into a patient's bank account could gain access to insider information.

Are there any circumstances in which it is appropriate to balance a patient's checkbook? It can be appropriate to do so as part of assessing the functional capacities of a developmentally disabled person and training the person to live more independently. Likewise, this may be one of many such tasks performed by a case manager, who might help a patient fill out applications for disability insurance, Medicaid, or residence in a group home. It is not, however, part of the training or job description of a psychotherapist. The therapist's role is to help the patient understand the problem he or she is having with finances and to identify resources (e.g., a calculator) for solving the problem.

The Limits of the Role

Sometimes the question of whether a therapist has stepped out of role is a subtle one, requiring a discriminating assessment, as in the following example:

> A male psychologist was treating a female patient whose diet consisted largely of junk food. The therapist noticed a cracking at the corners of the patient's lips (cheilosis) that is a sign of vitamin deficiency. Getting an orange from an adjoining room, he told the patient, "Eat this now."
> The psychologist presented this case anonymously at a professional conference. Those who heard him agreed that the boundary crossing was justified. He had acted clinically in response to a clear, immediate need, as with giving sugar to a diabetic patient having an insulin reaction. In a subsequent session with the same patient, he told her about the presentation. He related the story in an offhand, somewhat self-congratulatory way, with no therapeutic exploration of what it meant to the patient. In the absence of such exploration, the patient began to think about how the therapist was a pretty special guy to be speaking at a conference and how she herself must be special to be the subject of his case study. What did it mean, she thought, that he had singled her out for this attention?

As this case illustrates, it can be difficult to sort out questions of role maintenance in practice. This therapist acted appropriately first in the clinical role and then in a quasi-academic role. But it is hard to find a therapeutic rationale for his telling the patient about his presentation. He might have processed therapeutically with the patient what it meant when he gave her the orange ("What did you learn from this?"). Instead, his motivation appears to have been to show what a well-connected and recognized professional he was. Not surprisingly, his revelation fed the patient's fantasies of having a special relationship with him.

Contrast this with the following case:

> A therapist sought a patient's permission to include in an article an anonymously written vignette about the patient's sexual involvement with a previous therapist. The therapist explored the implications of this request with the patient: "How do you feel about this?" He showed respect for the patient by asking her permission in advance, and the patient thanked him for it.

In this case, it was easier to maintain clear role boundaries, because the vignette was not about the present therapy and the exercise had the therapeutic purpose of helping the patient understand why her previous therapist had been unethical and what she had experienced as a result. There was no guarantee that being in this spotlight would not feed the patient's fantasies, but the therapist's conduct minimized this risk while maximizing the chance that the patient would benefit. It is precisely this kind of therapeutic risk–benefit analysis that needs to be carried out whenever role definitions and boundaries are in question.

Role Reversal: The Patient as Caretaker

A patient was surprised to hear her therapist ask her how he should respond to a false accusation another patient had made against him. The patient's immediate response was to commiserate, "How could anyone do that?"—but before long she sued him, too. This therapist tried to cope with one boundary violation by inviting another. For a therapist to consult a patient about a professional or personal problem is an inappropriate role reversal. It opens a door that should not be opened, undermining the secure structure of the therapeutic frame.

Therapeutic role playing is a standard technique, appropriate in many therapies. One therapist, for example, used it in an inpatient setting with a patient who insistently demanded a pass to leave the hospital. The therapist invited the patient to switch roles, and so put the patient in the position of setting limits.

> THERAPIST: *(imitating patient's sometimes whiny tone)* Why can't I have a pass?
>
> PATIENT: *(gruffly, parodying the therapist's typical brusque responses)* We'll talk about it.
>
> *(Both burst into laughter.)*

This role-play exercise is an example of a deliberate therapeutic role reversal designed to help the patient put his or her desires and behavior in perspective. It dispelled the tension that had built up with this difficult patient. Role playing is also used to rehearse challenging life situations the patient will face. Role reversal becomes a boundary violation only when the therapist begins to seek gratification of his or her personal needs.

> A senior therapist resigned from his local professional society and surrendered his license after admitting he had an improper relationship with a patient. Having been diagnosed with cancer, this therapist was confronted with a patient who was acting as a dedicated caretaker for a friend with cancer. The therapist confessed to her that he wished he could be taken care of as fully as she was taking care of her friend, but that his wife could not fulfill this need because she also had cancer. The therapist–patient relationship evolved into an intimate personal one, until the patient left treatment and brought her concerns about the therapist's conduct to the professional society.

Problematic role reversals typically begin with an inappropriate self-disclosure (see Chapter 5). This needy, vulnerable therapist invited the patient to interact with him person-to-person, outside the frame, an invitation many patients are all too happy to accept. It was as if the therapist said, "I envy the care that your friend is receiving from you. I have the same illness, the same mortality as your friend. Won't you please take care of me, too?" The therapist and friend became rivals, competing for the patient's devoted support.

A surprising number of patients have been somebody's caretaker in their family of origin, perhaps pulling a drunken father or mate out of the gutter, absorbing abuse in a mother's place, or protecting siblings. Indeed, this role and its impact on the patient's life may be part of what the patient needs to examine. In the service of the "golden fantasy"— that is, the patient's wish that the therapist can meet all of the patient's needs (Smith, 1977)—the patient may shift into this familiar caretaking role. If a patient says, "That plant on your window sill needs dusting," the patient may be mounting a hostile challenge, as if saying, "If you can't keep your plants clean, how do you expect to take care of me?" Alternatively, the patient could be expressing a caretaking impulse: "Let me dust your plants for you." Patients bring all sorts of needs and desires to therapy ("I'll do anything for you; I'll clean your office; in fact, why can't I just *move in* to your office?"), but those goals cannot be allowed to drive the interaction. The vigilant therapist who remains in role and at task can say, "I notice that you seem to be trying to take care of me." This response, by maintaining structure and control, keeps the therapy on track. It closes the door to role reversal and opens the door to therapeutic exploration.

A therapist with a conscious or unconscious personal agenda or life-stage-specific needs (e.g., midlife crisis) can tap into a patient's instinctive caretaking tendency. Intentionally or not, the therapist extends a welcoming, even imploring, hand to the patient, whether by verbal or nonverbal cues. For example, by double-booking appointments the therapist may appear disorganized, overwhelmed, unable to handle the professional role without help. Or the therapist may display messy hair or rumpled, disheveled clothing (see Chapter 7). Verbally or behaviorally, the therapist is letting something hang out. Then the patient can say, "Don't you have a wife (or office assistant) to help you with that? Here, let me help you." From taking care of the therapist's need for dependency and nurturing, the patient may eventually move to taking care of the therapist's sexual needs. Role reversal is often a pivotal event that can begin a slide toward sexual misconduct.

TIME

Setting and maintaining clear limits on the frequency, timing, and length of sessions gives the therapeutic frame structure, stability, security, regularity, consistency, and predictability—qualities lacking in many patients' experiences with previous caretakers (Epstein, 1994, pp. 121–122). Out of respect for the value of the patient's time and as a model for the patient's commitments to others, the therapist must always be on time except in an emergency. The time boundary conveys to the patient that this relationship is a professional one, with a specific serious purpose. It is not a friendship or a parent–child relationship, even if it sometimes feels like one. From a risk management standpoint, working within a scheduled rather than irregular time frame makes the statement that even unconventional approaches are being practiced in a planned, purposeful, therapeutic context.

Extended Sessions

Trying to hold on to a therapist's caring attention beyond the scheduled end of a session is a common form of limit testing by patients. Gabbard (1982) catalogs a number of "exit lines" patients use to prolong or redirect the interchange after it is formally concluded. Therapists need to allow for occasions when a patient's immediate distress calls for flexibility in ending a session. This should be viewed as an emergency intervention, like making a special appointment for an acutely suicidal patient, and should be documented as such. Patients with dissociative identity disorder (multiple personality disorder) may need flexibility in session length to allow for the emergence of various alters (Simon, 1992). On the other hand, treating a patient as "special" can play into the pathology of a patient with narcissistic, borderline, or dependent personality disorder (Gutheil, 1989). There is all the more need to maintain boundaries with patients who have more difficulty recognizing boundaries.

Therapists, too, experience a separation at the end of the hour, and therapists have been known to speak their own exit lines (Gabbard, 1982). When a therapist feels so involved with a patient as to lose track of time or to allow the patient repeatedly to extend the session, it is the therapist's boundaries and self-discipline that must be restored (Gutheil, 1999a). When sessions regularly run over their scheduled time, it is necessary to consider what therapist or patient needs may be contributing to this pattern.

In setting limits with patients, it is generally considered unnecessarily rigid and alienating to have an alarm clock go off at the end of the session except when a contract to this effect is mutually desired. Instead, the therapist can explain that it is inconsiderate to the next patient to go over time. A patient who routinely falls apart at the end of a session is meeting his or her needs at the expense of other patients. Negotiating this give-and-take is part of therapy, part of the patient's learning that respect and consideration can be mutual rather than mutually exclusive.

If more work is needed to deal with a patient's separation anxiety, the therapist can prepare the patient explicitly for the end of the session (Gutheil & Simon, 1995). The therapist might say, "We will be stopping in about 20 (15, 10, 5) minutes. Do we need to talk about anything else, arrange anything else, before next week?" Then, if the patient raises additional questions as the session is ending, the therapist can reply, "I guess that can wait until next time." The patient and therapist can also try to anticipate special circumstances that may call for additional sessions, or longer sessions, so that these deviations can occur in a planned rather than erratic way. When a session is extended significantly (e.g., to 2 hours instead of 1), the full time should be billed. Consultation is helpful in assessing and documenting the need to cross time boundaries, especially when a patient's acute or chronic resistance to ending sessions may indicate a need for hospitalization.

Scheduling Sessions at Odd Hours

"The last patient of the day" has become a code phrase signifying trouble, and not only among clinicians. For some attorneys and boards of registration, seeing a patient at the end of the day has become virtually presumptive evidence of sexual misconduct. From a risk management perspective, a patient with an intense erotic transference to the therapist is best seen during normal business hours when a receptionist is present and there is high traffic at the beginning as well as the end of the patient's hour (Gutheil & Gabbard, 1993).

Where there is smoke, there is sometimes fire. Permissive scheduling can feed the fantasies of a vulnerable patient or therapist. Without a line of patients waiting to be seen, both parties may feel a sense of limitlessness, as if they did not have to take seriously the end of the appointed hour. Letting "the time fly by" is analogous to letting a patient's debt accumulate. These two boundary violations may occur together, since spending more time with a patient should increase the patient's bill. In both cases there is a breakdown of the therapeutic frame. As time is allowed to expand, both the physical space and the financial space lose their shape as well and no longer serve to structure the relationship.

In one case a patient had achieved some success, and the patient and therapist went out for a celebratory dinner after their session. Role, time, and place were all implicated in this ill-advised indulgence. The spirit of celebration need not be an unwelcome guest in the therapy hour, but why not simply say "Congratulations"?

When a patient is scheduled outside of normal working hours, there must be a demonstrated necessity, a documented risk assessment, and an alternative structure put in place to maintain boundaries. These precautions were not followed in the following case:

> A male psychiatrist came to a hospital for sessions beginning at 2:00 A.M. with a female inpatient diagnosed with borderline personality disorder. He rationalized that this odd arrangement, made possible by the hospital setting, was necessitated by scheduling problems. For the patient, the timing gave the sessions an irresistibly adventurous flavor, and she began to shower and perfume in preparation for her therapist's arrival. In-depth sessions lasting 2–4 hours, with intensely romantic content, led, not surprisingly, to an overtly sexual relationship.
>
> This therapist's extraordinary, and extended, lapse of judgment had severe consequences for both parties. Feeling exploited in the aftermath, the patient became phobic about medical care. Without the

benefit of timely examinations, she developed a cancer that reached an advanced stage by the time it was diagnosed. Before she died, her husband sued the psychiatrist for loss of consortium, winning a multimillion-dollar settlement.

It should be noted, once again, that patients with borderline personality disorder, given their need for definition and structure, are at the highest risk for problematic reactions to overly fluid boundaries (Gutheil, 1989, 2005b, 2005c).

Phone Calls between Sessions

Telephone calls between sessions are to be expected, especially from patients with personality disorders, posttraumatic stress disorder (PTSD), or dissociative identity disorder and those experiencing acute distress for any reason. It can be difficult to draw the line between limit testing that needs to be restrained and an emotional crisis that calls out for an empathic response. Even borderline patients, who are notorious for limit testing, behave that way in part because of difficulties with evocative memory that drive them to seek reassuring confirmation that the therapist is still there for them (Gutheil & Gabbard, 1993).

Therapists of different schools, philosophies, and styles of practice vary in their receptiveness to such calls. When does a clinician's availability provide an atmosphere of security, and when does it indulge regression and inhibit growth? Dialectical behavior therapists distinguish between an off-hours "coaching call," in which a patient asks for guidance in applying skills learned in therapy to an immediate situation, and a "heart-to-heart," in which a patient seeks ventilation, reassurance, support, or historical exploration. Whereas the latter is not encouraged, the former is supported to the extent that some DBT practitioners give patients their cell phone numbers, a practice clinicians generally are well advised to avoid (Linehan, 1993).

This clinical assessment notwithstanding, every therapist has a personal and professional need to keep the calls down to a manageable volume. If you don't protect your patients' access to you by the way you conduct yourself, you may get driven away and burned out by a patient's insistent needs. Thus, it is protective of therapy to build in reasonable expectations early in the relationship by setting gentle, firm, nonrejecting limits. When necessary, for example, you might say, "We can't keep having you call me at 4 A.M. between every session." Such a remark opens for examination the conflict between the patient's childhood needs and an adult's needs for reliability and mutual consideration. Therapy begins with the effort to negotiate boundaries that will meet both the patient's and the therapist's needs. The patient then experiences a give-and-take in which both parties' needs are respected. The therapist, even with a case-load of challenging patients, can aim to hold down the evening calls to a reasonable level.

Calls by a therapist to a patient should be made only for documented clinical reasons and should be conducted professionally, without personal chatting. Even when these precautions are followed, an air of impropriety may surround after-hours telephone contacts with patients, as the following case illustrates.

> A male therapist was seeing a female patient who had recently suf-fered the deaths of several family members. During one session the patient became grief-stricken, sobbing uncontrollably. That evening the therapist called her at home to see how she was feeling and to ask whether she needed additional support. "I'm fine," the patient told him. Subsequently she reported the therapist to the licensing board for what she characterized as the intrusive act of calling her at home.

This case was a by-product of public hypersensitivity to therapeutic boundary violations—a regrettable condition of practice today. For the therapist it was disheartening to be brought before the board for a simple gesture of concern, even though his documentation of his rationale for the call spared him from censure. For her part, the patient's reaction to this benign boundary crossing was conditioned by revelations of other thera-pists' misconduct. In this atmosphere, the best-intended interventions may bring about discomfort rather than healing support (Gutheil, 1994b).

PLACE

"Place" in this chapter refers to the physical settings in which therapeutic and related encounters occur. Accidental meetings in personal settings in the community will be discussed in Chapter 6. Our concern here is with where a therapist chooses to conduct therapy, as well as with where a therapist may encounter patients routinely or as an outgrowth of the ther-apist's role.

The Office

As a rule, therapy is conducted in the therapist's office or in a suitable in-stitutional setting. Like the limits set by the clock, the physical boundaries of the office emphasize the specific, serious purpose of the session. Therapy is not the kind of activity that is conducted at lunchcounters or in cars, except in planned programs of exposure and desensitization or in treatment of eating disorders. The office provides a consistent, private, professional setting, in contrast to the inconsistency and intrusiveness that many patients have experienced in other relationships and environments.

The office should convey a professional image, avoiding self-revealing displays of personal paraphernalia. It is appropriate to respond flexibly to the patient's expressed preferences—for example, to turn the heat up or down, or to draw the blinds if the patient fears being exposed to the outside world. Such routine accommodations can reach a limit when the patient's requests threaten to compromise therapy.

Space boundary issues can arise even within the office, as when the patient and therapist are placed in uncomfortably close physical contact by a cramped office, a narrow entrance space, or the therapist's inadvertence or unexamined motives. Based on the concern that small offices, dim lighting, and the absence of windows increase the likelihood of inappropriate intimacy, the American Psychological Association has published recommendations with respect to office dimensions and ambience (Yenney & American Psychological Association Practice Directorate, 1994). However, clinicians have little or no control over these setting variables in inpatient and agency settings.

Boundaries of space as well as time are blurred when the patient moves through the transition zone "between the door and the chair" at the beginning of a session and "between the chair and the door" at the end. Other boundary crossings and violations may result if the therapist is complicit in the patient's attempts to communicate "informally" or "off the record" while in this no-man's land. On the other hand, an alert therapist can observe, in what the patient says and does in this space, the beginnings of such potential boundary excursions, and use those insights for therapeutic exploration (Gutheil & Simon, 1995).

Accompanying the patient beyond the office door—to the restroom, the cafeteria, or outside the building—extends this ambiguous space into even more treacherous territories. Unless there are clinical reasons to do otherwise, it is best for patient and therapist to separate at the office door (Gutheil & Simon, 1995). One case of sexual misconduct began when a lesbian therapist regularly went to the restroom with a female patient and continued to talk with her from an adjoining stall (Gutheil & Gabbard, 1993). Given the outcome, the therapist's behavior can be understood as a goal-directed effort to break down normal barriers and groom the patient to take the therapist into her physical space. It also foreshadowed the pathological bonding the therapist subsequently manifested when she would wear the patient's clothes to the office after they had spent the night together.

Home Offices

Although professional acceptance of home offices may vary by community and region, home offices are generally acceptable as long as there is a clear boundary between the areas of the home devoted to personal and professional use (Hundert & Appelbaum, 1995). There should be a designated office space separate from the therapist's living quarters, with (whenever possible) an entrance exclusively or primarily for the office and a separate bathroom for patients' use. Even with these precautions, patients will see (in a general way, from the external setting) how the therapist lives. Occasionally there will be inadvertent self-disclosures when a patient sees members of the therapist's family near the entrance or in the vicinity of the home. How to deal with such accidental boundary crossings will be discussed in Chapter 6.

Not all practitioners can afford a spacious home with a separate entrance for patients. When, for example, patients may observe residential areas in the house or apartment from a hallway on the way to and from the clinician's office, close attention must be given to any messages that may be conveyed by the less than fully private setting. Moreover, the risk of unintended boundary crossings should be reduced by visual and aural barriers (e.g., closed doors, curtains, noise machines) and by keeping family members out of the proximity of patients as much as possible. If a bedroom is visible, the door must be closed, and no one should go into the bedroom in sight of a patient. If patients must use a bathroom also accessible to residents or visitors, it must have a locked cabinet for personal belongings (including, obviously, sharp objects such as razors). The setting should appear comfortable but professional, with no clothing or other revealing objects thrown around.

Give thought to what any visible accouterments might communicate to a patient. To take an easy example, displaying a copy of *Playboy* on a magazine rack in the hallway would clearly be inappropriate. Whether *Field and Stream* would likewise be inappropriate might depend, say, on whether you are offering patients practical assistance and counseling or deep personal exploration. In psychodynamic therapy, patients might perceive you as hunting them, or reeling them in. As a precaution against such associations, some clinicians stock their waiting rooms with magazines that appeal to a wide range of interests.

If you don't maintain a professional atmosphere in the face of a somewhat penetrable boundary between your working and living environment, you may unintentionally encourage a patient's conflicted wishes to be part of your family. Furthermore, even if you do observe all the recommended guidelines, good clinical practice as well as risk management call for not seeing patients who present a foreseeable risk of problematic reactions in such a setting. Home office issues can be incorporated into the informed-consent process, and patients who are likely to feel uncomfortable or inhibited in this setting should be referred elsewhere. In the following vignette, merely seeing his therapist in a home office (as opposed to anything about that setting) was more than the patient could tolerate.

> Early in her career, a psychoanalytically oriented psychiatrist moved from an office in a hospital to a home office. Subsequently, one of her male patients terminated prematurely. His therapy with this female psychiatrist did not survive the uncomfortable feeling of intimacy he associated with the home office setting.

This was not a case of impropriety, since the therapist followed professional guidelines in setting up her office at home. This patient's therapy was a casualty of the changed setting, but preventing that outcome, had it been possible at all, would have required adjustments in analytic technique rather than in ethical behavior.

Meeting outside the Office

Professional mores have changed since Freud analyzed people while walking along the Danube. Now, when a Jungian therapist advertises therapy conducted while jogging, the predominant profession reaction is: "Who is this for? Why should this therapist be paid for time he spends exercising?"

Conducting therapy over lunch is the quintessential example of what to avoid. This practice has given rise to the joke that "it might work if you don't talk with your mouth full." A restaurant, with staff and patrons passing by, is not a confidential setting, and a lunch meeting doesn't look like therapy—not to the people in the vicinity and not to a subsequent fact finder. It looks like a date or friendly chat. More important, it can feel like that, too. Whereas the office setting reminds both parties to keep to the business at hand, an eating place encourages informal social conversation with casual mutual revelations. That is why lunch with a patient is a common way station on the path to serious boundary violations.

There are, of course, legitimate exceptions to conducting therapy in an office setting. Going outdoors to play "catch" with an adolescent with developmental problems can be a vital step in engaging the adolescent in therapy. Active interventions such as "play therapy" are more typical in the treatment of children, as in the use of natural learning environments in applied behavior analysis. Still, there are contexts in which one can remain within role while leaving the office with adult patients. Religiously oriented therapists may accompany patients to a house of worship, and in some circumstances one may go with a patient to a court hearing. Caseworkers can render practical assistance such as driving a patient from home to the welfare office. As the last step in a desensitization program, a CBT practitioner may accompany a patient on an elevator, in a car, on an airplane, or even to the bathroom in the treatment of paruresis, the fear of urinating in a public restroom. The patient has contracted for this and knows what to expect. Gutheil and Gabbard (1993, p. 192) explain that "a body of professional literature, a clinical rationale, and risk–benefit documentation will be useful in protecting the clinician in such a situation from misconstruction of the therapeutic efforts." In some cases, effectiveness studies will be part of this documentation.

However, neither one's professional discipline nor school of practice is an all-purpose excuse for stepping outside the normal physical frame of therapy. The social worker as case manager is different from a social worker doing psychotherapy, where there is clinical benefit to maintaining the therapeutic frame. Likewise, not every kind of cognitive-behavioral treatment requires leaving the office. If treatment for anorexia calls for eating in the presence of the therapist, that can be done initially in the office. In some cases eating in public with the therapist is the next step, but this is a planned, documented intervention with a clinical rationale, not something done casually on impulse.

Informed consent is an essential part of the ethical and professional framework that supports departures from the usual boundaries. Samuel and Gorton (2001) give this example of how a psychotherapist might verbally involve the patient in considering the therapeutic rationale of a proposed "field trip":

> "While it is not typical for a psychodynamic psychotherapist to go outside of the office with a patient, in this situation we might want to try a visit together to your old boarding school so that we can refresh some of your memories and pursue further in-depth work on your feelings about having been 'abandoned' there at age six, but we should first carefully weigh what this might mean to you and to our work together." (p. 68)

A change of therapeutic venue may also occur in an emergency. The day after a fire in your office, do you see patients in another office in the building (perhaps a less secure setting with distracting stimuli) or cancel the day's patients? The question is one that requires clinical judgment. Some patients can handle a change of setting more easily than others, and some patients will suffer more than others from an interruption of therapy.

The following, regrettably common, case involves more than a temporary interruption of therapy.

> A social services agency announced that it was closing and instructed the therapists it employed to terminate their patients with little notice. Referrals were offered in an impersonal, bureaucratic manner that did not seem to meet patients' needs, especially given the sudden transition. Some patients were traumatized, and a few therapists considered whether they should continue to see their patients at home.

This poignant situation strains the general principle that good clinical and ethical care constitutes good risk management. These therapists have worked to create an alliance with their patients, but that relationship loses its legal standing and recognition once the therapists' employment is terminated. Personally, the patients feel attached to their therapists. Legally, however, the therapists have no direct relationship with their patients; they cannot be charged with abandonment. If the patients have a cause of action, it is against the agency. Seeing the patients at home under a makeshift, ad hoc arrangement leaves the therapists open to being characterized as predators seizing the opportunity to exploit patients who have been cast adrift. To minimize this risk, the therapists need to open a chart for any patient they continue to see once the agency's charts are closed. They should set up the formal apparatus of a home-based private practice as quickly as possible so as to reestablish a legitimate therapeutic frame and boundaries.

The Therapist as Samaritan

> A male therapist in a small town was treating a female patient with a possible diagnosis of multiple personality disorder. The therapist, who was planning to attend a conference about this disorder in a nearby city, thought it might be beneficial for the patient to attend as well so that she could learn about the illness. However, there was no public transportation to this city, and the patient did not have a car or the wherewithal to rent one. The therapist contemplated the propriety of offering to drive the patient to the conference.

Driving the patient to the conference is problematic, because it would be a deliberate boundary crossing rather than just an emergency measure—as giving a lift in a blizzard would be. A safer course for the therapist would simply be to give the patient a flyer about the conference and leave it to the patient to get there. If the patient is eager to attend the conference despite the obstacles, the therapist and patient might discuss how the patient could get there. Perhaps the patient could borrow a car from a friend or relative or arrange to ride with someone other than the therapist who was planning to go.

If these options are not feasible, the therapist might consider driving the patient to the conference if the potential benefit to the patient justified the risk of getting the therapy off the track. The risk–benefit analysis is patient-specific. For example, how might the excursion together play upon this particular patient's fantasies? In the context of a lawsuit, it will be easier for a jury to believe an accusation that the therapist "came on" to the patient if it is admitted that they went somewhere together in a car. For this and other reasons, documentation, debriefing, and a consultation—in this case *before* as well as after the fact—are clearly called for. One advantage this situation has over an emergency is that the therapist can lay the groundwork in advance, not only with a supervisor or consultant but also with the patient. The patient and therapist need to explore the purpose and meaning of the boundary crossing as well as to plan what they will and will not do (e.g., not sit together at the conference). Should the patient later bring a complaint, the therapist will have a strong defense if the therapist has documented therapeutic intent and consideration of risks and benefits. Although clinical as well as legal considerations dictate caution about undertaking such a boundary crossing, fear of liability need not absolutely rule out an unorthodox gesture intended to benefit the patient.

An emergency that can lead to out-of-office contact occurs when a therapist feels a need to intervene directly to help a patient in real or perceived danger. For the therapist, the danger lies in not being able to separate the patient's actual clinical needs from the therapist's desire to help. There are legitimate emergencies that call for direct intervention outside the normal boundaries of therapy. A rule of thumb would be: "Don't touch your patients, but if one has a cardiac arrest, you'd better pump the chest." Likewise, the humanitarian act of giving a patient a ride in a storm is justifiable as a therapeutic boundary crossing, as long as the therapist behaves professionally toward the patient and documents the therapeutic intention. However, driving a patient to a conference from which the patient could gain useful insights is not an emergency; usually there would be time to make other arrangements for the patient. In a similar vein, a therapist would not take a patient to a movie, but (as with giving a patient a book to read) a therapist might say, "I recommend that you see this movie, and then we'll discuss it."

One of the more difficult dilemmas a therapist may face occurs when a patient calls and indicates (directly or otherwise) that he or she is suicidal and in need of immediate hospitalization. As a rule, transport should be made by ambulance or by police, not by the therapist. In a true life-or-death emergency, when no one else can get to the patient in time, the therapist may need to take direct action. However, documentation and consultation as to clinical necessity are especially important in this situation, since the therapist's motives are likely to be scrutinized to determine whether this boundary crossing constituted a boundary violation. Any susceptibility on the therapist's part to take on the role of rescuer could encourage a patient to stage suicidal episodes to get the therapist's attention and assistance.

Boundaries of physical and interpersonal space are sometimes violated when a therapist's rescue fantasies get out of control, as in the following case:

> During a housing crisis a male psychiatrist invited a female patient who had difficulty finding shelter to stay temporarily in a guest room in the psychiatrist's house. He then slept in front of the door of the guest room to prevent the patient from leaving this protective environment and going back out on the street. When questioned about his unusual conduct, the psychiatrist explained that he had acted only out of a desire to help a destitute patient. The psychiatrist sustained criminal and civil penalties. (summarized from Gutheil, 1989)

Especially with patients who have difficulties with boundaries and limits, a therapist's conflicts about his or her own limits and/or about setting limits for the patient can have disastrous consequences. In this extreme case, the psychiatrist's violation of the boundary of place was part of a larger transgression of role boundaries. Having prescribed medications for himself (an illegal act in some states), he manifested a fusion of identity with this patient by giving her his own medications, as if to say, "What's good for me is good for you." He also gave her money. Yet, even such bizarre behavior as this arose from a misguided impulse to help the patient. Colluding in the patient's fantasies about him, the therapist allowed himself the personal gratification of being the patient's all-powerful benefactor rather than limiting himself to the appropriate professional role.

Therapy in Institutions

Therapy is regularly conducted in institutional settings as well as in private offices and clinics. In consultation rooms in psychiatric hospitals and residential facilities, the physical frame should reflect the same professionalism and respect for privacy as in a freestanding practice. This principle may be compromised in a setting such as a prison, where one may be required to interview an inmate in a cell. In such a setting the goal is to negotiate, to the greatest possible extent, a safe but confidential environment. The same is true with dangerous patients in a psychiatric hospital. Thus, when a patient has acted out violently, a therapist may see the patient first in a seclusion room, then in a quiet room, then in the ward, and finally back in the regular consultation room. These variations in the inpatient therapy setting depend on the patient's condition.

Clinicians employed in residential or all-day settings such as hospitals, inpatient addiction treatment centers, halfway houses, or day treatment programs may find it difficult to avoid fraternizing with patients, particularly in the cafeteria. There it is best to sit with other staff members when possible. Failing that, sit with patients other than your own. If you go to an empty table and one of your patients sits down next to you, handle the situation just as if you found yourself with a patient in an elevator, or in your car in a blizzard. Maintain a polite, professional demeanor. Do not reveal confidential information or turn lunch into a therapy session. Avoid inappropriate self-disclosures. If a patient makes a habit of sitting with you in the cafeteria, raise the issue for exploration—back in the office.

Whether to call or visit a patient in a general medical hospital (or in prison after an arrest) is a question that requires careful case-by-case judgment. Document the clinical or humanitarian benefits of the out-of-office visit(s), including maintaining the continuity of therapy, versus the risk that the patient will feel exposed or intruded upon or that the visit will reinforce destructive or self-destructive behavior (Linehan, 1993). Relevant considerations include the patient's history, the seriousness of the illness and length of hospitalization, the nature of the therapeutic alliance, whether the hospitalization is related to psychiatric issues (e.g., a drug overdose or suicide attempt), and the patient's preferences. When there is time to prepare, a frank discussion with the patient can help resolve the dilemma (Gutheil & Gabbard, 1998).

Home Visits and Treatment in the Community

House calls by physicians are an honored tradition that have been undermined by time and resource issues. It is more convenient to bring the patient to a facility with laboratory and x-ray departments than to bring today's medical technology to the home, but such developments do not negate the benefits house calls have had for patients, their families, and clinicians (Bursztajn, Feinbloom, Hamm, & Brodsky, 1990). Some primary care physicians have revived home visits, but in an era when physicians are sued for alleged improprieties in office visits, unchaperoned physical examinations in a patient's bedroom are fraught with risk. Yet, it is a well-established practice for members of the Visiting Nurses' Association to perform routine medical procedures at home. Psychotherapy in the home is considered an especially sensitive area, although it is not clear why this is so, since talking with a therapist at home would seem less threatening or compromising than having a gynecological examination in one's bed.

In what circumstances might traditional office-based therapy be extended to the patient's home? Home visits may be called for with patients who are homebound because of severe medical illness or disability. A last visit to a dying patient can be an appropriate gesture. Then there are the patients who are kept at home by the psychiatric disorder for which they are treated, such as agoraphobia.

> A patient with severe body dysmorphic disorder was seen by his therapist at home for several years. This patient suffered from the delusion that his face looked so hideous to others that he had to stay hidden at home. As his therapy progressed, he eventually felt able to go out and face people.

The criteria for determining the legitimacy of a home visit are the same as for any other treatment intervention. Is it an exploitative intrusion on a patient's personal space or an attempt to deal with an issue clinically? This assessment is most usefully viewed in four dimensions: (1) the therapist's intentions (clinical rationale); (2) foreseeable impact on the patient; (3) consistency with therapy contract or informed-consent process; (4) appearance to third parties. All of these questions lead back to the therapeutic contract. Unlike nursing or social work—or behavioral treatment of agoraphobia—dynamic psychotherapy usually does not include house calls. Changing the venue, therefore, requires informed consent, which is obtained through therapeutic exploration. When patient says, "I want you to come to my house," an appropriate response is: "What would it mean if I did? What would it mean if I didn't?"

A home visit may be perceived by the patient, and subsequently by licensing boards or courts, as an unwelcome advance on the therapist's part or as intentionally or unintentionally encouraging the patient's fantasies of nontherapeutic intimacy. For this reason, it is prudent to have two therapists, one of each gender, visit the patient together to neutralize any disruptive patient interpretations. In addition to documenting thoroughly the reasons for the home visit, it is advisable to get a consultation *before* making the visit. The consultant can then help estimate the likelihood that the patient will misunderstand the therapist's intentions.

Home visits are well established in community psychology and community psychiatry, which emphasize the need to observe patients in their actual living and working conditions rather than in the office, where a patient's presentation is seen as an artifact of the clinical setting. Workplace visits are also justified by the rationale of "taking down walls," or deliberately blurring boundaries between the therapy environment and the patient's home and work environment. Questions of confidentiality may arise, however, in either the home or workplace. Community psychology and psychiatry refute the claim that home visits are antithetical to therapy; again, context and purpose are critical. However, even in this context the current professional and legal climate calls for caution and prudence.

The New Frontier of High-Tech Therapy

Simon (1992, p. 281) wrote, "Psychotherapy cannot be conducted effectively over a telephone." As psychotherapy traditionally has been conceived, this injunction still makes sense, although (as discussed earlier in this chapter) telephone communication is necessary for off-hours emergencies and when a patient is physically unable to come to the office. In recent years, however, the definition of psychotherapy has become more elastic not only procedurally but geographically as well (Canning, Hauser, Gutheil, & Bursztajn, 1991), including expanded use of the telephone for psychotherapy (Simon, Ludman, Tutty, Operskalski, & Von Korff, 2004). In the global village of cyberspace, therapists with national and international reputations or highly specialized methods attract clients on their websites. The Internet, by facilitating long-distance contacts, has made personal counseling by telephone as well as online increasingly commonplace. Telepsychiatry, using computer-based videoconferencing equipment, is another form of long-distance therapy that has shown initial promise, especially for people in remote rural areas and prisons (Johnson, 2006; Ruskin et al., 2004).

E-mail and the Internet are bringing about profound changes in the nature of psychotherapy and therapeutic boundaries (Berg, 2002; Norcross, Hedges, & Prochaska, 2002). Evidence of the effectiveness of computer-assisted treatments for depression, anxiety, loneliness, and eating disorders has stimulated interest in e-therapy (the provision of mental health treatment through the Internet) (Recupero & Rainey, 2005a). E-mail can give agoraphobic, physically disabled, and other homebound patients an opportunity to establish a therapeutic alliance without having to travel to the office. The body-dysmorphic patient (described earlier in this chapter) who required home visits by a therapist until he was able to tolerate face-to-face contact exemplifies the kind of patient who can benefit from e-therapy.

Yet, the potential benefits of e-therapy, as well as websites maintained by psychotherapists and ordinary e-mail communications with patients, are associated with a number of practical, ethical, and legal difficulties (Recupero, 2005, 2006; Recupero & Rainey, 2005a). These include verifying the patient's and clinician's identity, maintaining clinician availability in the event of a system breakdown, ensuring timely responses, protecting confidentiality and information security, and dealing with unsolicited e-mails requesting professional advice. Advertising on a website may be held to constitute explicit warranties in a fiduciary relationship. E-mail addresses posted for use by colleagues may be accessed by patients and prospective patients. By analogy with telephone communication, professional advice given via e-mail (even without a fee) may be held to establish a clinician–patient relationship and a duty of care when it is foreseeable that the patient will follow the clinician's advice. Posted disclaimers to the effect that the service provided is merely educational or informational rather than clinical, or that it is only "personal coaching" rather than psychotherapy, may not be accepted by courts or licensing boards. Clinicians may be held accountable in court for diagnoses and treatments based on insufficient or misleading information given them by patients they have never seen. In the regulatory sphere, clinicians who provide services to out-of-state patients through e-mail or an interactive website risk prosecution for practicing without a license in their patients' home states. Third-party reimbursement and malpractice insurance coverage may be restricted to states in which a clinician is licensed, although insurers increasingly are reimbursing clinicians for online visits. Psychiatrists who prescribe medications online may find themselves caught up in the Drug Enforcement Administration's scrutiny of Internet pharmacies.

Clinical issues are raised by the rapid-fire, depersonalized character of e-mail, a form of communication characterized by "the stripped-down cool neutrality of letters combined with the hotter immediacy of an ongoing dialogue" (Gutheil & Simon, 2005, p. 953; cf. Mallen, Day, & Green, 2003). Physically separated from each other, deprived of the informative sensory data that accompany face-to-face meetings and (in the aural though not visual dimension) telephone conversations, clinicians and patients are susceptible to unchecked fantasies and the development of intense transference and countertransference. An informal tone and otherwise unexpressed wishes for closeness may enter into such communications. These boundary problems occur not only in e-therapy but also in e-mails exchanged by clinicians and patients who see each other in normal office sessions. In one instance a patient who called her therapist "Dr. Jones" in the office sent her e-mails beginning "Dear Jane." In the following case, e-mails served as a "wedge" for the introduction of classic boundary-breaking dynamics:

> A male therapist was treating a personality-disordered female patient. At one point the patient wished to show the therapist something she had written, and asked for his e-mail address. Although the therapist had never given out his e-mail address, with this patient he felt moved to make an exception. The patient sent him some writings that were not actively explored in the session. The patient continued to send more and more autobiographical and journal material without its being explored. The relationship deepened "outside the office," with an eventual sexual relationship resulting. In ensuing litigation, the therapist lost his license. (Gutheil & Simon, 2005, p. 954)

Here a familiar "red flag"—a therapist's rueful admission that "I don't usually do this with my patients, but in this case . . ."—appeared in the unfamiliar territory of electronic communication.

Given this mix of opportunities and hazards, clinicians are advised to consult published guidelines for appropriate, prudent use of e-mail and the Internet (Federation of State Medical Boards, 2002; Kane & Sands, 1998; National Board for Certified Counselors, 2007; Recupero, 2005; see Drude & Lichstein, 2005, for an extensive list of professional organizations' guidelines) and handbooks for online practice (Derrig-Palumbo & Zeine, 2005; Goss & Anthony, 2003; Hsiung, 2002; Kraus, Zack, & Stricker, 2003; Maheu, Pulier, Wilhelm, McMenamin, & Brown-Connolly, 2004; Tyler & Sabella, 2003). We note here a few fundamental principles (not meant to be an exhaustive list). First, as with any other clinical intervention, informed consent (either to e-therapy or to e-mail communication with existing patients) is essential (Recupero, 2005; Recupero & Rainey, 2005b). Second, clinicians should consider their rationale for using e-mail in any particular instance and should maintain the same professional tone and language in e-mails as in the office. Third, all e-mails (except inconsequential procedural exchanges), like other extratherapeutic communications, should be explored in subsequent office sessions so that those communications are incorporated into therapy instead of remaining outside it (Gutheil & Simon, 2005).

Finally, all e-mails should be made part of the patient's electronic and printed records, and the subsequent discussions with the patient should be documented in the chart (Drude & Lichstein, 2005; Gutheil & Simon, 2005; Kane & Sands, 1998; Maheu & Gordon, 2000; Recupero, 2005). Clinically, this precaution makes all relevant information available to subsequent caregivers. (Harm to the patient resulting from failure to convey such information can be the basis of a malpractice action.) From the perspective of boundary maintenance, inclusion of e-mails in the record underscores the need to process the content of e-mail communications in therapy. For risk management purposes, clinicians need to be aware that e-mails constitute written evidence that, especially when inconsistent with the clinician's records and testimony, can be produced in court to support allegations of malpractice or ethical violations. This developing area of clinical ethics, case law, and administrative regulation bears close watching in the years ahead.

KEY REMINDERS

- A fundamental principle of boundary maintenance is that the clinician needs to stay in the therapeutic role, avoiding role reversals, extratherapeutic interventions, and (as far as possible) multiple relationships with the patient.
- Informed consent and adherence to a contract for therapy are foundations of effective clinical and ethical treatment.
- Secure boundaries of time and place give the therapeutic frame structure, stability, security, regularity, consistency, and predictability.

CHAPTER 4

Money, Services, Gifts

For most people, the term "boundary violations" calls to mind sexual relationships between therapists and patients, or the kinds of extracurricular social contacts that typically lead to sexual misconduct. In fact, the dual relationships that result in disciplinary or legal action against mental health professionals often have to do with things of material value: money paid or not paid, gifts given or received, and services performed by a patient for a therapist. Such dual relationships occur at all points on the continuum: innocuous boundary crossings, errors that risk compromising therapy, and outright exploitation of patients.

MONEY

Regular specified payment for services contributes to structuring the therapeutic frame for both patient and therapist. The exchange of money indicates that therapy is work, a difficult task at which the therapist assists the patient, rather than love or friendship. Defining the meaning of this exchange involves setting appropriate limits. Maintaining these boundaries can strengthen other boundaries in the patient's life.

This section is concerned primarily with the direct exchange of funds involved in fee-for-service payment (or copayments for insured services). For treatment of a wider range of monetary and business issues, such as specific billing practices, third-party reimbursement, managed care, institutional conflicts of interest, and publicly subsidized mental health services, the reader is referred to other sources (Appelbaum & Gutheil, 2007;

Epstein, 1994, pp. 159–179; Reamer, 2001, pp. 143–147, 181–190; Simon, 1991a, 1992). It is, however, a generally accepted clinical and ethical principle that to collude with a patient in fraudulent billing of an insurer, even with the intention of helping the patient, is a boundary violation that models corrupt, maladaptive behavior.

The Meaning of Payment for Services

It used to be a standard joke in analytic circles that therapists are prostitutes, because they take money and use a couch. Indeed, a patient may say to you, "You're just like a prostitute. I pay you to care about me. If I didn't pay you, you wouldn't see me or do anything for me." There is a kernel of truth in that complaint. "Yes," you can tell the patient, "this relationship is fee-for-service, but that's exactly why a therapeutic relationship can be helpful." As Freud (1913/1958b) made clear, a therapist provides a relationship for which there is no model in real life, one that is different from all other relationships. Because a fee is charged, the focus is entirely on the patient's concerns. Unlike in any other area of life, you attend fully to another person, to the exclusion of yourself (except insofar as understanding your own reactions helps you understand the patient). That is an atmosphere in which a great deal of valuable work can be done.

Nonetheless, even a straightforward exchange of payment for time and services is far from conflict-free (Krueger, 1986; Langs, 1973). The patient derives positive meanings from the exchange when he or she looks admiringly at the therapist's car or house and thinks, "My money helped pay for that." Here the patient connects with the therapist around their mutual indebtedness. The patient is beholden to the therapist for help, and the money, a concrete expression of gratitude, balances the books. There is, of course, a thin line between paying out of gratitude and out of a wish to be important to the therapist. "I can pay the full fee," a patient may think, "so I'm special and more deserving than other patients." Some wealthy patients have been known to cross over that thin line by offering, sometimes insistently, to add a tip to a therapist's fee. In one such case, when the therapist declined to accept a tip, the patient indignantly retorted, "I can give you a tip if I want, just as I tip the waiter at a restaurant!" This equating of a therapist with a waiter is significant clinical material, ripe for exploration. The therapist might appropriately respond, "This may be something we need to think about—why you see this work we're doing as equivalent to being served food in a restaurant."

On the negative side, each monthly bill is a grim reminder that the therapist's interest in the patient is not a spontaneous, personal one. A therapist does not "love me for myself"; rather, the therapist's time and attention are for hire, a setup derisively referred to by critics of psycho- therapy as "rent-a-friend." Thus arises the patient's wish to pay nothing: if therapy comes free of charge, then "it really is love." The wish not to have to pay for therapy can also express narcissistic entitlement, as in the case of a patient who blurted out during a session that her previous thera- pist, instead of charging a fee, should have paid her because her case was so interesting (Gutheil, 2005c). When a patient precedes the amount writ- ten on every check to the therapist with the commonly used words "Pay only . . .," he or she can be understood at another level to be minimizing the value of the therapy or his or her need for it.

The therapist, too, may have conflicting wishes—on the one hand, to charge as much as possible so as to obtain the patient's acknowledgment of and gratitude for what really is hard and beneficial work; on the other hand, to charge nothing for what is an inherently enjoyable and high- minded effort. Many helping professionals have difficulty dealing with payment because they want to see themselves as humanitarians—altruistic healers (Welt & Herron, 1990). Those who are strongly motivated by a "rescue fantasy" may have difficulty maintaining boundaries in this area. Consequently, clinicians need to examine the conscious and unconscious meanings that payment by patients has for them (which ultimately is an examination of why they do what they do), even as they explore what it means to the patient to pay or not pay (Blatt, 2001; Gutheil, 1986; Pope, 1994, pp. 70–73).

Setting the Fee—or No Fee

Therapists who receive payment directly from patients need to take the same care in this as in any other aspect of the relationship, so that therapy is not compromised by unexamined conflicts and fantasies. It is legiti- mate to set up a sliding-fee scale, keyed to the patient's income, as long as the therapist does not suffer undue hardship and feels properly rewarded for his or her efforts. Many clinicians, having learned their trade by work- ing with indigent patients, also feel a responsibility to repay this debt by seeing their most needy patients without charge. This form of "tithing" is also appropriate as long as it represents a deliberate decision based on the patient's need rather than simply acquiescence in the patient's nonpay- ment of bills. Seeing patients at a reduced fee or no fee at all requires that the therapist's and patient's reasons for entering into such an arrange- ment be discussed and documented, that there be no explicit or implicit quid pro quo, and that all normal boundaries of the therapeutic frame be respected.

From the patient's viewpoint, the benefit of making treatment affordable needs to be weighed against the pitfalls of "getting something for nothing." A patient who is treated for little or no charge may feel uncomfortable and even guilty. The patient may feel that he or she has no right to express anger or disappointment or that he or she owes the therapist something in return (Gabbard, 1999a, 2005). A patient's guilt, combined with a therapist's unconscious desire to reject or punish (or reassure) the patient, creates a combustible mixture that increases the risk of serious boundary violations. There is no simple way to resolve these dilemmas, beyond adhering to the principles of good clinical and ethical practice: ongoing exploration, alertness to problems, consultation, and documentation. It can, however, be helpful to charge even a very needy patient a nominal fee so that the patient will be more likely to respect the value of the time spent and the work that needs to be done.

Kanter and Kanter (1977) have outlined a systematic, provocative approach to setting a fee with a patient at the beginning of therapy. We summarize their approach, which some clinicians regard as extreme, not as a recommended procedure, but for its heuristic value in opening up for examination the anxieties and ambivalences associated with the monetary exchange. In Kanter and Kanter's model, the therapist says to a new patient, "I want to charge you a lot, and nothing. You want to pay me a lot, and nothing. Given these wishes, which define the bounds of the playing field, we need to settle on what's fair to you and to me." Some patients—not to mention therapists—will find it anxiety-provoking to be confronted with the responsibility for addressing the question of mutual fairness. Instead of being presented with a fee as a matter of routine, the patient is forced to struggle constructively with his or her greed, altruism, wishes, entitlement, and all the other subjective and subconscious factors that enter into the monetary transaction. In this way, the question of the fee is taken out of the calculus of numbers and into the realm of the personal and experiential, where it sits at the nexus of a complex pattern of feelings, thoughts, and memories. The patient's and therapist's anxieties, thus made available, become a takeoff point for exploration.

A therapist who issues this challenge to patients can obtain valuable clinical information. Until you get to know a patient, you don't know whether your standard fee will bankrupt him or her within weeks. Is the patient paying you the food or rent money? At the outset the patient may not be able to be open about this, but when you say, "Now we're going to talk about your whole financial picture—how you earn, how you spend, how you save—to determine what would be a fair fee," you are opening up the issue as one that requires exploration.

Although this kind of inquiry may seem intrusive, many clinicians do not adequately explore a patient's financial condition, reflecting Krueger's (1986) observation that money "may be the last emotional taboo in our society" (p. vii). In fact, such exploration can give you an early entry point into the patient's therapeutic issues. For example, one patient with self-defeating personality disorder would not reveal to her therapist for a long time that she owned a car—not because she was trying to justify a lower fee, but because having a car contradicted her carefully constructed self-image as a victim. Although not many therapists may follow Kanter and Kanter's rubric in the uncompromising way presented here, the example is useful to keep in mind so as not to go naively into billing transactions with patients.

Limit Testing by Patients

Patients will test limits in the monetary realm, just as they will make repeated after-hours phone calls, try to meet the therapist outside the office, or flirt with the therapist. For example, a patient may say, "Here, I'll pay you in cash; then you won't have to declare it," or "Could you write down a full hour even though we've been meeting for only half an hour?" By inviting the therapist to be corrupt, the patient is testing the safety and integrity of the therapeutic environment. In varying degrees, the patient may wish to corrupt the therapist, but also may wish the therapist, and the process, to be proved incorruptible—the point at which progress can begin.

> A male patient seeing a male therapist in a clinic setting would regularly say to the therapist when he paid the bill, "Here's some money to buy groceries for your children." In this way the patient rationalized the transaction not as a fee for service but as a donation to the therapist as a needy parent. This absolved the therapist of any wish to have the money for personal gratification. Through this maneuver the patient extended the therapeutic frame to include the therapist's family, in which the patient may have wished to assume the role of a mother feeding her children. When this behavior persisted, the clinic called in a consultant, who advised the therapist about the need to explore the behavior with the patient. "By letting this sit there unexplored," the consultant explained, "you may be giving this patient a confusing message. The patient may hear your silence as saying, 'You're right. I am a father, and every time I feed my kids I think of

you.' Especially in a patient with a personality or character disorder, you may be encouraging a fantasy that will block the patient's progress in therapy and perhaps encourage more serious limit testing."

This patient's characterization of his payment for therapy as a contribution to the therapist's family was as clear a manifestation of transference as anything short of calling a therapist "Daddy." But should it be viewed as a boundary problem? Here there is no impropriety, no exploitation. The monetary transaction is entirely legitimate. Yet, the patient's wish to turn it into a gift calls out for exploration. If the patient's construction of the meaning and function of his payment goes unchallenged, he can continue to deny that he is receiving a service for his money. Likewise, he can continue to harbor the fantasy that he is exerting control over the therapist by telling the therapist what to do with his money. He is also not presented with the need to resolve whatever emotional conflict he is expressing. This blurred definition of the therapeutic frame may embolden the patient to further acting out in the financial, social, physical, or sexual sphere. Thus, the patient can be seen as subverting the therapeutic contract at the level not of action, but of feeling. Failing to set an early limit on such fantasies could ultimately compromise the relationship at the level of action as well. This dynamic exemplifies the principle that *boundary violations often are, or can be understood as, or can originate in, technical errors in therapy.*

Dealing with Lapsed Payments

A common form of limit testing by patients is nonpayment of bills. A patient who falls behind in payments may be having financial difficulties, expressing anger or entitlement, or seeking confirmation of the therapist's love. For a therapist to fail to confront this situation in a timely manner is a serious error, as Gutheil and Gabbard (1993) make clear:

> Consultative experience also suggests that the usual problem underlying a patient's mounting debt is the clinician's conflict about money and its dynamic meanings. Initially reluctant to bring up the unpaid bill, the clinician may soon become too angry to discuss it. Explorations of the dynamic meaning of the bill are more convincing when they do not take place through clenched teeth. A clinician stuck at this countertransference point may simply let it slide. In the minds of fact finders, this raises a question: "The clinician seems curiously indifferent to making a living; could the patient be paying in some other currency?"—a line of speculation one does not wish to foster. (p. 192)

As with other repeated, disruptive challenges to the therapeutic frame, tactful confrontation is called for (see Epstein, 1994, p. 174). The clinician can take the following sequence of steps:

1. Discuss the matter when the opportunity arises to tie it in with therapeutic material. If the patient is not paying, there is likely to be a connection with the content of therapy, for example, with the theme of people taking advantage of others. The therapist can make the parallel explicit by connecting the patient's actions to clinical material as it emerges: "You just described how you've been taking advantage of people. On that subject, I notice you haven't been paying your bills here." In effect, the therapist is allowing the patient to bring up the payment issue unconsciously. Once the issue is out on the table, it can be explored. For example, the patient may be testing his or her value to the therapist, whether as an especially intriguing case or as a love object.

2. If the issue is not resolved by therapeutic exploration, after a reasonable time the therapist can bring it up actively.

3. Later the patient's delinquency can be made the only issue: "I wish we could talk about your mother, but since you haven't paid your fee for _____ weeks, we have to talk about that and see if we can resolve it. The therapy itself is in jeopardy."

4. At a certain clinical and ethical threshold that each therapist needs to set individually, nonpayment becomes a deal breaker. "If we don't resolve this in the next 2 weeks, our contract for continuing therapy will terminate."

This scheme can be used as a model for responding to other boundary challenges as well. A therapist can confront such challenges by saying, "We can't spend every session on your asking me to have sex with you," or "We can't keep having you call me at 4 A.M. between every session." With any pattern of ongoing provocation on the part of a patient, the therapist explores the meaning of the behavior therapeutically and then, if necessary, raises the question of whether the therapeutic frame can be maintained. Note that all "deal breaker" terminations should be accompanied by appropriate referral to clinic, low-fee, sliding-scale, or free care; such referral counters the charge of abandoning the patient.

Inside Information and Conflicts of Interest

One of the introductory case vignettes in Chapter 1 was that of a therapist who was prosecuted for insider trading after he bought a large amount of stock on the basis of a "tip" inadvertently given him in therapy. Dual relationships of a financial nature, which create a clear conflict of interest for the therapist, are as much to be avoided as sexual relationships with a patient. Entering into business transactions with patients violates the principle of therapeutic abstinence and the therapist's fiduciary duty to act in the patient's best interest and not for personal gain. A therapist who has business dealings with a patient, including giving or receiving investment advice, is stepping out of role and not keeping to the task at hand. Such dual relationships not uncommonly lead to disciplinary action, civil lawsuits by patients, and/or criminal prosecution.

In a case that combined sexual and monetary transgressions, a clinical psychologist treated a patient for multiple personality disorder for 5 years. During the course of the treatment, the two married and had a child. In addition, the psychologist staged public performances in which he hypnotized his patient/wife before paying audiences and contracted with a video production company to produce tapes documenting her case. The patient's condition deteriorated, and she was diagnosed with posttraumatic stress disorder requiring long-term therapy. She sued the psychologist she had married, alleging boundary violations and other forms of professional negligence. The defendant argued that he had discontinued treatment of the plaintiff before their marriage and that she had consented to his publicizing her case. In a bench trial, the judge, visibly disturbed by the image of the psychologist selling tickets to events at which he put his patient on display, awarded the plaintiff $465,000 (*A.B. v. C.D.*, 1996).

Cases of outright exploitation or gross misjudgment are readily identified. With training and experience, a clinician can learn, for example, to avoid giving patients information or gratuitous advice about investments. Without using a therapeutic session to elicit information from the patient from which the therapist can derive personal gain, the therapist can still encourage brief, nonexploitative conversation that reinforces the patient's self-confidence in areas of the patient's special expertise and mastery (Reamer, 2001, p. 14). Nonetheless, even an ethical, experienced clinician may face unintended potential conflicts of interest that require sensitive clinical judgment—and, often, consultation—to resolve. The following case examples illustrate these clinical and ethical dilemmas.

> A therapist deposited her patients' checks in a money market account. One patient, seeing that particular endorsement on the back of the check, began to volunteer information and advice about the money market fund, such as which types of accounts earned at a

higher rate. The therapist initially disregarded these remarks. By the time the therapist recognized a pattern of behavior that needed to be addressed, the patient announced that he had transferred funds to the same money market fund so that he, too, could deposit his checks into that account.

Without committing any impropriety herself, this therapist was ensnared in a boundary challenge on the part of the patient. The incident brought home to the therapist that many small forms of self-disclosure are unavoidable (see Chapter 5) and how readily a patient can seize on such routine, unintended disclosures to gratify the fantasy of an extratherapeutic relationship with a therapist. Any patient who pays by check can identify the therapist's bank, but not all patients act on this available knowledge. After consulting with her supervisor, this therapist realized that timely exploration of the patient's unsolicited financial advice might have prevented the patient's escalation to the fantasy of shared finances. Once recognized, the wishes underlying the transfer of funds could be explored.

> In therapy, a patient who worked in the electronics industry referred to what he was working on only as "the product." When the therapist questioned this indirect locution, the patient explained that he feared that if he identified the product the therapist would rush out and buy it. Knowing that this sort of concern, expressed so obtrusively, often masks or coexists with its opposite, the therapist explored the patient's ambivalence. When the patient asserted, "I'm afraid you'll do it," the therapist countered, "Maybe you're afraid I won't." Ostensibly protecting both himself and the therapist from the possibility that the therapist would improperly come under his sway, the patient also was defending himself against his fear that the therapist would not gratify this fantasy. Once the patient became aware of this conflict, he was able to progress in therapy.

Not all clinical and ethical dilemmas involving inside information are so smoothly resolved. In another case (Dewald & Clark, 2001), a therapist learns from a patient during a session that a particular company has engaged in corrupt practices that are likely to bankrupt the company. The therapist's family happens to be considering investing in this company. If the therapist advises his family not to invest in the company, neither the patient nor government regulators would ever be made aware of a transaction not made; nor would the patient's name be revealed. Still, the therapist is left to ponder the potential impact on his own feelings and therapeutic stance, and therefore on the patient, if he advises his family to pass up what might turn out to have been a valuable investment opportunity, or if he refrains from intervening and his family suffers a loss (pp. 38–39). In another variation, a patient gives a credible account of an impending technical breakthrough that is likely to result in a major expansion of his company. The therapist, who has not said or done anything with this information, then hears from his financial adviser that there are rumors of the very development his patient has talked about and of the profits likely to result from it. How can the therapist avoid being influenced by his patient's confidential confirmation of valuable information already in limited public circulation? (p. 40).

A case adapted from the authors' consultative experience raises similar issues.

A clinical psychologist who managed the funds of a large condominium association began to see a patient who, it turned out, had a responsible position in the bank where the funds were invested. During the course of therapy the patient revealed that the bank was in unsound condition and might be forced to close. The psychologist did not see this disturbing situation as an opportunity to profit from insider trading. Rather, as she put it, she felt "as if I've been told that the ground under my house isn't safe anymore." She struggled with the competing claims of her fiduciary responsibility to her fellow depositors and her fiduciary responsibility as a psychotherapist to refrain from misusing a patient's confidential disclosures for any purpose outside of therapy. Did the former responsibility extend to acting on information which, being privileged, the psychologist might be said not even to "know" outside the therapy setting? Did the latter responsibility extend to considering specific harms the patient might suffer if his therapist withdrew funds from the bank? Would a large withdrawal cause the patient (as one of a small number of individuals possessing the "inside information") to come under suspicion as the source of the disclosure, which he had made in the expectation of safety and confidentiality? Would the withdrawal make it more likely that the bank would close, or close sooner, thereby costing the patient his job? Finally, if the psychologist's withdrawal of funds were to be traced to her therapeutic relationship with the bank manager, not only would this patient suffer a damaging loss of trust in therapeutic confidentiality, but other patients might be discouraged from speaking openly with therapists. On the other hand, if the psychologist adhered strictly to her ethical duty to her patient and did not make the withdrawal, her distress at her fellow depositors' losses might damage or destroy the very therapeutic alliance she was struggling to protect.

A dilemma such as this one calls for consultation or supervision to help the therapist apply an ethical perspective to the unique facts and circumstances of the particular case. Since therapists, like patients, are susceptible to exaggerated fears and forebodings, it is useful to begin by clarifying the nature, scope, and severity of the problem and the anticipated consequences. As a general rule, consider the simplest possible solutions first. For example, if the deposits were insured, depositors would suffer little or no harm from the bank's insolvency. At the other extreme, if the patient threatened to blow up the bank, the therapist's duty to maintain confidentiality would be outweighed by the duty to warn prospective victims. A consultant can help set a threshold of danger that would justify taking action outside of a therapist's normal role. If that threshold is not reached, the therapist will need to put the patient's interests first and work through her own losses with ongoing support from her supervisor, consultant, and, as needed, her own therapist. In especially difficult cases, termination and referral to another therapist can be considered, but once therapy is well under way this is not a preferred solution.

An alternative approach suggested by this case is, whenever possible, to anticipate and extricate oneself from potential conflicts of interest before such conflicts become manifest. By treating a patient who was in a position to reveal inside information about a bank in which she and her associates had invested money, the psychologist was placing herself at significant risk of ethical compromise. If she had already been treating this patient, she might have declined to accept the fiduciary role of managing the association's funds. If she were already managing those funds when she began to see the patient, she might then have turned over that responsibility to someone else. Or, as soon as she learned the nature of the patient's employment, she might have referred him to another therapist before he had a chance to form a therapeutic alliance with her.

There is, however, no way to anticipate all potential conflicts of interest that may arise in the course of therapy, especially in small or isolated communities (geographical or ethnic) where everyone knows and observes one another and there are limited choices of people to do business with (see Chapter 6). It may, then, be worth expanding the informed-consent process at the beginning of therapy to take into account such unanticipated dilemmas. Clinicians already inform patients of limits to confidentiality (e.g., information provided to insurers, threats to identified victims, and mandated reporting of child abuse). Clinicians might also add, "If problems come up, we'll discuss them and figure out the best solution."

SERVICES AND BARTERING

In a letter to *Psychiatric News*, a practitioner reported that a patient in treatment for years was struggling financially and might not be able to continue to pay for treatment. The letter continued:

> She has asked if she could, on a temporary basis, work off a portion of her charges for each session. She has suggested cleaning my office, doing my shopping, office filing, and so on. Initially I was opposed to her suggestion, but several of my colleagues do not think there would be a problem with such an arrangement. Am I right or are they? (Psychiatrists' Program, 2002)

What *is* wrong with exchanging services for therapy? Among other things, the patient may feel trapped, or coerced, into doing work he or she doesn't want to do, or into working at a rate of compensation that seems inadequate. A patient who shops or babysits for a therapist is likely, through various forms of disclosure, to come into inappropriate contact with the therapist's personal and family life. A patient who is handed "office filing" will thereby gain access to confidential information about other patients. All of these scenarios, in addition to the ethical compromises they involve, risk undermining the patient's therapy with disruptive information and issues. For these reasons, the Psychiatrists' Program (a liability insurance program endorsed by the American Psychiatric Association) advised the letter writer to avoid barter arrangements with patients or patients' relatives. The group recommended instead that psychiatrists consider working out a monthly payment plan with a needy patient or terminating treatment and referring the patient to community mental health services.

There is a long historical tradition of barter for medical care, especially in small towns and rural areas. If you couldn't pay the midwife or doctor to attend your baby's birth, you would give them a chicken or a bushel of peaches, mow their lawn, or fix their Model T Ford. However, this tradition of exchange did not encompass psychotherapy as a specialized professional service (Pope, 1991). Although not intrinsically unethical, barter has ceased to be normative with the increasing specialization of society and compartmentalization of relationships. In today's professional context, barter arrangements are easily corrupted and have a highly exploitative potential. Malpractice suits resulting in large damage awards have resulted when therapists have had patients regularly doing favors and running errands.

Patients have offered to barter not only services but also goods, such as jewelry, antiques, works of art, and even cars and real estate, for psychotherapy. As Simon (1992) cautions, "Patients who desperately feel they need treatment, or who experience intense, positive transference feelings toward the therapist often are unable to render an arm's-length assessment of the monetary value of their possessions" (p. 284). Dewald and Clark (2001, pp. 51–52) present a hypothetical arrangement in which a young artist whose professional recognition exceeds his earnings (he works as a waiter) agrees to pay a psychoanalyst $5 per session plus one painting every 6 months. In this scenario the analyst is, in effect, investing in his patient's career. If the paintings appreciate greatly in value, is the analysis, or the analyst's ethical position, compromised? What if the artist, in the course of his analysis (or any kind of therapy), considers giving up painting and changing careers? The therapist (especially one who speaks more directly to the patient's issues and choices than a psychoanalyst would) might then have a conflict of interest. Epstein (1994, p. 173) even suggests that the patient might produce inferior work for the therapist out of resentment or to get the best of the deal.

With these considerations in view, Hundert and Appelbaum (1995) explain why the Massachusetts Board of Registration in Medicine, while not ruling out the possibility of an ethical barter arrangement, strongly advised physicians practicing psychotherapy to avoid this practice.

> Barter raises the danger that therapists will take advantage of patients' dependency and desire for further treatment by placing unrealistically low valuations on the property or services being exchanged, or will deprive patients of possessions whose importance to patients transcends their market value. Moreover, when patients provide services in return for therapy (e.g., secretarial services, house cleaning, babysitting, home repairs), therapist and patient are brought into contact in settings that may result in further breakdown of boundaries. One egregious Massachusetts case involved a psychotherapy patient who performed clerical work in the psychiatrist's office in exchange for treatment, including billing the psychiatrists' other patients. Disagreements over whether the services agreed to in fact were rendered or rendered adequately can cause serious disruption to treatment. (p. 349)

Professional organizations in the fields of psychology, social work, and counseling have taken similar positions in their codes of ethics, allowing for bartering only in very limited circumstances and setting strict standards to ensure that any such arrangement is uncoerced, is entered into with the patient's fully informed consent, and does not exploit or harm the patient (Reamer, 2001, pp. 12–14, 122–128). Woody (1998) provides specific risk management guidelines for those considering such an arrangement. Moreover, although in some circumstances it may be difficult or impossible for a therapist to avoid purchasing goods or services from a patient, there are virtually no conceivable circumstances justifying a therapist's selling goods or services (other than clinical) to a patient. Given the tendency of some regulatory boards to apply rules mechanistically, without regard to context, clinicians who participate in barter or other exchanges of goods or services with patients can expect to bear the burden of proof if a complaint is made.

GIFTS

In an earlier vignette, a patient regularly spoke of his fee payment as providing food for the therapist's children; he was offering his money in the guise of a gift. Most boundary challenges by patients can be thought of in the same way. The patient is offering the therapist a gift, some variety of "forbidden fruit" outside the standard therapeutic dialogue, whether it be unscheduled contact, personal friendship, or an invitation to view or touch the patient's body. Such gifts come with strings attached for the therapist and (although the patient often does not realize it) for the patient as well. Thus, the question of accepting or giving gifts can be treated as a model for virtually all boundary issues.

In appropriate circumstances, a gift may constitute a boundary crossing—not harmful and perhaps helpful to therapy—rather than a boundary violation. Indeed, Gabbard (1999a) notes that "certain kinds of gifts may signal a turning point in the treatment and that to decline the gifts can be a devastating technical error" (p. 155). More often, it can be a serious error to accept a gift from—or give one to—a patient. In all cases, it is the therapist's responsibility to consider the meaning of the offered gift, to explore that meaning with the patient when called for, and to distinguish between boundary crossings and violations in this area.

The Meaning of Gifts in Therapy

In the television series *South Park*, a character gave a party for himself, assigning each guest a gift to bring him. Powerman dolls being the rage at the time, he told his friends, "You give me a blue one; you give me a yellow one," and so forth. As he opened each gift, the host said, "Thank you, Kyle, for the blue Powerman figure. You may now have cake and cookies." The skit was an amusingly concrete, literal representation of the feelings some people have about gifts as part of an exchange, a ticket to the goodies behind the door. In therapy, this kind of bargaining is referred to as a form of *acting in.* Whereas "acting out" means taking an issue from therapy and acting on it outside of therapy, "acting in" means taking an issue from outside of therapy and acting on it inside therapy.

> At the beginning of a weight reduction group for women, one woman walked around offering Life Savers candy to everyone, including the group leader as she came through the door. The group leader said, "Please sit down, and let's talk about this." The leader then asked the group to consider what it meant, in a group focused on overeating, for a member to attempt to give the therapist, as well as other group members, something sweet and pleasant that was called a "life saver." At first, as often happens, the group saw this as an overreaction. The therapist was being too punctilious. Why make such a big fuss about a little piece of candy?

To this group therapist, the meanings implicit in the act of offering Life Savers were evident. A member of a group that addressed the dynamics of eating was "feeding" the therapist. Was she expressing the hope that the group would save her life? Did she see the therapist as a life saver? Was she trying to save the therapist's life? In psychodynamic therapy, these questions needed to be explored for the group to make progress. Even in types of group or individual therapy that do not explore such questions directly, it is useful to recognize that seemingly uncomplicated behavior can have layers of meaning, for patient and therapist alike, that need to be dealt with—or not dealt with—carefully. This is particularly true of gifts in therapy (Smolar, 2002; Talan, 1989).

A patient's gift to a therapist may represent a conscious or unconscious effort to suppress the expression of aggression or anger (the patient's or the therapist's) in the therapeutic dyad. "If I buy off the therapist with a gift," the patient may wish, "maybe we won't have to get into all that messy, unpleasant stuff." A gift from a patient can be seen as a potential bribe, with an explicit or implicit quid pro quo (Gabbard & Nadelson, 1995). For example, a patient being treated by a resident in a psychiatric hospital gave the resident a gift. In their next session, the patient asked, "Will you be here next year in therapy?" By preparing the ground with a gift, the patient reduced the anxiety associated with the question by (at the level of fantasy) obligating the therapist to stay on for another year of residency.

If you are offered a gift by a patient, consider whether you are being asked to recall something, to look at something, or not to look at something. Are you being asked "to accept me through this token," "not to confront me about painful issues," or "to keep me in treatment"?

More broadly, is there something the patient wants to elicit or get from you, such as a favor or an expression of "special" appreciation, gratitude, and even indebtedness? Does the patient have a mental image of a proposed exchange ("Here's a gift, for which you'll agree to . . . ")?

Most broadly, is the patient trying to keep alive and even actively implement the "golden fantasy" that a therapist can satisfy all of the patient's needs, not just therapeutic needs (see Chapter 2)? At one level, the patient may simply be trying to maintain a warm, glowing feeling about the therapist that feeds the fantasy of a sexual or substitute-parent relationship. At another level, the patient may actually hope to bring about such a relationship.

For your part, do you have any feelings about this patient that might make you susceptible to these appeals? Here is how one therapist learned, through awkward experience, to ask these questions.

A male therapist in training was leading a group of male schizophrenics. One patient proved especially needy and difficult; he phoned the therapist frequently and required additional sessions outside the group. On Christmas Day the therapist was called to his office to see this patient, who claimed to be suicidal. The patient brought a bottle of scotch as a Christmas gift, adding that he realized he had caused the therapist a lot of trouble. The therapist hesitated but felt inclined to accept the gift. It might improve the therapeutic alliance, he reasoned, and this patient really was troublesome.

In supervision the therapist was told that he should give back the bottle of scotch because the patient had given it to him outside the group as part of a continuing effort to bypass the group process in order to create a special one-to-one relationship with the therapist. His supervisor also explored with him his desire to keep the gift as payment for the disruption of his Christmas celebration with his family ("the S.O.B. owed it to me"). Stressful as he found it to do so, the therapist returned the gift in the next group session, apologizing to the group and tying the incident to the dynamic issues with which the group was engaged. In so doing, he showed the group, including the gift giver, that he was fallible but not corruptible.

This gift was not only an attempted bribe but also an end run around the group, something the patient had tried repeatedly but unsuccessfully. Up to that point, the therapist had discussed every emergency individual meeting with this patient in group. The patient had then resorted to a concrete gift. The therapist's accepting this gift could, on the surface, have improved the therapeutic alliance. But how would the group have recovered when the other group members found out about the special treatment accorded one member? Moreover, the patient would not have benefited therapeutically from being able to think "I'm special to you—now I've got something on you." This case exemplifies the narcissistic dimensions of the gift exchange. The patient, through his offer of the gift, was saying "I have something to offer you." By accepting the gift, the therapist said, "I deserve this because of how much this patient has made me suffer"—a combination of narcissistic feelings and victim entitlement.

A patient's gift may represent the *self* or the *therapist*. One patient gives her therapist a framed photograph of herself, with the fantasy of the therapist admiring her image hanging in his office. Another patient gives the therapist a nameplate: "Dr. Smith." This patient is giving the therapist himself. Either way, the patient is establishing a kind of ownership of the office. Even if it is the therapist's name on the door, the patient can believe that he will think of her every time he comes in.

The patient bearing gifts approaches the therapist from a superficial posture: "To accept my gift is to accept me. To refuse my gift is to refuse me." If the therapist leaves this posture unchallenged, the patient is left in the position of a suitor who wonders whether the woman he is courting is welcoming him for himself or for the flowers he brings. The patient misses the opportunity to get to a deeper realization: "If you refuse my gift, that means you're accepting me without added blandishments—not as a quasi-lover, quasi-child, or quasi-friend, but as a person with my own valid claim to your attention. When you turn down my gift, it means I'm enough by myself."

To an analytic therapist, a gift accepted is a fantasy validated and therefore lost to exploration. When, instead, the gift is kept "on the table" (literally and figuratively), neither accepted nor refused, the patient's continuing anxiety about what the therapist might do with it can generate useful therapeutic material. The clinical goal is not (as even some analysts think) to reduce anxiety but to work with it as fuel for exploration. There are, of course, exceptions, as noted in the following section. But with a patient capable of self-exploration, this end run around the therapeutic contract needs to be addressed.

Criteria for Accepting a Gift from a Patient

Recognizing that a patient's offer of a gift is usually problematic but unable to fall back on an absolute prohibition against it, how can a therapist decide when it is clinically and ethically appropriate to accept a patient's gift? As with other boundary questions, the answer lies not in a mechanistic formula but in an understanding of the context of a particular case. The following guidelines can help a therapist reach such an understanding.

Monetary Value of the Gift

Only 5% of the psychologists surveyed by Pope et al. (1987) believed that accepting a gift worth less than $5 from a patient is clearly unethical, and only 8.6% reported that they had never accepted such a gift. By contrast, about two-thirds of those surveyed believed that accepting a gift worth more than $50 either is never ethical or is ethical only under rare circumstances. Nearly three-fourths reported that they had never accepted a gift of such value. Inexpensive gifts are more likely than expensive gifts to be mere expressions of appreciation or personal consideration, although their potential symbolic meanings must still be considered. Expensive gifts, on the other hand, are more likely to be intended, consciously or unconsciously, as bribes and have a greater potential to exert undue influence over a therapist's judgment.

Handmade versus Purchased Gifts

If a patient makes you a ceramic bowl while in the hospital as an expression of appreciation, it may be best to accept the gift while exploring its meaning. A patient may be all the more disturbed by the rejection of his or her own handiwork. At the same time, the clinical significance of such a gift is that it was made with the therapist in mind and therefore tends to be loaded with personal meanings and active fantasies—including, perhaps, the assumption that the gift would be accepted, coupled with fear that it would not be. Thus, a handmade gift is all the more to be appreciated and all the more to be understood.

Characteristics of the Patient

It is common to see the walls of a therapist's office covered with appreciative drawings made by child or adolescent patients. This is appropriate and reflects differences in the kind of alliance a therapist forms with a child as opposed to an adult. Even so, the impact of such displays on other patients, including other children, needs to be considered. Clearly the clinical and ethical calculus with respect to giving or receiving gifts is different when the patient is a child. Likewise, since gifts have different meanings in different cultures, the patient's cultural background is another contextual factor to be evaluated.

The nature of the patient's disorder is also a factor. For example, in the case of a patient diagnosed with panic disorder, the therapeutic benefits of the increased anxiety generated by refusing a gift must be weighed against the risk of triggering a panic attack. To minimize this risk, the therapist might accept a gift that is not clearly problematic and then discuss it.

Thought disorders also pose a challenge in this area. A distinguished senior clinician gave trainees the following rule of thumb: "With a neurotic patient you reject the gift and discuss it; with a schizophrenic you accept the gift and discuss it as far as possible." Although any simple formula such as this does not take the place of a deep understanding of the individual patient, this patient-centered rule can be viewed as a useful heuristic on the way to a deep understanding. That is, the terms "neurotic" and "schizophrenic" are a convenient shorthand for conveying that the patient's overall condition and ability to tolerate and (with the therapist) manage the interaction are the decisive factors. For a patient with primitive capacities and serious problems, accepting the gift while exploring it may be clinically and therefore ethically appropriate.

Type of Therapy

Giving and receiving a gift is a form of action. Where the contract between clinician and patient does not limit their interaction to words, as may be the case with a social worker or case manager, a gift is not necessarily a breach of contract. If the gift is of an inappropriate kind or is offered as a bribe (as in the examples below), the therapist needs to confront the ulterior motive but does not cite the therapeutic contract as the basis for refusing the gift.

Appropriateness of the Type of Gift

A homemade Christmas fruitcake is generally regarded as innocuous. Likewise, books or articles relevant to the therapy can be accepted when offered in a spirit of mutual investigation or simply goodwill. (In psychodynamic therapy, the question of what the patient may think the therapist needs to learn would arise for exploration.) At the other extreme, sexually suggestive gifts are obviously inappropriate. Whether psychoanalyst or case manager, a clinician would not accept an X-rated video or a Victoria's Secret teddy from a patient.

Stage of Therapy

Early in therapy, considerations of trust and alliance building may argue for accepting a gift, at least provisionally, in marginal cases. On the other hand, early in therapy it is also critical to establish and maintain a therapeutic frame strong enough to withstand the patient's wishes, fantasies, or bribes. This is when the patient is most in need of clear communications as to what therapy is and is not.

Gifts at termination also raise special issues; these are considered in a later section.

Red-Flag Contexts

Anything out of the ordinary about the situation in which a patient offers a gift should be documented and explored, and usually will rule out accepting the gift. For example, if the patient seems to have put a good deal of thought and angst into the gift or shows conflicted feelings about it, then the therapist is dealing with something other than a routine gesture of appreciation. Any circumstances indicating an expectation of a quid pro quo also change the nature of the gift. Even a book that a client gives a case manager is no longer innocent when it is followed the next week by a request for a letter to the client's parole officer.

Incorporating a Patient's Gift Offer into Therapy

A patient's offer of a gift can be incorporated into therapy by holding the gift in a "neutral zone" and tentatively exploring what it would mean to accept it. For example, when the patient is too fragile for therapeutic goals to be accomplished by outright refusal, the therapist leaves the proffered gift wrapped and puts it in a desk drawer. When relevant material is brought up during a session (i.e., when the patient may be unconsciously expressing interest in exploring the meaning of the gift), the therapist brings out the gift and asks, "Is there anything more we need to learn about this?" How long to hold a gift in suspension in this way is a clinical judgment. Eventually, the patient understands what he or she was trying to do and takes back the gift, still wrapped and untouched.

This scenario can have many variations, such as the following, in which the gift is left visible on top of the desk:

A patient brought in a 10-foot-long scarf as a gift for her therapist. The therapist left the scarf on top of his desk in a bag. He did this as a positive challenge to the patient to understand that her act was about something other than the concrete object given. The patient periodically looked at the bag, but took a number of weeks to ask why it was still sitting on the desk. Once she did, she and the therapist could begin to explore the meaning she attached to the gift. For example, did she think the therapist needed warmth and insulation from a cold world? Was she suggesting that he hang himself?

Therapists have their own conflicts about patients bearing gifts, and these conflicts, too, can cause problems if not explored and understood, as in the following example:

A resident in psychiatry was seeing an alert, thoughtful, well-functioning woman in outpatient therapy. One day the patient brought in a white bag. She explained, "I bought four brownies on the way over here, and when I finished three I realized I wouldn't be able to eat the fourth, so I saved it, and here it is. Think nothing of it; it's just a harmless extra, nothing real. I just happen to have it with me." The patient's devaluing and "de-meaning" of the gift (i.e., stripping it of meaning) were evident. However, the inexperienced resident took an unnecessarily severe posture toward her. Instead of saying, "Let's see if we can understand the meaning of this gift for the benefit of the therapy," he reacted sternly, as if to say, "Now see here, young lady. What is the meaning of this?" The patient, who missed the next two sessions, subsequently acknowledged that she had done so because she was offended and distressed by this hostile confrontation. By that time the resident had received sufficient supervision to apologize for his harshness, and he and the patient were able to explore the meaning of the gift.

The offer of the brownie needs to be considered in the context of the patient's having asked the therapist the previous week, "What do you think of me? How am I doing?" The patient could be understood to be putting something sweet in the therapist's mouth in the hope of getting something sweet from his mouth in return.

The experience of gift giving is a complex one for both the patient (giver) and therapist (recipient). A therapist, such as the resident in this case, may feel anxious and resentful at being challenged to deal with something beyond the limits of the classic psychotherapeutic verbal exchange. Caught between the wish to accept the gift and the wish to make it go away, the therapist may either be drawn into the patient's dynamic or react in a way that leads the patient to feel devalued and rejected. A therapist can avoid these errors by thinking of the situation in terms like the following (parallel to the framework suggested earlier for exploring the fee to be charged):

> "There's a part of me that very much wants you to give me this gift, and there's a part of me that wants you not to do it. Likewise, there's a part of you that very much wants to give me the gift, and a part of you that wants not to do it. What we need to do is explore those factors and understand them."

Whether it is appropriate to say exactly these words to a particular patient is a matter for clinical judgment. But a therapist should be aware of people's normal ambivalence about material exchanges and the productive anxiety this ambivalence can create when it is laid out on the table for examination. Recognizing that the two parties have symmetrical wishes, what matters clinically and ethically is not what the therapist wishes, but what the therapist does, which is to stay in role and not become either coopted or defensively rigid.

Patients often resist exploration of their gift offers; such resistance is part of the content and process of therapy. For example, when a patient gives a therapist a pair of gloves and the therapist begins to explore the fantasies this gift may express (such as keeping the therapist warm or holding the therapist's hand), the patient may say, "Why don't you just take the damn gloves and stop making an issue of it?" The following is an appropriate response:

> "I wish I could just do that. If this were not therapy, I could give you gifts, you could give me gifts, and we'd have a social relationship. But you have hired me to help you explore these things. If I just took the gloves and said, 'Thanks,' I wouldn't be fulfilling my responsibility to you to stick to my job and help you understand your feelings and wishes."

When a gift is kept on display for therapeutic purposes, it may affect the dynamics of the therapist's relationship with other patients, as in the following case involving two difficult patients:

> A therapist on an inpatient unit was treating a seriously disturbed adolescent who was devaluing and paranoid. This girl had had a traumatic experience that she associated with the novel *Lord of the*

Flies. When talking with other teens on the ward, she referred to the therapist, who wore glasses, as Piggy, the name of a character with glasses in the novel. Two years into her therapy she gave the therapist a small ceramic pig. Because this was an adolescent who had spent the first 2 years of therapy hiding behind her hair, the therapist left the figurine on the desk where, although it was not obviously in view, she could see it if she looked. For this patient, looking for her gift meant peeking out from her obsessive internal preoccupations and fears and engaging, in an elementary way, with the outside world. The therapist sought to engage her further by discussing what the gift meant to her.

Subsequently, the same therapist began to treat a tough, dangerous woman with borderline personality disorder. Noticing the ceramic pig on the therapist's desk, this patient figured out that it was a gift from another patient. After the therapist had succeeded in staying out of trouble with her for a long time, the patient gave him a ceramic owl, implying that he was a "wise old owl" for avoiding trouble with her. The therapist placed the owl beside the pig and used it as a point of departure for exploration.

On an inpatient ward this kind of competitive striving is common: "If another patient gave you that, I want in. I'll know you have my owl next to her pig." Both of these patients were giving the therapist his "self"— that is, their subjective conceptions of him. Both were inpatients who might have had difficulty doing abstract exploration, but both gifts (by virtue of their very concreteness) were discussed successfully. By accepting and displaying these small, inexpensive gifts, the therapist succeeded in generating a dialogue that opened up the feelings associated with the objects.

In contrast to this therapist's skillful navigation of boundary challenges, the following vignette highlights the potential consequences of an inability to confront such challenges therapeutically:

A high-functioning patient with borderline personality disorder (a kind of patient commonly encountered in practice) gave his therapist $80,000 worth of gifts over a period of years. The therapist, who was made uncomfortable by the patient's largesse, repeatedly protested, "You don't have to give me these things." What the therapist, lacking a firm grounding in clinical dynamics, could not bring himself to say was: "This thing isn't going home with me; it's staying in this desk until it goes home with you." The gifts did go home with the therapist, who found himself setting aside an entire room for them. Subsequently the patient sued, alleging mismanagement of the therapy, of which the therapist's accepting the gifts was the most signal example.

Some boundary issues are hard to get across to lay people. This jury found in favor of the defendant therapist. Despite the therapist's inability to set limits, the jurors perhaps concluded, "What's the problem? The therapist didn't ask for these things. The patient gave them voluntarily." Even so, this therapist had to go through the extended trauma of a lawsuit, which in another jurisdiction or region might have had a different outcome.

The therapist might have avoided this personal trauma, as well as the lost opportunity to help this patient, if he had understood the gifts as statements: "I don't feel good about myself. I know you don't want to see me; you want to get rid of me; you can't stand me. The only way I can be sure to get what I need is to bribe you. I have to give you gifts or you'll lose interest in me." Borderline patients such as this one do not feel entitled to ask straightforwardly for what they need. They are unable to enter into an adult transaction: "I pay you for your services, and you treat me to the best of your ability."

At the outset, the therapist might have been reluctant to make the patient's gift giving a "deal-breaker" if he believed that he was creating an alliance with a difficult patient and that the patient was beginning to make gains. (Even then, the therapist should have tested this perception in supervision or consultation.) Even after accepting one or more gifts, the therapist could have regained control of the situation and put the therapy back on track by saying "You've now given me so-and-so many gifts. It's not necessary to reward me in that way, wherever that's coming from. So, let's see now if you can tolerate the experience of not giving me anything and of telling me instead about your feelings about giving me things."

Termination Gifts

When is it appropriate to accept a small, innocent gift at the end of therapy when exploration is over? Patients often bring a small gift at the end of therapy, when it is too late to explore its meaning. It is customary to accept such gifts if they are of insubstantial value and of an appropriate nature. Even at this stage, however, there are issues to be assessed in each case, as in the following example:

A male patient had been seeing a male therapist for years in the evenings. On the last scheduled day of therapy the patient brought in champagne and two small glasses. To celebrate their termination, the therapist took a sip of champagne with the patient. This had two unfortunate consequences. First, the next patient picked up the scent of alcohol. Second, the mood of celebration the patient took pains to create reflected the fact that his termination was premature; in retrospect, it was a flight from the next subject to be explored. When the patient came back to resume therapy, it was with a sense of anticlimax.

In an appropriate termination, the patient needs to be free to come back if necessary. If the patient does not need to come back, ongoing guidance from remembered dialogue with the therapist can be disrupted by crossing professional boundaries at the time of termination.

The following example shows how a clinician can maintain clear boundaries at the conclusion of therapy.

A social worker conducted a long, intensive, and generally effective course of inpatient therapy with a schizophrenic child and his family. When the child was about to be discharged from the hospital in preparation for his family's move to another city, his parents, who were in the home furnishings business, gave the social worker their company catalogue and said, "Why don't you select something nice from here; that will be your termination gift." Asked, in effect, to request a gift of her own choosing from the family, the social worker gave the appropriate response: "Thank you. I get my salary from the institution. I don't need anything more. I appreciate your offer, which I must kindly decline."

At first sight, this offer may appear innocuous, because it was made by the patient's parents, not the patient. However, the social worker was working with the parents as well as the child. Thus, the meaning and intention behind the gift were ambiguous. Furthermore, they chose to express their gratitude to the social worker in a detached, indirect way, through a kind of "bridal registry." They placed the burden of choice on the recipient, thereby eliciting from her, had she accepted the gift, an expression of acquisitiveness and entitlement.

Bequests and Gifts to Institutions

Grateful patients commonly make substantial donations and bequests to hospitals and medical schools. In nonpsychiatric medicine the propriety of such gifts usually is not questioned. A psychotherapist, on the other hand, may face serious questions of undue influence if a patient leaves money to an organization with which the therapist is associated. Whether the therapist knew about or agreed to the bequest and whether the therapist benefited directly from it are considerations for forensic evaluators and judges or juries, but there is no guarantee against professional or legal sanctions. The type of therapy also enters into consideration; donations or bequests to an analytic institute are more likely to be scrutinized than similar gifts to a community health center (see Dewald & Clark, 2001, pp. 56–57). In any case, when a patient indicates a desire to donate or leave money to, say, a research foundation or training program, the therapist would do well to consider all of the implications, just as if the patient were handing money to the therapist. Independent consultation, for the therapist and for the patient as well, may be called for to avoid the appearance or the reality of undue influence and exploitation.

Gifts from Therapist to Patient

When Freud learned that a patient was planning to buy a set of his complete works, he gave the patient the set as a gift. Afterward, the patient found himself unable to use his dreams productively in his analysis as he had before. Freud used this case as a cautionary example of the hazards of gift giving in psychoanalysis (Blanton, 1971). Although gifts from therapists to patients are no longer absolutely proscribed in today's diverse therapeutic environment, it is still important to be aware of the dynamics Freud observed (see Smolar, 2003).

Context-dependent guidelines for giving or not giving gifts to patients are similar to those for accepting gifts from patients. A therapist should never give gifts of substantial value or of a sexual or intimate nature to a patient. Therapists who give patients expensive gifts may arouse suspicion (on the part of both the patient and subsequent evaluators) as to whether they are trying to make the patient feel obligated to the therapist. If you give a patient a substantial gift over and above your professional services, what does the patient now owe you? Patients who have been abused in the past can be highly sensitive to such unsettling implications.

There are, on the other hand, clinical contexts in which gifts of small value can be appropriate. Examples include therapy-related materials such as medication samples (for indigent patients) or educational texts related to the patient's condition. Small gifts can help establish therapeutic relationships with adolescents or severely regressed adults (Hundert &

Appelbaum, 1995). Gifts may be offered to a dying patient or to mark important occasions in a patient's life (Krassner, 2004). For example, when a patient who has struggled with infertility finally gives birth, a therapist may wish to acknowledge the meaning of this event by sending congratulatory flowers or giving a small baby gift. In any of these circumstances the rationale for and manner of giving the gift should first be discussed with colleagues and documented, and an appropriate gift should be chosen.

Still, an appropriate gesture, such as offering a tissue to a crying patient, can, in a moment of inattention, escalate into an inappropriate one, as in the following case:

> A patient became very upset during a session with her therapist and began to cry. The therapist, proffering a tissue, held out a hand-tooled Florentine leather case in which a pocket pack of tissues had been placed. After the patient had withdrawn a tissue, the therapist impulsively said, "Why don't you keep the case?" In subsequent supervision the therapist came to understand that this "gift" to the patient was an unconscious bribe designed to avert the anger that the therapist sensed just below the surface of the patient's sorrow. (Gutheil & Gabbard, 1993, p. 193)

This gift was also a boundary violation, obligating the patient to the therapist beyond the limits of the therapeutic exchange.

In the following case, a therapist who failed to maintain clear boundaries got into trouble with a well-intentioned gift.

> A young woman who had had great difficulty with relationships with men was seeing a male therapist for depression. Early in therapy she gave the therapist a pair of socks for Christmas. The therapist accepted the socks (but did not wear them) to help the patient engage with treatment at that early stage—a reasonable rationale if properly documented. Subsequently the patient asked the therapist to give her a pair of his socks. The therapist quite properly declined to do so. But the request, in retrospect, should have prompted further exploration of her reasons for giving him socks.
>
> A few months later, in an effort to give her life more structure, the patient started a used clothing store just when the therapist's wife was giving away some ill-fitting men's shirts she had purchased abroad. In what he regarded as a gesture of encouragement, the therapist gave one of the shirts to this patient to add to her inventory. To his dismay, the therapist later discovered that the patient was sleeping with the shirt, which he had never worn.

This outcome was hardly unforeseeable. When the therapist gave the patient his shirt, he created "unfinished business" by encouraging the fantasy the patient had expressed when she asked for his socks. A patient's gift to a therapist may be a concrete representation of the patient's conception of the therapist. In the same way, a patient may see a therapist's gift, especially an article of the therapist's clothing, as a talisman conferring the therapist's imagined power and love. The kind of magical thinking that led the patient in this case to sleep with the shirt is quite common. It can, for example, lead a patient to make repeated telephone calls just to hear the therapist's voice on an answering machine. In cognitive-behavioral therapy, patients have made fetishes out of audiotapes on which their therapist's recorded voice teaches relaxation methods. In one such case, a patient refused to use a tape made by a therapist who had abruptly terminated with him. The patient said that he never wanted to hear that therapist's voice again. In another idiosyncratic variation, a patient whose previous therapist had terminated with her listened at bedtime to a tape the therapist had made for her and masturbated to the sound of his voice. If patients can attach such meanings to objects properly given them for a therapeutic purpose, it is foreseeable that they will do so with garments taken from a therapist's personal wardrobe. It is not within a therapist's role to contribute directly to a patient's work project by donating clothing any more than by investing money in her store. The proper role of a therapist is to say, "I support your going into the used clothing business. I support your becoming a working person, because it's good for your mental health and furthers your life's goals." Leaving the field undistracted by any concrete objects, the therapist keeps the therapeutic issues in focus.

In the vignette that follows, a patient asked for—and got—an article of clothing worn by her therapist to cling to at night.

> An adolescent who exhibited serious behavioral dyscontrol developed a paternalized relationship, not sexual but with romantic overtones, with her therapist. When the patient said, "I want one of your shirts with your cologne on it to sleep with," the therapist gave her the shirt. The patient's behavior escalated until the therapist's insurer had to settle a civil lawsuit brought by her parents.

By giving the patient the concrete object she demanded, the therapist closed off the patient's fantasies to examination. Instead, it would have been therapeutic to air the fantasies, to explore what the patient was looking for: "What if I gave you the shirt? What if I didn't?"

In contrast, Reamer (2001, pp. 149–151) presents a case that is a model for anticipating and preventing the boundary confusion seen in these cases.

> In a residential program run by the county child welfare department, a 17-year-old client had progressed to the point where she was ready to move into a subsidized apartment. The client invited her primary counselor to come to her housewarming party. The counselor wanted to accept the invitation and to bring a small housewarming gift such as a utensil, but was not sure whether it would be appropriate to do so. The counselor consulted her supervisor, who suggested that they take the matter to group supervision. The group concluded that there were good clinical reasons for the counselor to make the visit in order to reinforce and encourage the client's progress, bolster her self-esteem, and avoid hurting her by turning down her invitation. This discussion and clinical reasoning were documented in the case record, and the counselor planned to explain to the client in advance why she accepted the invitation and what her visit would mean. Finally, it was decided that the counselor would bring a gift consistent with social custom, also documented in the record, with a card stating that the gift was from the agency and its staff, so that the client would not misinterpret it as a personal overture from the counselor.

This plan, conceived to protect and benefit the client, also provided effective risk management for the counselor and the agency. Still, the resolution Reamer outlines might not be the same in the case of a clinician doing psychodynamic therapy in solo practice, since it was the agency's structure and mission that allowed for shared (but still clear) responsibility for serving the patient's interest.

KEY REMINDERS

- In fee-for-service practice, regular specified payment for services contributes to structuring the therapeutic frame for both patient and therapist.

- Clinicians need to attend to the conscious and unconscious meanings that the financial transaction may have for both patient and therapist.

- Bartering with patients for services is potentially exploitative and is to be avoided except in very limited circumstances.

- The giving or receiving of gifts has layers of meaning, for patient and therapist alike, that warrant careful examination.
- When offered a gift by a patient, the clinician is advised to stay in the therapeutic role and address the clinical dimensions of the gift offer. In most cases this entails exploring the meaning of the gift rather than accepting it.

CHAPTER 5

Self-Disclosure

Some degree of self-disclosure by a therapist is inevitable, but when do routine, inconsequential revelations become boundary violations? Self-disclosure has been the subject of much recent reconsideration (see, e.g., Aron, 1996; Bridges, 2001; Derlega, Hendrick, Winstead, & Berg, 1991; Derlega, Metts, Petronio, & Margulis, 1993; Farber, 2006; Geller, 2003, 2005; Kroll, 2001; Leahy, 2001; Maroda, 1994; Psychopathology Committee of the Group for the Advancement of Psychiatry, 2001; Renik, 1995; Stricker & Fisher, 1990; Wachtel, 2007). On the one hand, intimate self-disclosure by therapists can be a step on the path to sexual misconduct; such deeply personal self-disclosure may promote role reversal, wherein the patient is drawn into serving as a kind of caretaker for the therapist. On the other hand, numerous forms of self-disclosure are inescapable in all therapies, beginning with the therapist's appearance, speech, clothing, office decoration, and professional background.

Complicating this analysis, and the clinician's dilemmas, is the fact that regulatory agencies, aware that self-disclosure does sometimes lead to sexual misconduct, often tend to see any self-disclosure (that is, any knowledge by the patient of extratherapeutic data about the therapist) as evidence of wrongdoing, even in treatments that involve only prescribing of medications. In this forbidding atmosphere, what are the proper functions and limits of self-disclosure on the part of a therapist? How much do these functions and limits vary with different schools of therapy or different types of patients?

INEVITABLE DISCLOSURES

The following are all ways in which therapists unavoidably communicate information about themselves to patients:

- The therapist's name
- Speech (e.g., accent, volume, tone of voice)
- Dress
- Religious symbols worn and religious holidays observed
- Office decor (including family pictures)
- Books on the bookshelves
- Diplomas and certificates on the wall
- Information on the therapist's website
- Information provided by the therapist's employer (e.g., HMO) or affiliated hospital
- Nonverbal reactions
- Laughter or refraining from laughter
- Verbalized reactions or silence

Patients are entitled to information about a therapist's background, training, credentials, therapeutic orientation, and method so that they can give informed consent to treatment. Patients may learn a great deal more when they look into a therapist's professional experience and accomplishments. A list of publications on the Internet may reveal the therapist's specialized interests, with implications for the patient's diagnosis, or it may lead to inferences, accurate or not, about the therapist personally. In a hypothetical instance, a patient is referred to a therapist who has published a series of articles about borderline personality disorder; the patient then wonders "Am I borderline?" If a therapist has published regularly about working with gay patients, a patient may infer, rightly or wrongly, that the therapist is gay.

In the office, the patient sees a certificate on the wall honoring the therapist for excellence in his or her profession. This may give the patient an expectation of success and act as a positive self-fulfilling prophecy. However, if the patient fails to improve, the patient may blame himself or herself: "What's wrong with me that such a hotshot expert can't help me?"

Everything a therapist does or does not say is a disclosure, but not necessarily an inappropriate one. If, for example, the therapist perks up when the patient mentions a dream, this unintended disclosure of interest may encourage the patient to bring up other dreams. From a cognitive-behavioral perspective, the therapist is reinforcing the patient's dream-reporting behavior. Likewise, by laughing or not laughing in response to something a patient says, the therapist shows something of him- or herself as a person. It may be reassuring and therapeutic when the therapist laughs at an appropriate moment, but disturbing and alienating when the therapist laughs at an inappropriate moment. Such revelatory words, looks, and gestures are all part of a sea of self-disclosure, like the innumerable tiny pieces of plankton on which ocean fish feed, most of which disclosure passes by without notice. Patients do notice a great deal. As one recalled: "A patient searches for clues about his shrink. For me, in the early days, they were the map of Jerusalem on his office wall and his bookshelves lined with the work of Thomas Mann—the writer who embodied the nobility of reason for a generation" (Evanier, 2002).

Another layer of complication is added by the astonishing amount of information about anyone that has become available on the Internet. A litigious patient can use this and other sources to claim inappropriate self-disclosure.

> In support of a specious claim of misconduct brought by a patient as "revenge" against being terminated from treatment, the patient claimed detailed knowledge of the therapist's home. It was later revealed that the therapist had offered the patient's unemployed husband the opportunity to make some home improvements on the therapist's house. Through this work the patient's husband possessed blueprints of the entire house, which turned out to be the actual source of the knowledge the patient claimed had come from inappropriate disclosures and visits.

This case demonstrates (per Chapter 4) the inadvisability of hiring a patient's spouse to perform services and also shows how real or fabricated disclosures can be used to discredit a clinician.

ROLE REVERSAL

Given that some self-disclosures are unavoidable, when does disclosure become burdensome to the patient and detrimental to therapy? A clear indication of a boundary violation is when self-disclosure leads to role reversal, with the patient becoming an emotional caretaker. In cases of sexual misconduct, a key turning point (identified retrospectively) commonly occurs when the relationship shifts from a therapeutic exchange to one of "sharing" personal confidences and feelings. The therapist's stepping out of role to confide personally in the patient seems to break down the last barriers to a personal relationship, as well it might when the privacy and intimacy of the consulting room turn into a stage for "pillow talk."

Role reversal occurs in situations far short of sexual misconduct. In the following vignette, a medical student on a psychiatric rotation has been talking with a patient about the patient's weekend plans.

PATIENT: What about you? What are you going to do this weekend?

MEDICAL STUDENT: I'm going to go out and get drunk.

PATIENT: Do you think that's such a good idea?

With one ill-advised answer, this clinician-in-training has become the patient's patient. As part of his training, the student needs to be counseled that such a disclosure is inappropriate.

THERAPISTS' SELF-DISCLOSURE
IN THE "REAL WORLD"

The psychotherapeutic universe has evolved a great deal since the heyday of psychoanalysis more than half a century ago. Limits on reimbursement, the growth of health maintenance organizations (HMOs), and the advent of outcome research in psychotherapy have accelerated the development of practical therapies with more directive methods and expeditious procedures. Alternatives to psychodynamic psychotherapy have arisen, each with its own rationale for setting its own boundaries. Leahy's (2001) treatment of self-disclosure as part of the relational character of cognitive-behavioral therapy is particularly informative in this respect. Meanwhile, the health consumer movement, emphasizing informed choices by "empowered" patients whose satisfaction is sought and measured, has altered the traditional power balance between therapist and patient. People with different cultural backgrounds have different expectations of their therapists as to the sharing of personal information.

In this pluralistic, pragmatic, and somewhat chaotic environment, there can be no single standard for appropriate self-disclosure except the universal ethical standard that it be for the benefit of the patient rather than for the satisfaction of the therapist (Psychopathology Committee of the Group for the Advancement of Psychiatry, 2001). In some circles, both within and outside of analytically oriented therapy, the notion of intersubjectivity—of "real people" connected with each other in relationships—has supplanted the "blank screen" model of therapeutic anonymity discussed below. Indeed, some contemporary schools of psychotherapy advocate self-disclosure as a powerful therapeutic intervention (Miller & Stiver, 1997; Stricker & Fisher, 1990).

Self-disclosure as a tool to instruct or illustrate has had a place, albeit a limited one, even in analytically oriented therapy (Lane & Hull, 1990). As Gutheil (1994b) explains:

> A therapist in an exploratory therapy who discloses to a patient in crisis an inspirational perspective offered by the therapist's coach in college is crossing a boundary—discussion in therapy should focus on the patient's issues and history, not the therapist's—but the goal is obviously to support and encourage the patient. The patient here may well feel these desired effects, and the therapy may be advanced. (p. 219)

Psychodynamic therapists (e.g., Winnicott, 1965) have long recognized that children and people with impaired capacity for abstract thinking may require more direct answers to questions. Especially (but not exclusively) with children and adolescents (Barish, 2004; Gabel, Oster, & Pfeffer, 1988; Gaines, 2003; Gardner, 1993), self-disclosure can be useful in building a therapeutic alliance, as in the following example:

> A senior male therapist treating a 19-year-old young man who finds it difficult to talk may use conversations about sports to engage the patient at a level where he feels comfortable about relating to the therapist. In the course of this conversation, the therapist may reveal a great deal about his interests in sports, his preferences for a certain team over another, and his activities during the past weekend (if he happened to attend a sporting event). While he is self-disclosing, he is also adapting the frame to connect with the patient in a way that facilitates a therapeutic alliance. (Gutheil & Gabbard, 1998, p. 412)

In the rough-and-ready arena of frontline counseling in public agencies, where there is little opportunity for extended exploration, a simple rule of thumb for self-disclosures can serve a clinician well. One experienced social worker acknowledged his willingness to establish a relationship with a client by revealing "what teams I root for, what movies I like, what food I enjoy." But he drew a line at more personal information: "My sex life, how much money I make—these are no one's business" (Edelwich & Brodsky, 1991, p. 143). Cognitive and behavioral therapies, for example social skills training, use self-disclosure to model coping strategies (see

Leahy, 2001, and Linehan, 1993, for comprehensive discussions of appropriate self-disclosure in CBT).

Glasser (1965) developed reality therapy through his work with delinquent adolescent girls. The therapist and patient speak about a wide range of subjects—nearly anything the patient wants to talk about—to build an alliance that differs from that formed in analytic therapy. They might talk about jobs, movies, sports, or hobbies until they reach a key intervention point at which the therapist tells the patient that her behavior is not serving her long-term interests. The therapist might say, for example, "I can't support your drug use," or "I can't support your hanging out with a self-destructive guy. That's an example of your not taking responsibility. You need to take responsibility so that you can meet your needs." Both the disclosures and the directive statements made by the therapist are part of the contract and are for the benefit of the patient, according to reality therapy's theory of modeling. Self-disclosure likewise plays a part in rational-emotive behavior therapy (Dryden, 1990; Ellis, 2001; Walen, DiGiuiseppe, & Dryden, 1992).

Different schools of therapy involve different levels of disclosure, which in turn serve the needs of different patients. For example, a highly inhibited patient may become uncomfortable with a highly self-disclosing therapist and may change therapists. Another patient who finds an analytically oriented therapist too withholding may do likewise. No therapist or therapy is right for everyone. What is right—and necessary—for every patient is to be able to make an informed choice based on knowing what to expect.

THE "BLANK SCREEN"

Freud (1912/1958a) wrote, "The doctor [practicing psychoanalysis] should be opaque to his patients and, like a mirror, should show them nothing but what is shown to him." This classical psychoanalytic approach came to be embodied in the image of a "blank screen" (Arlow, 1969). The less factual information the analyst projected onto the screen, the more clearly the patient could experience his or her transference fantasies about the analyst. It has long been recognized, even by psychoanalysts, that the "blank screen" is only an ideal construct, since therapy by its very nature is interactive and the definition of the therapeutic frame varies from patient to patient as well as from clinician to clinician (Aron, 1996; Greenberg, 1995; Singer, 1977). As Gabbard (1999b) notes, "With the demise of the blank-screen stereotype, virtually all clinicians acknowledge that they make self-disclosures of various types on an ongoing basis" (p. 14; cf. Farber, 2006; Johnston & Farber, 1996).

Before dismissing the blank screen as an antiquated relic of ivory tower psychoanalysis, it is useful to understand what this ideal of the therapist's relative anonymity contributes to effective therapy in the service of the patient. The primary rationale for remaining anonymous— "behind the screen"—is that knowledge about the therapist may burden the patient and constrain or even foreclose certain areas of free discussion by interfering with the flow of the patient's material. In some cases it is the particular information revealed that is inhibiting. For example, knowing that you are Roman Catholic may make it more difficult for a patient to talk about having an abortion. If a patient knows that you have recently lost a parent, the patient may be less able to express his or her negative or even positive feelings toward parents. In certain cases, some personal knowledge about the therapist can be humanizing, demystifying, and de-idealizing in a manner that fosters the therapeutic alliance. With some patients, indeed, a useful alliance can be forged by the therapist's acknowledgment that he or she is familiar with the kinds of painful experience the patient has had (Viederman, 1991). It is healthy to be able to realize that the therapist is a human being. A patient who is not severely debilitated may be able to separate his or her transference fantasies about this neutral party from a realization that "this guy goes home to his house, and is tired at the end of the day, and gets sick, and has the same family conflicts as anybody else." However, it cannot be assumed at the outset that a patient is sufficiently well constituted to make this reality-based distinction. Idealization, after all, interferes with perception of reality. Giving the patient a window into one's life may simply arouse erotic fantasies in a patient predisposed in that direction.

As discussed below, these decisions need to be made on a case-by-case basis in the context of the type of therapy offered. As a rule, though, clinical experience indicates that detailed autobiographical vignettes (i.e., more than a couple of sentences) are usually counterproductive in exploratory therapy (as opposed to, e.g., client-centered, existential, or reality therapy). Whether or not there is anything in the information divulged that inhibits, distracts, or distances the patient, the very dynamics of exploratory therapy argue for withholding personal disclosures. It is a watchword of psychodynamic therapy that "a question answered is a fantasy lost." When a patient asks a question such as "Are you married?"—or, more pointedly, "What about *you*? Don't *you* ever get fed up with your husband? Have *you* ever been divorced?"—answering the question relieves the very anxiety that could otherwise fuel productive exploration of the conflicts that underlie the patient's curiosity.

The less information you supply, the more the patient fills in the missing data with transference material. Denied "the answer," the patient reaches into past experience to find it. Thus, the "truth" the patient and therapist are seeking is not fact, certainly not the facts of the therapist's life. In this form of therapy, the ultimate truth is transferential truth—that is, truth about the patient's subjective experience of his or her past. In cases where disclosure is deemed desirable, therefore, instead of answering directly the therapist can begin by saying, "Before I answer your question, what do you imagine about this and why?" This way of responding has a better chance to elicit the whole fantasy, powered by the anxiety of not knowing the answer. The purpose of the "blank screen" is to allow this transference to be brought to the surface and articulated.

SELF-DISCLOSURE IN THE ANALYTIC TRADITION

When the Psychopathology Committee of the Group for the Advancement of Psychiatry published its article "Reexamination of Therapist Self-Disclosure" (2001), Weiner (2002) expressed surprise at the revival of interest in this subject. As he reminded readers, the role of self-disclosure in psychotherapy, including indications and contraindications for self-disclosure by a therapist, had been studied decades earlier by Jourard (1971) and by Weiner himself (1983). Likewise, Maroda (1994) lamented the failure of psychoanalysis and psychoanalytic therapy to follow up on early explorations of the benefits of actively using and expressing the countertransference to advance the therapy (e.g., Gitelson, 1952; Little, 1951; Tauber, 1954).

Maroda's challenge to orthodoxy in the service of a less authoritarian, more reciprocal, working alliance between patient and therapist is thoroughly grounded in the analytic tradition (cf. Burke, 1992; Gill, 1982; Lomas, 1987; Racker, 1968; Tansey & Burke, 1989). Empirically, Maroda notes that analytic practitioners regularly deviate from the classical model of nondisclosure. Moreover, she asserts, "Many of us know in our hearts that patients have left us, often in depression or rage, because we could not or would not give them what they were asking for in terms of access to us" (p. 114). On the basis of a careful theoretical analysis, Maroda advocates revealing countertransference feelings, in appropriate circumstances, for several reasons. First, "The patient is aware of his therapist's feelings and he suffers from the distortions and confusion that arise when his therapist denies or circumvents his reactions to the patient." Second, "The patient's opportunities for delineating, understanding, and taking responsibility for his own motivations and behavior are limited by the therapist's refusal to do the same" (p. 110). On the positive side, "Therapists' intense emotions, when managed intelligently, have the potential for completing the much-needed cycle of affective communication between patient and therapist" (p. 156). Failure to allow appropriate expression of the therapist's feelings for therapeutic purposes, Maroda believes, can result in unsuccessful outcomes such as long impasses and premature terminations.

This reconfiguration of the patient–therapist relationship is not a license for indiscriminate, uncontrolled emotional expression on the therapist's part. As with other boundary questions, the assessment of appropriateness, rationale, and efficacy must be patient-centered. Self-disclosure may facilitate authentic engagement in one context, whereas it may intrude destructively on the patient in another. With some patients it can resolve an impasse and restore or strengthen the alliance; with others it can weaken or rupture the alliance. In making this assessment, the critical question is: For whose benefit is this being disclosed? In some cases the therapist may be motivated by his or her own feelings of discomfort at disclosing (e.g., anxiety about maintaining privacy or a narcissistic unwillingness to reveal weakness and show human frailty). In other cases the therapist may be uncomfortable about not disclosing, for fear of appearing to be withholding, even sadistic. In either case the therapist is not acting therapeutically in the interest of the patient. Disclosing to unburden yourself or for exhibitionistic motives is not serving the patient. Always look for possible narcissistic underpinnings of an ostensibly altruistic maneuver.

In some circumstances, self-disclosure can be a valid technique for getting "unstuck" in therapy. It is widely recognized that therapy sometimes reaches an impasse in which neither party will give an inch. Such an impasse usually requires a consultation or an ice-breaker, such as the deliberate role playing dramatized in a brief vignette in Chapter 3, where the therapist role-played the patient asking for a pass. In Maroda's (1994) analysis, some impasses are produced by the patient's needing to know that a problem occurred because of the therapist's dynamics, not the patient's. If the patient thinks it is his or her own "fault," the exploration stops. In a best-case scenario, therapeutic gains can resume when the patient can say, "Now I understand what happened; I realize it was you and not me. Now I can learn something from what I've stirred up in you." Here the patient owns a role in the therapist's countertransference, which the patient seeks to understand just as the therapist does.

For Maroda, self-disclosure can help preserve or repair the alliance in a special set of circumstances—namely, where exploration has made clear that the patient is not simply curious but, for dynamically understand-able reasons, *needs* to hear about the therapist's side of the exchange. Among the patients who request disclosure (e.g., "Why did you call me by that other patient's name?"), some do not really want to hear the answer. Others cannot get past not knowing. They reach a point where they no longer trust you, no longer feel sure who you are and what you are doing. These are the patients who may leave therapy without a special intervention to bring them back into an alliance posture. Always with a patient-centered focus, Maroda calibrates the clinical situation to assess the patient's suitability for disclosure of the therapist's dynamic process and the patient's authentic wish to know. This procedure distinguishes necessary self-disclosure from distracting and potentially noxious self-disclosure. For example, the patient's requests must be serious, heartfelt, and repeated. Sometimes it is necessary to ask, "Are you sure you want an answer?" If the patient is satisfied or loses interest, the therapist must overcome his or her own wish to disclose and drop the subject. While acknowledging that there are no absolute rules, Maroda emphasizes that the patient will make clear when self-disclosure is called for. Still, the therapist must remain in control, both of the emotions being expressed and of the limits of the therapeutic frame.

The following case shows how one therapist applied Maroda's model to a commonly encountered request for disclosure:

> A gay male patient repeatedly made remarks to a male therapist such as, "I'm really wondering whether or not you're gay." The therapist replied in a manner appropriate for exploratory therapy: "What would it mean if I were gay? What would it mean if I weren't?" The therapist did not answer the question directly as long as he sensed that the patient was struggling with it, waiting to see if the therapist would take the initiative. Only much later, when the patient asked directly "Are you gay?" was the therapist satisfied that the patient was no longer testing and probing him, but really was ready to discuss the issue. At that point the therapist addressed the question directly with the patient.

Like Maroda, Renik (1995) finds the principle of analytic anonymity honored more in the breach than in the observance. Renik believes that the ideal of the anonymous analyst *"has permitted us implicitly to solicit and accept idealization even while we are ostensibly involved in ruthless analysis of it"* (p. 479, emphasis in original). "By pretending to anonymity," Renik observes, "an analyst increases the constraint he or she exercises. Far from diminishing the analyst's presence, a stance of non-self-disclosure tends to place the analyst center stage" (p. 484). This idealization as an authority, while a legitimate and necessary stage in some analyses, can be personally gratifying for the analyst, just as self-revelation can be, and therefore is likewise susceptible to exploitation. By contrast, Renik finds, "When an analyst tries to communicate his or her thinking in full, respect for the patient as collaborator is conveyed" (p. 484). In the "atmosphere of authentic candor" that Renik advocates, "when my patients experience me as saying what I really think—about them, myself, us—they respond in kind" (p. 493). Renik's position, like Maroda's, is far from a no-holds-barred stance. Unlike the patient's free association, the analyst's self-disclosure is selective, purposeful, and focused on the analytic process. Such disciplined self-disclosure can be a springboard for productive analysis that furthers the patient's self-understanding (see Renik, 1995, for examples).

BOUNDARIES OF DISCLOSURE

When, what, and how to self-disclose are individualized situational decisions. Therapists will always face dilemmas in this area. The universe of possibilities is defined by two limiting cases.

On the one hand, it is generally regarded as useful to validate reactions that a patient observes or senses. When a patient says, "I think you're angry at me," if you answer "No, I'm not" while the anger is visible on your face, then a patient who already has an angry therapist to deal with now has a dishonest therapist as well. A more useful response is to say "I think you're picking up something that's really going on here. What's happening here is making me irritated. Let's see if we can figure out what that's all about." One experienced clinician uses a variation of this response: "The way you're acting would make a lot of therapists angry. What could be in it for you to behave this way?" This locution expresses the therapist's reaction while distancing it from the therapist, so that it is clearly about the patient.

Another example comes from an inpatient setting far away from the subtleties of analytic practice:

> [A] hospitalized patient lied to her therapist and the nursing staff about possessing a razor blade and delighted in having won their trust only to flaunt her power to deceive them. The therapist felt betrayed and hopeless as to his ability to help someone so deceitful and mean. He was encouraged by his supervisor to see his patient briefly at their next scheduled meeting to inform her that he was too angry to be helpful to her for

the moment and that he would need some time to think about what had happened and whether he would be able to go on being her therapist. Such a period of reflection allowed him to explore his emotional reaction, while affording the patient an opportunity (with the help of the skilled nursing staff) to consider the consequences of her behavior. (Gutheil & Gabbard, 1998, p. 412)

Maroda (1994) summarizes this approach as applied to a range of emotions:

> I believe it is worse than useless to hide from patients and to refuse to let them know that they have "gotten to you." Therapists should convey the feelings that provocative patients stimulate in them. This means having therapists show anger rather than sitting white-knuckled in their chairs while appearing to remain unmoved. Or it may mean shedding a tear, or expressing affection or respect. The idea is for therapists to respond to their patients' affect on a regular basis, rather than trying to remain impervious to them. There are no rules, except to let the patient be the guide. (p. 27)

This clinical honesty about the patient's impact on the therapist in the immediacy of the session can be especially helpful to severely disturbed patients, such as those with borderline or dissociative disorder. As Gabbard and Wilkinson (1994) explain: "Many patients do not experience themselves as 'real.' They may gain a sense of the real impact that they have on others when the therapist uses self-disclosure" (p. 143). (For an extended example of how such an interchange can work therapeutically, see Gabbard and Wilkinson, 1994, ch. 7.) It may also be necessary to disabuse a patient of disruptive fantasies—for example, that the patient has transmitted an infectious disease to the therapist, that the therapist would marry the patient if only she were free to do so, that the therapist is involved in a plot against the patient, or that the therapist couldn't care less if the patient lives or dies (Epstein, 1994, pp. 199–200).

At the other extreme, even therapists who favor more open self-disclosure agree that it is rarely useful and often burdensome for the patient to hear details (financial, emotional, sexual) of the therapist's personal and family life, or to be told about the therapist's dreams, fantasies, or emotional conflicts unrelated to the therapeutic interchange. Such disclosures, especially when they involve sexual feelings, are nearly always considered boundary violations. (For case vignettes showing how both female and male patients have been burdened, alienated, or intimidated by therapists' disclosure of erotic feelings toward them, see V. W. Hilton, 1997, pp. 190–193. For the rare exception, see Maroda, 1994, pp. 135–138.)

DISCLOSING TO DIFFERENT TYPES OF PATIENTS

Experienced clinicians learn to self-disclose differently with different kinds of patients. For example, it may be difficult to preserve strict anonymity with traumatized patients. A person who has been abused may not feel safe with someone he or she knows nothing about. When the therapist is too remote, a caricature of technical neutrality, the patient may not feel accepted, and the interaction is sterile. You need to be more real, more tangible, but you do that by expressing yourself with a wider affective range and making emotional contact with the patient over the patient's issues, not by talking about your own life. There is a delicate balance to be struck here, since patients who have been abused, especially by a previous therapist, need to have their boundaries respected.

Whether and when it is appropriate to answer a patient's questions about a therapist's personal life can also depend on the nature of the pathology and the primitiveness of the patient's defense mechanisms, together with other contextual factors, as in the following vignette:

> A clinician answering calls on an emergency hotline was speaking with a depressed, possibly suicidal, patient whom he had never seen or spoken with before. Noticing the clinician's accent, the patient asked, "Where are you from?" The clinician answered, "A long time ago I came from Italy, but right now I'm at Central Psychiatric Hospital, and I'm here to help you." This direct answer, followed by redirection to the present time and to the business at hand, was appropriate, given the telephone contact, exigent circumstances, and lack of a contract or alliance permitting psychodynamic exploration.

As noted earlier, clinicians are sometimes taught this simple rule of thumb: whereas a neurotic patient can tolerate the anxiety of not knowing the answer, a psychotic patient may not be able to do so (Winnicott, 1965). In some cases, therefore, when a psychotic patient asks, "Are you married?" it may be appropriate to say simply "Yes" and then to explore further. If the patient asks follow-up questions, you can gently redirect: "I appreciate your interest, but we are really here to talk about you." Context (including the state of the alliance) and tone are critical here, because the patient could take this redirection as pulling rank.

This rule, although obviously mechanistic, works in many cases. The ego-boundary problem expressed by the psychotic patient's question reflects the patient's inability to form a clear impression of who you are. To come into proper focus, you may need to tell the patient more. Thus, if you display some minor physical discomfort, a schizophrenic patient may attribute it to his or her pathology. Schizophrenics' feelings of reference and influence may lead them to conclude, for example, that you came down with the flu because the difficulty of working with them affected your immune system. To counter such fantasies, it may be appropriate to explain, "Listen, I didn't get a chance to go to the bathroom before I came in here. Either you can watch me squirm, or we'll take a break for a minute." Likewise, "I may have a little preoccupied look on my face. I'll pay attention the best I can, but it's not you that this is about." These are specific disclosures related to the therapy process, rather than to the therapist's life outside of the dyad, and used to improve the alliance.

Such patient- and diagnosis-centered decisions about self-disclosure are most difficult in the case of people with personality disorders. Typically, these patients present with an outward self-control resembling neurotic patients, yet their unstable ego boundaries, sometimes manifesting in provocations that call for limit setting, can reflect a deep anxiety about not knowing where the therapist's boundaries lie. Throughout this book we highlight areas of special concern with borderline and other personality disorders. For a focused treatment of this subject, see, for example, Gabbard & Wilkinson (1994) and Gutheil (2005b, 2005c).

AVOIDING COERCED SELF-DISCLOSURE

The film *Silence of the Lambs* gave many therapists cause for concern as patients began to echo Hannibal Lecter's demand for "a quid pro quo"—that is, "I'll answer one of your questions if you'll answer one of mine." Such demands may be made in the name of mutuality, reciprocity, fairness, or the patient's expectation that the therapist live up to a certain image (e.g., that of a "nice guy"). Contrary to some clinicians' concerns, it is possible to withhold a direct answer in a tactful, nonrejecting manner, such as the following:

> "I'd like to hear about your interest in this and to know more about it and any other questions you have, but I prefer not to reveal information about my personal life to you. Doing so could alter my special professional role with you, which is for me to listen to your thoughts and feelings rather than for me to burden you with mine." (Epstein, 1994, p. 203)

The therapist then needs to follow up to see whether the patient continues to be troubled by the nondisclosure. If the patient is not sufficiently reassured by the initial disclaimer, Epstein (1994) suggests an elaboration such as the following:

"It's really OK with me for you to ask me questions. It's just that sometimes I have to handle them as if they were like any other thought that
comes into your mind. Some of them I can't answer because I have rules I
have to follow, so that I can do my best job in my effort to assist you."
(pp. 203–204)

Patients sometimes seek to extract self-disclosures (all too often successfully) by lapsing into a chatty tone while the therapist is occupied
with prescription writing, appointment scheduling, or bill paying—or,
most commonly, in the transition zone "between the chair and the door"
(Gutheil & Simon, 1995). If the patient can elicit the therapist's tacit,
unconsidered agreement that the session is indeed over and that the
contract no longer applies, the therapist may respond with unguarded
matter-of-factness to remarks such as "Where are you going on vacation?" or "That's a beautiful necklace." It is as if the final whistle has
blown, the game is over, and the players are free to hang out and frater-
nize. In the face of such challenges, the therapist needs to maintain a professional stance, including awareness of the relevant dynamics and exploration during the next session.

Even when a therapist feels "put on the spot," there are other options besides dissembling or forced disclosure. For example, when a
patient asks "Do you find me sexually attractive?" the therapist can respond by saying "What would it mean to you if I said 'yes' and what
would it mean to you if I said 'no'?" This neutral position refocuses attention on what really matters, which is not what the therapist thinks of
the patient but what the patient thinks of himself or herself. Gabbard
(1999b) recommends any of the following responses to this provocative
question:

1. Inquire why at this particular time and on this particular day that information has become so compelling.
2. Point out how others have answered that question for the patient
   but how the answer does not seem to help the patient's fundamental
   problem with self-esteem.
3. Address the patient's insistence and coerciveness and point to how
   they may undermine the patient's getting the kind of answers that
   he or she wants.
4. Disclose the personal dilemma in which the patient is placing the
   therapist. The therapist might, for example, respond: "You place me
   in a dilemma when you demand to know whether I find you
   sexually attractive. Either way I answer the question could lead to
   significant problems for the therapy. If I say that I do not find you attractive, you may feel devastated. If I say that I do, you may feel that
   the therapy is not as safe a place as you previously thought." (p. 16)

This last response requires some tact and discretion, since it could well sound accusatory to some types of patients.

EXPLORING SPONTANEOUS SELF-DISCLOSURES

Boundary crossings sometimes occur when a therapist spontaneously discloses personal information that normally would be kept out of therapy. A therapist who is alert to and prepared to explore such crossings not only can recover from the error but also can help generate useful insights for the patient. The following illustration involves a female therapist and a male patient.

> At the end of a long and frustrating session, a therapist felt as though nothing she had said had been helpful. She had been preoccupied with the fact that her own mother was ill, and she had not been as available to the patient as usual. As the therapist and patient got up from their chairs, the patient asked, "So where are you going next week?" Without thinking, the therapist responded, "I'm going to visit my mother in Colorado. She's very ill." The patient said, "Oh, I'm sorry," and left the office looking worried. The therapist instantly recognized that she had revealed information that might have burdened the patient with her own problems. As she reflected on her enactment, she recognized that she had been feeling guilty about not having been very helpful because she was so preoccupied and that she had unconsciously tried to gain some sort of absolution or forgiveness from the patient by explaining the situation to him.
>
> After her 1-week absence, the therapist brought up what had happened at the end of the session with the patient and explained that she probably should not have burdened him with the information she offered. She went on to suggest that they might beneficially explore his reactions to it. In the course of sharing some of his thoughts about what had happened, the patient noted that his mother had always confided her problems to him, and he thought something like that was repeating itself in the therapeutic relationship. In this instance no lasting harm was done to the patient, and the event turned out to be a useful focus for further exploration. An important factor that led this enactment to be constructive is that it was *discussible* by the therapist and patient. (Gutheil & Gabbard, 1998, p. 410)

INESCAPABLE REVELATIONS: ABSENCE, ILLNESS, PREGNANCY

Unlike most "parting shots" directed at therapists by patients, the question "By the way, will you be in the program next year?" is a legitimate one for a patient to ask a clinical trainee, whose presence in the program is the basis of the treatment contract (Gutheil & Simon, 1995). Likewise, patients need to be informed when a therapist is planning to retire or move from the area during the anticipated period of treatment, or when a therapist has a terminal illness. When and how a therapist makes such disclosures will vary with each therapist and each patient, but the principle is to avoid unnecessarily burdensome detail, or emotional content that is personal to the therapist, while giving the patient enough information to grieve the loss, cope with the impact on treatment, and arrange for transfer of care as needed (Epstein, 1994, pp. 198–199).

Short of these treatment-ending contingencies, a therapist may need to miss one or more sessions for various reasons, including medical treatment, surgery, convalescence, death or illness in one's family, on-call service, a clinical consultation or emergency, or a court appearance. In such situations, how specific does the therapist's disclosure need to be? Should you say, "I'm going to be out for 2 weeks for medical reasons" or " . . . for minor surgery" or " . . . to have my gallbladder taken out"? The "answer" depends on the individuals involved and the type of contract and alliance they have. If there is a general guideline, it is to keep the patient's interests foremost by disclosing only as much as the patient needs to know or would in any case discover, as opposed to disclosures that are inappropriate, intrusive, and potentially damaging.

Therapists who are made vulnerable by illness or family problems may be tempted toward exhibitionism and/or an implicit appeal for help, thereby inviting role reversal. For example, a therapist may feel the urge to blurt out "I'm going to be missing next week's session to have life-threatening surgery, and I need your help and support." Instead, it is best to stick to the facts as they affect the patient—"We're going to miss a session"—and to the practical necessities. As a rule, the emphasis should be on coverage, not explanation. The patient needs to know whom to call during the therapist's absence. (For helpful suggestions for facilitating timely patient notification and coverage in the event of planned or unplanned incapacitation of a therapist, see Pope & Vasquez, 2007.)

The following brief vignettes exemplify dilemmas that arise in normal practice concerning disclosure of absences:

A therapist told a patient that he had to postpone their next session because of illness in his family; another postponement followed when the therapist's relative died. After each of these absences the patient said, "I'm not going to ask you anything about this, but are you all right?" That was an appropriate thing for the patient to say, but in retrospect the therapist felt that he had burdened the patient unnecessarily by sharing his personal misfortune with the patient. It shifted the focus of need, of care, from the patient to the therapist.

A therapist was called on short notice to testify as an expert witness in a malpractice case. Feeling uncomfortable and guilty about having to inconvenience one of his patients, the therapist explained his uncertain schedule. "I'll be in court the day before, and my testimony may run over to the next day," he said. "Let's reschedule now to make sure this doesn't cause us to miss a session." As he reached for his appointment book, the patient smiled and said, "Go do what you have to do." On reflection, the therapist reminded himself that people generally understand what it means for a clinician to have an "emergency."

Some disclosure is unavoidable in the case of illness involving visible disfigurement (see Pizer, 1995). If you are having a melanoma removed from your stomach, no one will see it. If it is on your cheekbone, patients will react to it. Whatever the site of the cancer, treatment that causes baldness will attract patients' attention. Although these problems cannot be resolved prescriptively, it helps to anticipate potential pitfalls. For example, more disturbed patients can be told, "I'll be having minor surgery on my face, so next time you come in you'll see me with a bandage."

An ill or injured therapist is in danger of regressing, and therefore of seeming to call out for caretaking. A patient who has been someone's caretaker at home may be all too ready to assume that familiar, reassuring role. The patient may think, "I've been in this scenario before. It's my alcoholic mother. *Déjà vu* all over again. I know how to do this job." Thus, the more you disclose about your illness, the more you risk shifting the focus of caring to yourself. On the other hand, as Munn (1995) has described in the case of a therapist with multiple sclerosis, a chronic illness that becomes part of the landscape of therapy can, at least with some patients, enrich the alliance and stimulate significant exploration.

Pregnancy is another visible condition that can have a substantial impact on therapeutic boundaries (Bienen, 1990; Fenster, Phillips, & Rapoport, 1986; Imber, 1990; Nadelson, Notman, Arons, & Feldman, 1974; Penn, 1986). Not only is there an expectation of missed sessions, but patients may sense in the therapist an actual or perceived shift of energy and concern from their needs to her own, while therapists worry about patients' actual or perceived feelings of destructive envy toward the baby. These dynamics are especially disruptive in the treatment of seriously disturbed patients, such as those with borderline personality disorder

(Bridges & Smith, 1988; Gabbard & Wilkinson, 1994). For useful guidelines for disclosure on the part of the pregnant therapist, see Gabbard and Wilkinson (1994, pp. 139–140).

DISCLOSING SHARED EXPERIENCES
OR AFFILIATIONS

Therapists' disclosures that they have had experiences and suffered difficulties similar to those of their patients, while not permitted in classical analytic therapy, are fairly commonplace in therapies that place less emphasis on therapist abstinence. Reamer (2001, p. 167) presents the case of a counselor at a community mental health center who told the parents of a 6-year-old child that she had found certain behavior management techniques to be effective with many children, including her own. Later the parents told the counselor that her brief mention of her personal experience as a parent had encouraged them by showing that she understood their frustration and had overcome similar challenges. This disclosure was appropriate in a context where the parents were not the identified patient and where the counseling (in the case of the parents) took the form of practical guidance rather than deep exploration of feelings.

Whether such a personal disclosure is appropriate in individual therapy depends as always on the context (type of therapy, patient characteristics and diagnosis, and the nature of the contract and alliance) as well as common sense. Obviously, it is one thing for a therapist to tell a patient with social phobia that he or she sometimes gets anxious when speaking in public—a disclosure intended to destigmatize the patient's anxiety by placing it on a continuum of normal human experiences. It is another thing altogether for the therapist to reveal that he or she, too, has been diagnosed with social phobia and treated with Paxil.

Such personal disclosures by clinicians have come to be rationalized and even institutionalized in subcultures with specific agendas, on the model of substance abuse treatment (Mallow, 1998). In their commentary on the guidelines established by the Massachusetts Board of Registration in Medicine for boundary maintenance by physicians practicing psychotherapy, Hundert and Appelbaum (1995) note:

> This [i.e., therapists' disclosure of their own past substance abuse] is so much a part of the culture of addictions work that the guidelines acknowledge it as "common" practice. Moreover, this practice appears to be spreading to other subcultural groups in which potential patients seek

out therapists who have a common identity with them (e.g., gay or lesbian patients, or patients from particular religious orientations). (p. 351)

However, the fact that this practice has gained acceptance in many
quarters does not mean that it is free of problems and complications. The
appropriateness of therapists' disclosure of their substance abuse histories, especially through attendance at AA or NA meetings also attended
by clients, is a matter of controversy even within the substance abuse
field (Doyle, 1997; Reamer, 2001). A therapist who attends self-help group
meetings with clients in attendance may not feel free to share his or her
feelings and experiences fully in the group meeting for fear of compromising therapeutic effectiveness. This is especially true, for example, if
the therapist has relapsed or nearly relapsed, or is struggling with negative feelings toward clients or doubts about continuing to work in the
field. Likewise, a therapist's presence may inhibit normal sharing by patients in group meetings. The power sometimes exercised by substance
abuse counselors over clients' lives (e.g., through progress reports to legal
authorities) adds a layer of potential exploitation to what is already an
uncomfortable dual relationship.

Self-disclosure of shared personal experience within the therapeutic
frame also raises serious questions. Clinical treatment, whether in individual or group therapy, is not egalitarian. Even in a group for substance
abusers or for survivors of sexual abuse or violent crimes, a clinician acting in a professional capacity has a clearly demarcated role. To act as if
such a group were the same as a mutual-support group for laypersons
risks confusion of identities and purposes. A counterargument is that in a
treatment group with a specialized agenda the therapist's personal connection to that agenda is relevant to the content of therapy. Sharing this
pertinent experience can facilitate the alliance and build trust by assuring
patients that they will be understood, not judged. Indeed, many patients
come to such groups thinking "No one will understand me except someone who's been through the same thing."

Typically, then, self-disclosure of a counselor's or therapist's substance abuse experience is rationalized by the argument that substance
abuse is so demoralizing at its core, leaving such a residue of shame, that
some patients can be comfortable only with a therapist who has had the
same experience. Like some patients with psychotic or personality disorders (discussed earlier in this chapter), they "can't get past not knowing."
To which one might reply, "They can't or they won't?" That is, it is hard to
separate this particular rationale from the idiosyncratic historical development of the 12-step movement and substance abuse treatment in the

United States (Peele et al., 1991; Peele, Bufe, & Brodsky, 2000; Rudy, 1986). Beneficial as such mutual-support groups have been, the attitude that "only an alcoholic can understand another alcoholic" encourages a certain self-indulgent narcissism: "I'm special; we're special. I/we need someone who is special in the same way to be my/our therapist." To play into this emotional rigidity and exceptionalism may be, in many cases, to accept a relatively primitive resolution that sets a ceiling on the self-awareness, autonomy, and growth that the patient can achieve. The fact that people may expect therapy to be just like a self-help group does not mean that it has to be that way. As in other kinds of boundary confusion experienced by patients, it may be more helpful to stand firm and educate the patient as to what professional therapy is and how it has been found to work best. Therapy isn't sex, it isn't socializing, and it isn't an AA meeting.

A therapist and patient can be thought of as two people who have similar conflicts, dilemmas, and challenges but different ways of managing them. A therapist might say, "There, but for the grace of certain defenses, go I." In most therapies, however, the perceived bond between patient and therapist is limited to a general acknowledgment of their common humanity. We all must deal with loss, grief, aging, and mortality. Part of a patient's maturation and growth is to be able to separate the therapist as a vulnerable human being from the therapist's role in relation to the patient. Whether there is a legitimate exception to be made for more specific self-disclosures in, say, substance abuse therapy is open to question. Why is the experience of compulsive substance use necessarily more shameful than other emotional conditions that produce pain and anguish? Is this experience measurably more devastating than losing one's parents in childhood, suffering periodic psychotic episodes, or enduring the mood swings of bipolar disorder?

People also suffer severe pain and shame as a result of childhood sexual abuse, spousal battering, and other traumas. In these areas, too, as in the treatment of gay and lesbian patients and people with certain religious affiliations, some patients now demand a specific bond of identification with a therapist. As with substance abuse treatment, there are several reasons for exercising caution and careful consideration before making such personal disclosures. For one thing, a therapist with a general practice must decide whether to reveal his or her special background only to patients who share that background. A therapist who considers it useful to tell gay patients that he or she is gay faces the dilemma that, for other patients (e.g., those from conservative backgrounds), this information may be extraneous, distracting, and potentially intrusive. If the information reaches those patients through the grapevine, they may resent not having been told.

One may, of course, question the bias that raises these questions for gay therapists but not for heterosexual ones. The inevitable, inadvertent self-disclosures a therapist makes can include wearing a wedding ring, to which patients may react for good or for ill. Nonetheless, whatever one's sexual orientation or lifestyle, there is a significant difference between passive, environmental disclosure (e.g., wearing a ring or having family pictures on one's desk or wall) and making an issue of one's personal life by announcing it. In the first case, the disclosure is background information, part of a therapist's generalized presentation. In the second case, having been brought into the foreground of the therapist–patient relationship, it is more likely to have a disruptive impact.

At a gay counseling center a therapist's sexual orientation is not extraneous information. There, being gay may be a condition of employment, like being a recovering alcoholic or addict in some treatment centers. In those contexts this form of self-disclosure is taken for granted. The same is true for therapists in private practice who set out to serve a particular community. Gartrell (1992) has written that, in addition to her professional background and interests, "new clients are also informed that I am a lesbian feminist" (p. 33). In response to initial questions, Gartrell discloses information that is reasonably public and that may assist prospective clients in choosing a suitable therapist. One such question is whether or not she has children. Some lesbian mothers prefer to see therapists who are also mothers. This preference is shared by some heterosexual patients concerned with parenting issues, who want to be assured that their therapist "knows what it's like." (For further discussion of self-disclosure with respect to sexual orientation, see Pope, Sonne, & Greene, 2006.)

Even with a patient for whom such information is relevant, the implications the patient draws from it may or may not be helpful. In the case of a patient seeking treatment for anxiety resulting from having been raped, should her therapist reveal (if it is the case) that she, too, has been raped? This revelation can be reassuring, but it can also be burdensome if the patient feels she cannot talk freely about her traumatic experience for fear it will bring up the therapist's own memories of assault and violation. In other words, whatever benefit the patient may derive from the awareness of shared experience is countered by the burden of having to consider the therapist's feelings. Thus, if a therapist does decide to reveal that she is a survivor of assault (or alcoholic, or lesbian), it would be in the interest of full disclosure to add "I have some idea of what you're going through, and that may make me more helpful to you, or it may not."

A patient may look for some shared identification or affiliation with a therapist in order to be able to explore issues the patient feels unable to discuss with anyone else or in order to avoid raising issues that "you already know about." Shared religious belief, for example, can serve as a form of resistance. A patient may go to a clinician of the same religious persuasion either to be understood or to evade understanding (or, of course, both). In one reported case, a Catholic priest was referred to a priest-psychologist who practiced exploratory therapy with a clientele that consisted largely of clergy and deeply religious laypersons. Relating to the therapist in the latter's clerical rather than clinical role, this patient saw himself as being at the confessional and felt that the therapist was passing judgment on his sins. This perceived judgmental context, reinforced by the therapist's failure to realize that his inquiries were being misinterpreted as a kind of catechism rather than as an open-ended investigation, inhibited free exploration of the patient's individual experience (Kehoe & Gutheil, 1984).

The relationship between the two clerics in this case can be characterized as a pseudoalliance in which the rigidity of the shared belief system (however valid in its own context as religious faith) prevented both parties from freeing themselves to engage in the work of therapy. Other pseudoalliances of an outwardly more permissive form can occur when, for example, the kind of experience (and related belief system) shared by patient and therapist leads the therapist to accept and even reify the patient's assumption of a "victim role." In its own way, this kind of belief system can be as much a constraint on therapeutic exploration as religious doctrine. The cozy "we're on the same team" feeling that comes from the choice of a therapist ostensibly tailored to the patient's needs can turn into collusion to focus on familiar issues while looking away from other issues that would be threatening to bring to the surface.

The presumed understanding, trust, and confidence that can follow all too readily from a therapist's disclosure of a shared experience or affiliation with a patient can, by virtue of being unearned and untested, quickly turn to disillusionment. This dynamic was one component of a complex case in which a woman began to see a psychiatrist who was treating her son (which raises another boundary question). The mother had a history of substance abuse, including stimulants and prescription medications, and was attending 12-step programs to stay sober. The therapist told the patient that she, too, had been attending 12-step groups, in her case for overeating. This disclosure reportedly created an immediate bond of trust and a belief that the psychiatrist would understand the patient's problems. Diagnosing the patient with major depression, history of polysubstance abuse, and attention-deficit/hyperactivity disorder (ADHD), the psychiatrist prescribed Prozac as an antidepressant and Dexedrine for ADHD. Within a few months the patient began to show signs of excessive use of prescribed medications. After the patient entered an inpatient drug rehabilitation program for addiction to pain medications, she sued the psychiatrist for malpractice, alleging negligent monitoring of her medications. Despite the patient's reportedly having been prescribed pain medications by other physicians, including her family physician, a jury found the psychiatrist 90% negligent and awarded the patient a six-figure judgment (*Zagha v. Kroplick*, 2000).

RESEARCH ON SELF-DISCLOSURE

With all of the clinical interest and controversy surrounding self-disclosure, not surprisingly there has been considerable research on the subject as well. This research (reviewed by Farber, 2006, and Hill & Knox, 2002) has focused on the frequency and types of self-reported therapist self-disclosures, patients' and therapists' beliefs about and attitudes toward therapist self-disclosures, and the effects of such disclosures. To date, this has proved a difficult area for research. In addition to the methodological problems with self-report studies generally, there has been no standard definition of self-disclosure used across studies for purposes of comparison and replication. Indeed, some studies specify either no definition at all or a definition so broad and vague as to be susceptible to a range of interpretations on the part of both respondents and readers. It is difficult to generalize from the findings of any of the numerous settings, conditions, methods, and patient populations found in this research. In particular, as Farber (2006) emphasizes, neither frequency studies nor outcome studies can yield useful findings in the absence of a clear distinction between factual self-disclosures about the therapist (the main area of controversy) and the kinds of clinically focused countertransference disclosures, arising out of the process of therapy, that are widely accepted in the clinical literature (e.g., Gabbard & Wilkinson, 1994; Maroda, 1994).

In a departure from previous research, Barrett and Berman (2001) systematically varied levels of therapist self-disclosure to assess the impact of such disclosure on the outcome of treatment. The study employed only reciprocal disclosures (i.e., a therapist's disclosure of personal information in response to similar client self-disclosures). Each therapist who participated in the study saw two patients for four sessions each. With one client, the therapist increased the use of reciprocal self-disclosures; with the other client, the therapist limited the use of such disclosures. (The therapists were trained in giving the two types of responses, and blind observation confirmed that the experimental conditions were successfully implemented.) The researchers found that clients in the increased disclosure condition reported less symptom distress and liked their therapist more than clients in the limited disclosure condition. However, increased disclosure by therapists did not lead to greater frequency or intimacy of self-disclosure by clients. Despite its limited scope and generalizability (for one thing, it did not include therapist-initiated self-disclosures), this study did provide evidence that, in the particular context examined, self-disclosure by therapists can strengthen the therapeutic alliance and improve treatment outcomes.

Knox and Hill (2003) have developed preliminary research-based recommendations for therapists' use of self-disclosure. Nonetheless, as Farber (2006) cautions, "This line of inquiry is very much in its infancy" (p. 147). Research at this early stage of development will have little impact on either the ethical concerns or the risks of legal and regulatory liability associated with therapist self-disclosure. Still, if ongoing research strengthens the argument that particular forms of self-disclosure have beneficial effects in specified contexts, the findings could be used in defending against allegations of boundary violations.

KEY REMINDERS

- Some degree of self-disclosure by a therapist is inevitable, but such disclosures can become boundary violations when they are not made for the benefit of the patient.
- Different schools of therapy involve different levels of disclosure, which in turn serve the needs of different patients.
- Self-disclosures of a personal nature that do not have a clinical purpose, whether or not requested by the patient, may inhibit exploration and/or invite other boundary violations.
- Decisions about the therapeutic use of self-disclosure need to be made on a case-by-case basis in the context of the type of therapy offered.

CHAPTER 6

Communication and Out-of-Office Contacts

Therapists need to communicate appropriately with patients, but just what is appropriate varies from patient to patient. Therapists also need to maintain a proper clinical and ethical stance in the event of inadvertent (or patient-instigated) patient contact out in the community, away from the normal boundaries of the therapeutic frame. This chapter is concerned with these two boundary contexts that resist straightforward ethical or technical judgments.

COMMUNICATION

A therapist needs to consider the therapeutic implications of the language used in communicating with patients. A therapist's language is problematic when it is experienced by the patient as disrespectful or intrusive, when it becomes an unproductive springboard for the patient's fantasies, or when it expresses the therapist's conscious or unconscious desire for intimacy with the patient. To begin with, in therapies with a practical focus and no contract to explore the dynamics of the patient–therapist relationship, a reasonably mature, well-functioning patient may accept being addressed by his or her first name without a second thought. However, it might be inadvisable to address the same patient by his or her first name in psychoanalytic therapy. With the latter context in mind, Gutheil and Gabbard (1993) offer the following cautionary thoughts:

There are distinct advantages to addressing the adult in the patient, in terms of fostering the adult observing ego for the alliance. Trainees often do not see the paradox of expecting adult behavior on the ward from someone they themselves call "Jimmy," which is what people called the patient when he was much younger. Last names also emphasize that this process is work or business, an atmosphere which may promote a valuable mature perspective and minimize acting out. In addition, calling someone by the name used by primary objects may foster transference perceptions of the therapist when they are not desirable, as with a borderline patient prone to forming severe psychotic transferences. For balance, however, recall that use of last names may also sound excessively distant, formal, and aloof. (p. 194)

It may be difficult, and may feel unnatural, to insulate the clinical setting from the informality that pervades contemporary America, where one recent head of state called himself "Jimmy" and another called himself "Bill." (Both were from the South, where such informal address is most common.) On the other hand, just asking the patient how he or she prefers to be addressed does not resolve any underlying conflicts that may be present. Many clinicians see a patient's seemingly straightforward request to be called by his or her first name as innocent and benign. Yet, even such small boundary challenges can be problematic, as in the following case (adapted from Gutheil & Gabbard, 1993):

> Early in therapy a female patient persistently asked her female therapist to call her by her first name. Although she had agreed to do this with some patients, the therapist in this case resisted. Sensing that the patient might be threatened by the familiarity she requested, the therapist continued to call her "Ms. Jones." Later the patient acknowledged that if the therapist had acceded to her request, she would have left therapy because the familiar address would have felt like an intrusion, recapitulating the abusive family dynamics she had experienced.

Experienced analytically oriented therapists know that a request such as this one requires exploration. In this case the patient, consciously or unconsciously, was testing to see whether the situation was safe, whether the boundaries would hold. A patient may or may not be distressed and may or may not be relieved (or both) when the therapist refuses to cross the boundary. On the other hand, for a patient who is disposed to distort clinical material, the therapist's acceding to such a request may represent an imagined invitation to join the therapist's family. As in other meetings at the outer edges of the therapeutic frame, there is no rational limit to patients' fantasies. A therapist's innocent intentions do not ensure a comparably constructive reaction on the patient's part.

Other guidelines for appropriate use of language include the following:

- *Avoid unnecessary jargon.* Language should be used to further communication and understanding, not to impress, intimidate, or overpower the patient.
- *Use language appropriate for the type of therapy being practiced and the patient's cultural background.* Different schools of therapy vary considerably with respect to the formality or informality of the language employed. Likewise, patients' expectations and comfort levels with different forms of expression depend on various cultural, personal, and clinical factors. The key considerations are respect for the patient and ease and effectiveness of communication.
- *Where appropriate, use language consistent with the patient's language when referring to intimate matters.* Explorations of sexual questions can be experienced as violating boundaries when the therapist probes intrusively in areas the patient has not yet addressed. In particular, a therapist who introduces four-letter words can be perceived as verbally assaultive, especially by a patient who has been sexually abused. Since language can either exacerbate or alleviate the patient's feeling of being threatened by therapeutic exploration, it is good practice to adopt the patient's language, especially when referring to sex or genitals. If the patient uses words like "intercourse" or "lovemaking," the therapist should do likewise. The patient can then feel understood by a therapist who is talking at the same level as the patient about a difficult subject.

Whether the same guideline applies when the patient speaks in "four-letter words" is a more difficult question, one that might be answered differently by a psychoanalyst and a substance abuse counselor. Some approaches call for faithful mirroring of the patient's language, with the rationale that translating into euphemisms avoids the intensity of the patient's experience. In other contexts, a therapist's use of profanity might be regarded as colluding in and reinforcing the patient's aggressive or juvenile utterances, thereby sacrificing the therapist's authority as a model in a vain quest for authenticity. In any given case, the resolution of this question depends on the school of therapy, the standards of the relevant professional community, and the therapist's clinical assessment of the patient.

- *Maintain a professional tone.* Language is a matter of tone as well as content. In one case of alleged sexual misconduct, a therapist's intimate, seductive tone in a telephone conversation tape-recorded by the patient led to a settlement.

• *Avoid unintended verbal overtures.* Especially with a traumatized patient, a statement as innocuous as "Yes, I like you," or even the more distanced "I find you a likable person"—let alone "You're looking good today"—risks an unintended boundary transgression. Words can be an early step to seduction, arousing fantasies and expectations that can subvert therapy even if no overtly improper behavior occurs. The more a therapist can create an alliance through appropriate professional behavior rather than emotionally laden statements, an alliance in which the patient feels affectively held, the safer the therapy remains.

• *Avoid verbal abuse rationalized as therapeutic confrontation.* Occasionally it is necessary to speak firmly, even loudly, to a patient, but this must be done only for therapeutic purposes and with uncompromised respect for the patient. Even the most directive therapeutic approaches do not justify the aggressive, cruel, or contemptuous comments that analytically oriented therapists refer to as countertransference sadism.

Written Personal Communications

A common boundary pitfall is the greeting card a therapist may wish to send to a patient on a holiday, wedding, birth, graduation, or other important occasion (Reamer, 2001, pp. 112–115). In particular, many clinicians think it altogether normal to send a patient a condolence note after the death of a loved one. Whether the therapist's intentions are strictly proper or reflect an unconscious wish for a closer personal connection with the client, the patient will react not only to the sending of the note but also to the stationery and return address used, whether the note is typed or handwritten, and the language in which the greeting is expressed. Some patients will receive such a note as if they were playing a detective game, searching for half-hidden clues to the therapist's feelings. The therapist who is weighing, for example, whether to send a condolence note on agency or personal stationery risks giving the appearance of cold formality and impersonality versus that of undue familiarity. Such dilemmas must be resolved on a patient-by-patient basis, with consultation as needed.

The disruptive impact that an ill-considered personal communication by a therapist can have is dramatized in this account by a highly aware, articulate patient, a psychiatrist who began her analysis when she had just finished her residency:

"Distraught over news that my father had passed away, I called him [her analyst] at home one night. The talk was brief. He was supportive but not overtly encouraging of my calling. However, within the week, after I returned from the funeral, he sent flowers of condolence to my house, with a one-page handwritten note. I was stunned. Overwhelmed. My analyst had sent me flowers. With a note. In his handwriting. To me! He wrote of his thoughts about death and the preciousness of life. He shared his inner self. Stunned. That is how I felt. Like the time when I was 13, and a handsome boy, 2 years my senior, asked me to a special high school dance. How had he picked me? Was I indeed beautiful? I had done nothing, and suddenly a prince had appeared. What did this mean?

" . . . I treasured that note. I read and reread it and allowed myself only the feeling of safety and harbor contained within it. I did not let myself fantasize or associate in romantic ways. Only now, as I write this, am I aware of the clearly romantic associations that go so readily with the feelings experienced back then. At the very moment the most important man in my life passed away, a prince appeared to replace him." (Gabbard & Lester, 2002, p. 133)

Even when condolences over a loved one's death are the issue, we see how this patient's personal associations to those condolences lead to her being asked as a date to a dance. This leap captures the romantic associations that the patient initially disavows. The lesson here is obvious.

OUT-OF-OFFICE CONTACTS

In Philip Roth's novel *My Life as a Man*, Peter Tarnopol goes to a psychiatrist, Dr. Spielvogel, whom he had met casually at a few large summer parties. "I don't remember that the doctor and I had much to say to each other," Tarnopol comments. "I never even noticed which woman was his wife; I discovered later that he had noticed which was mine" (Roth, 1974, p. 202). In his first session as a patient, Tarnopol is astonished to hear Dr. Spielvogel describe his (Tarnopol's) wife from memory. He recalls, "My impulse was to get up and leave, my shame and humiliation (and my disaster) still my own—and simultaneously to crawl into his lap" (p. 203). Roth's vignette dramatizes the disturbing power of a psychotherapist's ever-vigilant, all-knowing intrusiveness as perceived by a patient. It thus highlights a dilemma virtually every therapist faces, namely, how to handle encounters with patients, usually inadvertent but sometimes planned, that occur outside the office and outside the therapeutic frame (as opposed to visits or outings conducted for a therapeutic purpose, which are discussed in Chapter 3).

Chance meetings with patients can occur anywhere. In small or geographically isolated communities or in communities united by interest or affiliation (e.g., religion or sexual orientation), such meetings will occur predictably. To minimize their occurrence, Langs (1973, 1976, 1982, 1984–1985), a psychoanalytically oriented psychotherapist, has advocated that therapists not live in the locality where they practice—an impractical solution for many clinicians. Planned encounters may occur by invitation (e.g., to a patient's performance, exhibition, or ceremony) or when a patient deliberately intrudes into a therapist's living space. These are all ways in which the patient's and therapist's personal worlds may intersect. When they do, it is not just the patient's feelings and behavior that are at issue. The therapist, too, may have various reactions to seeing and being seen out of the usual context—awkwardness, discomfort, curiosity, satisfaction. Both parties cannot help but process the situation at the levels of feeling, thought, and action. How should two people who normally limit themselves to a highly specialized, even ritualized, way of interacting face each other in the no-man's land? How much will a patient "notice" about the therapist? And how much is it the therapist's business to notice about the patient?

Probably no other profession (except the police) faces such an ever-present responsibility to maintain professional judgment away from the work environment, to the point of considering where to go, what places or events to avoid, and how to act in the community. Even in off hours, a therapist needs to be alert to the need to snap back into clinical demeanor and exercise clinical judgment. You can be out with your family at the zoo or a baseball game, and suddenly, unexpectedly, clinical, ethical, and perhaps legal responsibilities impose themselves.

What, then, is "the boundary of boundaries"? How far does a therapist's responsibility for setting, monitoring, and managing boundaries extend? Up to a point, the situation is analogous to taking phone calls from patients after office hours. When patients have your phone number, any call could be from a patient. Therefore, it is appropriate to answer in a professional manner even if you are not otherwise on duty. Likewise, when you "run into" a patient outside the office, whatever else you end up doing or not doing, it is appropriate to maintain a professional bearing and consciousness. The difference is that when what connects you with (and separates you from) the patient is a telephone line, it is a relatively simple matter to stay in role and limit the communication to the task of treatment, just as if you were in the office. By contrast, when you meet out in the community, both you and the patient are exposed in your personal lives.

Meeting by Invitation

Patients often invite a therapist to a celebratory event that they feel might not have occurred without the therapist's support. The following vignette shows one therapist's response:

> After initially agreeing to attend his analysand's wedding, the analyst later declined, reasoning that his presence would be inappropriately distracting. Later, after the death of the analysand's first child, he attended the funeral service. Both his absence at the first occasion and his presence at the second were felt as helpful and supportive by the analysand. They both agreed later that the initial plan to attend the wedding was an error. (Gutheil & Gabbard, 1993, p. 192)

An invitation allows time to process the therapeutic implications before responding. As in this case, with proper consideration and discussion one can change one's mind in order to avoid a potential boundary violation. Moreover, some boundary violations can be minimized or undone after the fact by discussion with the patient. A therapist attended the wedding of a patient who had told him, "I wouldn't have made it to this point without you," only to find himself in line to kiss the bride, his patient. In such cases an apology by the therapist may be called for. Sometimes, it's best simply to say "I think that was a mistake" and then together explore the meaning the incident has had for the patient.

Some therapists believe that it is proper (in suitable cases) to attend a patient's wedding ceremony but not to stand in the receiving line or stay for the reception. (What if the patient asks you to dance?) A safer alternative is to "celebrate" privately with the patient by acknowledging the milestone in normal discussion during office sessions. It is a boundary violation when the therapist goes to the wedding to validate and get credit for his or her role in the patient's progress. This narcissistic emotional context makes the occasion exploitative. There is also a risk of a violation of confidentiality if the therapist is not careful to be discreet in explaining to others where he or she is going.

The same analysis applies to other ceremonial occasions such as a graduation, baptism, bar mitzvah, or housewarming. The therapist needs to ask "Who is this for? Is there a risk of exploitation?" Potential negligence lies in failing to think through the choices and their implications and to document that consideration.

Going to a patient's funeral, on the other hand, is generally found to be an appropriate gesture. Therapy is over and can no longer be compromised or complicated, and the patient is beyond being exploited. The family, on the other hand, can benefit from the therapist's being there to support them and share their grief. Families often feel they can unburden themselves to their loved one's therapist as they could to no one else.

With patients who are creative artists, a therapist may be invited to performances or exhibits. There are situations in which, after discussing the issue with the patient, the therapist can attend and then explore the patient's productions in therapy. This is most clearly the case when the therapist's presence is part of the treatment—for example, for performance anxiety. In other circumstances the therapist's observing presence may interfere with the patient's self-expression and relationship with the audience. In the case of an art exhibit, the therapist may choose to visit at some time other than the reception, so as not to intrude on the patient's personal space. Whether such data gathering outside of therapy sessions, even in the patient's absence, is within boundaries depends on various contextual factors, including the type of therapy.

Unplanned Encounters

More than most boundary challenges, inadvertent meetings with patients are fraught with unpredictable implications. When, for instance, you bump into the patient in the supermarket, you have all kinds of data on display, from the way you dress in your off hours to what your family eats. Your reality has intruded into the patient's world, and the patient may be inhibited from talking to you about, say, your having a child who is difficult to manage. Similarly, the patient may have difficulty talking about his or her own difficult-to-manage child on seeing that you have a child who is (at that moment) well behaved. An African American patient, seeing a white therapist with a spouse who is African American, may think "Where do I fit into this?" In such a chance encounter, therapist and patient are both out of role, and their interaction is not protected by the familiar structure of the therapeutic frame. For many patients it is interesting, even exciting, to see their therapist outside of the usual setting and learn something about the therapist's life. For other patients this is an embarrassing, upsetting, perhaps threatening intrusion. These patients may think "Here is this person who knows all these horrible things about me, popping up at a place where I came to have fun with my friends."

The therapist's dilemma, then, is whether a polite acknowledgment makes the situation worse or better. Do you greet the patient who walks by on the street or pretend you don't know him? Obviously, no one answer covers all situations. As mentioned earlier, a good starting point is Karl Menninger's dictum: "When in doubt, be human." A second principle is to respect the patient's privacy and anonymity—and, as far as possible, the patient's wishes. One way of handling this is to take your cue from the patient. Don't acknowledge a patient in a public place if the patient appears to be avoiding eye contact with you. This may be a patient who reacts to a mere acknowledgment that you know him or her as if it were a violation of confidentiality.

Of course, you cannot count on being able to read the patient's intentions quickly or accurately; indeed, the patient may be waiting for cues from you. Accordingly, some therapists prepare for this eventuality in advance by bringing it up at the beginning of therapy as a matter for informed consent: "If we run into each other on the street or in some other public place, and if one of us is accompanied by others, would you like me to say 'hello' or not?" In one case where a former patient moved into the therapist's neighborhood and was brought into contact with the therapist through their children's shared activities (a common occurrence), the patient and therapist agreed to maintain the fiction that they were meeting for the first time.

Meeting in Social Situations

Running into a patient at a social event such as a party or reception, as opposed to passing on the street, raises the ante by presenting the prospect of continued mingling or observation. (In addition, the therapist may be consuming alcohol in the patient's presence.) Is a therapist required to use clinical skills outside the office to determine the patient's comfort level and preferences in that situation? Do you ask, "Are you OK with my being here?" If not, are you obligated to leave, irrespective of your reasons for being there and obligations to others? If you decide not to leave for any reason, including the patient's saying, "Yes, I'm fine," does that give the patient a cause of action against you? What if the patient files an ethics complaint or a lawsuit, saying "My therapist came to this party and flaunted his lovely wife and family in my face"?

It is not clear how far beyond mere coincidental presence at a party a therapist would have to go to incur legal liability. A claim that "my therapist was overly friendly to me at that party" would need to be examined closely in the absence of a deliberate rendezvous between therapist and patient. Although it is unlikely that such a vague and benign allegation would actually result in liability, this detail might serve as one element of a broader claim. A therapist has clear clinical and ethical duties that in some cases have legal ramifications. The guidelines for "contact management" presented in Chapter 1 are applicable here and are worth repeating:

1. Behave professionally while together. Do not engage in personal revelations or exchanges that would be inappropriate in the office.
2. Do not attempt to conduct therapy outside the office.
3. Document the boundary crossing as relevant data.
4. At the next office session, debrief the patient and open up the incident for exploration.
5. Make note of the boundary crossing in supervision, or obtain a consultation.

At a social gathering the patient and therapist are not compelled to carry on a conversation. Unless it is a small dinner where everyone is eating at one table, the therapist can observe the requisite social niceties, stay out of the patient's vicinity, and consider the advisability of leaving early. Since the patient and therapist are not alone, the need to maintain confidentiality becomes critical. As would be true anywhere else, the therapist cannot identify the patient as such to others, including mention of this as an explanation for leaving. Of course, the patient is free to point and say, "That's my shrink over there." However, if the patient attempts to initiate a therapeutic dialogue, the therapist is well advised to caution, "That really belongs in the office."

Extracurricular Data Gathering

At a cocktail party or barbecue, as opposed to when giving a patient a ride in an emergency, the dictum "Don't carry on therapy outside the office" takes on another dimension. Just as a patient may intrude on a therapist's personal life at such a gathering, an inexperienced or inappropriately trained therapist may seize on the accidental meeting as an opportunity to gather therapeutic data, whether by simply observing the patient with his or her personal associates (as Peter Tarnopol, in Philip Roth's novel *My Life as a Man*, thought his psychiatrist had done) or by actually questioning the patient's family or friends. "Here's my chance to interview the wife and kids and find out what's really going on," the therapist may think. Ethically, such behavior may be regarded as intrusive in almost any form of therapy. It is clearly inappropriate and not very useful clinically in exploratory, psychodynamic therapy, where the data need to emerge from within the patient's world view.

Ongoing Involvements or Affiliations

One alleged boundary violation resulting in an ethics complaint to the American Psychiatric Association was a therapist's joining a book discussion group of which a patient was a member (J. Lazarus, 1993). Questions such as the following would be critical to the resolution of such a complaint: Did the therapist know that the patient was participating in the group? Did the therapist stay after finding the patient there? Did the therapist exercise clinical judgment, considering the potential impact of the incident on the patient, and process the interaction with the patient?

The prospect of ongoing extratherapeutic contact adds yet another level of complexity to the chance encounter between therapist and patient. How complex such cases can become is demonstrated by the following cases.

> A therapist and his patient were both invited to be on the board of directors of an art museum. Neither was aware of the other's presence on the board until they saw each other there. While realizing that serving on the board would bring him not only into contact but also into potential disagreements with his patient, the therapist was reluctant to sacrifice the opportunity to apply his interest in art in a meaningful and influential way (Dewald & Clark, 2001, pp. 54–55).

> In another case, a realtor unknowingly arranged to rent a therapist's vacation home for a month to a patient, thereby exposing the therapist to an invasion of privacy. It put the patient in the tempting position of turning fantasy into reality by living among the therapist's belongings and sleeping in his bed. The realtor brought the rental contract to the analyst to sign. The analyst could say, "I'd prefer not to go through with this rental, and I can't say why," but he was concerned that the realtor would infer that the prospective renter was his patient (Dewald & Clark, 2001, pp. 53–54).

If the analyst did not want to refuse the rental, he would need to follow the "contact management" principles above.

Both in this case and in that of the therapist and patient invited to join the museum board, exploration with the patient is called for before the fact (to assess the advisability of proceeding) and after the fact (to monitor the impact on the therapy and bring out what can usefully be learned from the boundary crossing). While there is no magical answer to these dilemmas, they raise the question of whether the therapy could survive those situations.

Processing the Contact

Bringing the matter back within the therapeutic frame by discussing it in the next session can preserve and even advance the therapy in the face of the unintended boundary crossing. Some patients may feel awkward about having intruded on the therapist's world; others may feel intruded upon; still others may feel shamed or humiliated by the therapist's avoidance of contact in a public place. Therefore, debriefing may need to begin with reassurance. Epstein (1994) recommends language such as the following: "If my failure to acknowledge you in public stirs up feelings of shame and embarrassment for you, let's talk about it so that it needn't be so secret or fearful an emotion" (p. 214).

Therapists, too, sometimes need to overcome resistance to exploring inadvertent contacts with patients outside of therapy. Even psychoanalysts who routinely ask patients about their associations to unexpected encounters with other individuals (e.g., a family member, friend, or employer) sometimes pull their punches when they themselves figure in the exploration. A therapist who would readily ask "What was it like to dream about meeting me out in public?" may not feel free to ask the same question when the meeting was real. Even though it is the patient's experience that is to be explored, therapists may feel sufficiently conflicted about having been "exposed" to the patient out in the world that they refrain from exploration, rationalizing that they do not want to call attention to themselves (Strean, 1991).

For a simple example of how to begin exploration, we can take the scenario of a female patient seeing (she assumes) her male therapist's children as she arrives for an appointment at the therapist's home office. This is an inadvertent boundary crossing occurring in conjunction with scheduled office therapy, where the patient's appearance is expected rather than a surprise. Some patients will not bring up this sort of "sighting," either because they really do think nothing of it, because they consider it impolite or prohibited to ask, or because they don't know, or resist knowing, what it brings up for them. When a patient does mention it, it may be as mere social acknowledgment ("Oh, how's your family?"); such casual reference may or may not mask deeper concerns.

Thus, a therapist who is aware of the extratherapeutic contact might bring it up even if the patient does not, to see whether it has relevance yet to be explored. The therapist's dilemma is whether to say nothing and risk dehumanizing the experience for the patient ("I see I'm not worth talking to") or to risk burdening the patient with a factual explanation ("So, you have this ideal Norman Rockwell family, while I'm so miserably screwed up"). In many cases these extremes can be avoided by exploring the encounter. Although the kind of extended exploration described here may not be practical in all kinds of therapy, it highlights underlying issues that may need to be dealt with, in one way or another, in any type of therapy.

PATIENT: I saw your kids outside as I was coming in.

THERAPIST: What was it like seeing them?

PATIENT: I wouldn't have expected you to have such young children. I would have expected to see grown children.

THERAPIST: What does that bring up for you? (In neutral exploration, one works to bring out the affect rather than dispute or clarify the content. It does not matter if the children the patient saw aren't actually the therapist's children—only the patient's experience matters. By contrast, in cognitive therapy the reality of the situation might be disclosed in order to check for cognitive distortions, such as magnification, minimization, or jumping to conclusions.)

PATIENT: Is your wife younger than you—a second marriage, perhaps? (Here the patient's persistence in seeking direct answers reflects resistance to exploring her feelings. Persistence equals resistance. So the therapist continues to explore.)

THERAPIST: What would it mean to you if it were?

PATIENT: I'd wonder if she's as young as I am.

Patients show different degrees of persistence in demanding answers. In general, the greater the persistence, the greater the resistance. Therefore, the therapist parries each question with an invitation to explore what this is all about. Once the patient moves into an exploratory mode and the therapist begins to sense where the patient is headed, the therapist can initiate more focused exploration, as in the following exchange:

THERAPIST: Does it bring anything up for you to see me as a parent?

PATIENT: You're as cold and vicious as my mother.

THERAPIST: What's it like to have a cold and vicious therapist? (Subtle distinctions in tone are important in this kind of dialogue. For example, "Why would you think I'm cold and vicious?" might sound plaintive and defensive, directing attention to the therapist, whereas the language actually used keeps the focus where it belongs, on the patient's experience.)

An incident such as the above can interrupt the flow of therapy. Whether ignoring the boundary excursion or dealing with it as literal fact, the therapy risks becoming stuck in the same place. However, by exploring the patient's fantasies around the intrusive event with the sort of dialogue sampled above, the patient and therapist can let go of it and get on with the flow of therapy, now made all the richer for the interruption.

The two cases that follow exemplify the range of issues revealed through exploration of extratherapeutic encounters. What emerges is often unpredictable, but—in part for that very reason—almost invariably useful.

A patient on a hospital inpatient ward who was diagnosed with paranoid schizophrenia was being treated by a resident in psychiatry. One day the patient saw the resident wheeling another patient on a gurney back to the ward from electroshock therapy. The expression of concern on the resident's face was the first indication the patient had seen that the resident might not be part of "the great conspiracy." From that day, the patient's alliance with the therapist improved.

In this case, the patient's observation of the therapist in an unguarded moment in a hallway humanized the therapist in the patient's mind. In the following case, also from inpatient practice, exploration yielded more complex material.

A female patient who had been abused in childhood experienced heightened anxiety and anger when she saw her therapist in the hospital coffee shop. Although the therapist obviously was committing no impropriety by being there, his presence felt extremely threatening and intrusive to her. She feared that, freed from the constraints of his office, he would turn harshly judgmental in a way that his clinical role precluded. This patient could be comfortable with her therapist only so long as she could imagine him confined to one place and one role. It was as if he was supposed to remain in his clinical office 24 hours a day, never showing up in unexpected places and, in fact, having no existence outside the therapeutic frame. In this restorative fantasy, the patient used a rigid caricature of therapeutic boundaries, as applied to the therapist, to contain otherwise unmanageable fears. In the course of therapy she gained insight into this fantasy as a reflection of her early experiences.

Debriefing after Embarrassing Contacts

An inpatient unit at a psychiatric hospital had one men's room with only a half-height marble barrier between the toilet and the urinal. The chief resident was sitting on the toilet when one of his patients walked into the bathroom. "What are you doing here?" asked the patient. "Pretty much what it looks like," the therapist replied. This was a highly charged encounter. The fact that it occurred in the course of daily routine on a hospital ward made it easier to process without damaging the alliance. It would be different if, say, a therapist and a patient of the same gender found each other stark naked in the locker room of a health club. In the face of such a major unintentional breach of personal privacy, the principles of "contact management" outlined above still apply: Behave professionally. Do not violate confidentiality. Do not attempt to do therapy. Document the incident and obtain consultation. Debrief it at the next session.

Debriefing can help determine whether the nude encounter means the end of treatment. One patient may say, "I'm glad I saw you naked in the locker room. It means you're real; you have a body; you're a person. I can handle that." Another patient may react very differently: "I will never be able to walk into your office without seeing you as I did that day. It's getting in the way. It stirs up so many feelings (sexual and anxious ones, and the like) that I can no longer continue this therapy." In the latter case, unless the therapist has reason to believe that the alliance can be repaired, the patient will need to be transferred to another therapist. Patient-specific characteristics may figure in this determination, such as whether the patient is gay or has a specific fetish or sensitivity.

What if, instead of giving a clear answer one way or the other, the patient says, "I don't feel comfortable talking about this. It's too embarrassing for me"? A psychodynamic therapist would attempt to elicit a normal therapeutic dialogue: "What about it is embarrassing to you?" If the patient says, "I don't want to talk about it now," you can reply, "I'll respect that, but it's something that really happened, and it may get in our way. So, we should think about it, and let's talk about it in the near future." Given the unconscious pressure the patient must be feeling, a trained therapist will be alert for cues to reopen the issue, as in the following exchange:

PATIENT: Oh, I was at a party where someone was wearing the same dress I was, and I was embarrassed.

THERAPIST: So, embarrassment comes to mind as you're sitting here talking to me. I guess embarrassment is on your mind these days.

The technique is the same as when a patient feels uncomfortable talking about anything essential to therapy, whether or not it has to do with patient–therapist boundaries, as in the following dialogue:

PATIENT: Yes, I had an unhappy childhood, but I don't want to talk to you about it.

THERAPIST: Why wouldn't a person want to talk to a therapist about something like that?

PATIENT: I just don't want to talk about it!

THERAPIST: Well, I'll respect that, but we need to understand that it may be directly relevant to what we're talking about here, and we have to be careful that you're not saying to me, "Take out my gallbladder, but keep your left hand tied behind your back." (This is a good reminder to the patient of what the therapist's role is.)

The therapist needs to stay attuned to the issue and try to keep it open, documenting each attempt to do so. With the passage of time there should be opportunities to come back to the issue, which may need to be addressed one way or another, even if the kind of therapy being practiced does not call for extended exploration. The issue may emerge again in a way that is less threatening for the patient because time has passed and because the current precipitating event is remote from the interaction in question. It may be more bearable for the patient to confront a feeling of embarrassment about a subsequent encounter with somebody wearing the same dress at a party than about seeing the therapist naked at the health club.

Similar questions can arise when a patient sees the therapist in circumstances that may be revealing or compromising. What if a patient encounters his or her therapist, heretofore assumed to be straight, in a gay club? What if a patient who is homophobic sees the therapist come out of a gay club? Can the patient manage this revelation, or will it overwhelm the alliance? In another variation, the patient may observe the therapist in a perceived impropriety. For example, the patient sees the therapist with a woman and projects that he is having an affair. The therapist could be the subject of a false accusation by someone else; in that case the patient may think, "If you're being accused of sexual misconduct with a patient, can I safely see you?" These situations need to be debriefed as outlined above. If the patient says, "It's no problem," but the next half-dozen sessions are flat and unproductive, a decision will need to be made about referral and transfer of care.

Debriefing cannot always solve the problems created by an inadvertent encounter. Reamer (2001, pp. 191–193) presents two examples. In one, a psychiatrist arrives at a family Thanksgiving celebration, only to find that her brother's new girlfriend is her patient. At their next session, she and the patient decide to terminate and transfer care, since they had begun therapy only recently. In contrast to this mutually satisfactory resolution, a female social worker finds a male patient working out in her health club. She has been concerned that this patient may be feeling attracted to her. After discussing the matter in peer supervision, the social worker decides that the clinical risks necessitate her changing to another health club. The patient takes this as a rejection, despite the therapist's best efforts to address the issue, and eventually terminates counseling. In each case, the therapist acts prudently in the patient's interest, even if she cannot guarantee a fully satisfactory outcome.

Intermingling in Small Communities

The probability of out-of-office encounters with patients increases significantly in small and/or geographically isolated communities, to the point where such encounters can be a fact of daily life (Barnett & Yutrzenka, 1994; Brownlee, 1996; Campbell & Gordon, 2003; Faulkner & Faulkner, 1997; Gates & Speare, 1990; Gottlieb, 1993; Reamer, 2001, pp. 173–181; Schank & Skovholt, 1997; Schetky, 1994; Simon & Williams, 1999). The same is true in "communities of interest" (e.g., ethnic, religious, political, cultural, military, feminist, gay and lesbian, parental, professional) (Gartrell, 1992; Gonsiorek, 1995b; Lyn, 1995). The inevitability of such contacts is acknowledged, for example, in the Massachusetts Board of Registration in Medicine's boundary guidelines for physicians practicing psychotherapy. The board's guidelines nonetheless caution that forming a personal relationship with a psychotherapy patient is inappropriate in any setting (Hundert & Appelbaum, 1995).

At the same time, in a setting where one's role is analogous to that of a "country doctor," being too punctilious about maintaining boundaries can have the opposite of the intended effect. As Smith and Fitzpatrick (1995) note:

> Denying help to a potential client because of a preexisting relationship could mean that the person gets no help at all. Moreover, in rural settings where mental health professionals might be regarded with suspicion, heightening one's visibility by way of involvement in community activities may defuse the suspicion and make the clinician appear more approachable (Gates & Speare, 1990) [citation in original]. (p. 502)

Likewise, Schetky (1994) observes that in self-contained communities (such as a small town or island) where most people know one another, going out of one's way to avoid seeing or acknowledging a patient may actually signal to others that a therapeutic relationship exists. Moreover, a patient may feel shame and humiliation from appearing to be shunned. Based on the experience of practicing in a small coastal community as well as visiting patients living on islands, Schetky gives examples of boundary dilemmas resolved through reflection, common sense, and respect for patients. These include being waited on in a restaurant by a former patient, attending a musical in which a former adolescent patient had a leading role, using a boat yard that employed a patient's parent, accepting tea in a patient's home, and, generally, accommodating to the "island ethos where everyone looks out for everyone else" (p. 18). With one patient the therapist discussed the possibility that the patient would have to draw the therapist's blood at the local hospital. The patient "enjoyed this brief role reversal and being able to help me for a change." As Schetky concludes, "There are times when psychoanalytic interpretations need to be tempered with reality" (p. 18).

Although inadvertent contacts with patients usually are thought of as occurring in small towns or rural areas, the same pattern can occur in densely populated urban communities. We are indebted to an anonymous reviewer of this book for the following case example:

> A street-based drug counselor lived downtown in the area where he worked. Many of his clients were sex trade workers (prostitutes). He described an amusing dilemma he faced: "When I walked down the street with friends, I'd often have sex trade workers say hello to me by name. I had to explain to friends that I could not divulge whether I was the sex trade worker's client, she was my client, or we were just friends or acquaintances. My friends knew about the type of work I did, so it was not a big issue to them. When I talked about these encounters with clients, most had no qualms about saying hello to me on the street, even if it meant some of my friends might infer they were my clients or vice versa."

Some of the most complex and difficult boundary challenges arise when the patient's and therapist's children are the focus of interaction around school or neighborhood activities, or when the patient has independent relationships with members of the therapist's family or vice versa. Gottlieb (1993) has developed a decision-making model with which clinicians can estimate the level of risk associated with these and other boundary dilemmas. The model has three main dimensions: the therapist's power over the patient, the duration of treatment, and the clarity of termination (i.e., the likelihood of future professional contact). In Schank and Skovholt's (1997) extensive survey of rural psychologists, respondents reported three criteria by which they decide whether to treat prospective patients despite potential boundary issues: the clinicians' comfort level with the dual or multiple relationships, the patients' attitudes toward and ability to deal with the boundary questions, and the nature and severity of the patients' problems. Based on the survey data, Schank and Skovholt provide practical guidelines for helping professionals faced with boundary issues. Acknowledging the inevitability of overlapping relationships in small communities, the guidelines recommend clear expectations and limits (in areas such as informed consent, confidentiality, documentation, and being explicit about overlapping relationships), ongoing consultation and discussion of cases to counter the isolation of rural and small-community practice, self-knowledge and having a life outside of work, and maintaining a consistent interpersonal style and authentic presence with clients.

Gartrell (1992) describes boundary dilemmas that arise for a therapist who, being active and visible in the lesbian community, can expect to run into patients in the normal course of her community activities (cf. Reamer, 2001, pp. 115–119). With experience, a clinician can develop workable, if imperfect, ways of protecting her own privacy and that of her patients without becoming a recluse. Yet, such accommodations remain always a work in progress. Specifically, Gartrell (1992) ponders what to do when a patient discusses her planned attendance at an event that the therapist also plans to attend:

> I have tried both announcing and concealing my plans in different situations, and neither has felt very comfortable. I once had a client who became so anxious about seeing me that she decided not to attend herself. I, on the other hand, feel deceitful going to an event knowing a client will be there who does not know that I will be. I tend to err on the side of honesty about my plans, because it gives me an opportunity to remind the client that I will just say "hi." (p. 42)

Patient-Instigated Contacts: Stalking

If a therapist's joining a patient's book discussion group can precipitate an ethics complaint, what if a patient knowingly joins a therapist's book discussion group? Since patients do not have an ethics code to observe, there is no strict reciprocity of duties. Still, it is cause for concern when a patient keeps track of a therapist's whereabouts in order deliberately to cross his or her path, especially when the patient escalates to showing up unannounced at the therapist's office, home, or outside activities.

We can begin with cases of relatively innocuous boundary violations by patients:

> When a clinical psychologist was hospitalized with a mild heart attack, one of his patients, who was diagnosed with borderline personality disorder, became very upset and called the hospital. She identified herself as a member of the psychologist's immediate family in order to get through to his room.

Patients with borderline personality disorder are among those who have the greatest difficulties with boundaries. In this case, a patient who normally did not act out in such a way suffered a weakening of boundaries under the stress of her reaction to her therapist's illness.

> A patient saw an advertisement for a lecture her psychiatrist was to give on "the bereaved therapist." The title referred to therapists who have lost a patient through suicide. The patient, however, attended the lecture in the belief that her psychiatrist would speak about his personal losses. At the lecture the light shining in the psychiatrist's eyes prevented him from seeing the audience as he spoke. Nonetheless, during her next therapy session this patient told him she had fantasized that he was either looking straight at her or avoiding meeting her eyes.

Patients often attend public appearances by their therapists, whether out of curiosity, a desire to see how the therapist speaks and acts outside the treatment context, or in an effort to gain insight into their own case. All such contacts of which the therapist is aware should be processed clinically. In this case, the patient's hope of eliciting personal revelations from her therapist and her fantasy that the therapist was reacting to her presence personally indicate a need to explore boundary questions with the patient.

The boundary challenges in the cited cases are mild enough to be dealt with through therapeutic exploration. Therapists must, however, assess at what point such intrusions risk damaging the therapy, violating the therapist's personal and family privacy, and perhaps threatening the therapist's safety. In one such case presented as a teaching exercise for psychoanalysts, a female patient of a male analyst made repeated attempts to turn the analytic relationship into a social friendship. Having resisted analyzing this behavior, she terminated with unresolved issues when she moved to a nearby community. The ex-patient then invited the analyst's daughter to babysit for her, while her husband offered the analyst's son a well-paying summer job at his country club. Upset by these intrusions, the analyst was concerned both to protect his and his family's privacy and to safeguard his ex-patient's privacy as well as the confidentiality of the analytic relationship. He also felt that the patient, who had not had a proper termination, might interpret reasonable protective actions on his part as a wounding rejection (Dewald & Clark, 2001, pp. 39–40).

As in this case, patients who seek to insinuate themselves into a therapist's life often use children to compel ongoing contact between families. Putting children together through play or school activities is an all-too-effective indirect way to create interaction between parents who must be a responsible presence in their children's lives. This is a deliberate attempt to create a type of situation that does, in fact, often occur accidentally—thereby, in some cases, making the contact appear coincidental and unplanned.

A therapist must consider when such conduct rises to the level of stalking and when it needs to be dealt with by extratherapeutic means. In what may be the first empirical study of stalking among psychologists, Gentile, Asamen, Harmell, and Weathers (2002) surveyed members of the American Psychological Association who provided clinical services. Of the 294 respondents, 30 (10.2%) reported having been stalked by a client, as they understood the term (stalking was not defined in the study). Harassing clients were more likely to be women (68%) and without a current intimate relationship (80%). They were characterized by high rates of diagnosed mood (62%) and personality disorders (over 75%). In reaction to the perceived stalking, 41% of the psychologists reported feeling fear, 70% experiencing anxiety and anger, and 50% modifying the way they conducted their practice, including screening new patients for potentially dangerous behavior and no longer listing their home addresses publicly. In a subsequent survey of a random sample of Australian psychologists (Purcell, Powell, & Mullen, 2005), 19.5% of the 830 respondents reported having been stalked for 2 weeks or more. Psychologists attributed the stalking to resentment (42%) or infatuation (19%). Most of the respondents altered their professional practice in response to the harassment.

When the risk or actuality of stalking is an issue, Epstein's (1994, pp. 223–236) guidelines for dealing with exploitative patients are helpful. Recommended measures include discussing all boundary violations with the patient as soon as possible, reviewing the patient's associations and behavioral reactions to any boundary crossings required in unusual circumstances, taking precautions (including setting firm, immediate limits) with patients who have a history of assaultive or other predatory behavior, and not allowing a pattern of intrusions into the therapist's personal space. The steps outlined in Chapter 4 of this book for addressing a patient's persistent nonpayment of bills can serve as a model for confronting stalking and other intrusive, boundary-violating behavior as well. Eventually, as with nonpayment of bills, the patient's nonresponsiveness to such progressive limit setting necessitates termination of treatment.

As Hilliard (2001) makes clear, a clinician has the right to terminate treatment of a patient who persistently violates treatment boundaries. Outside intervention may be necessary when the patient's behavior cannot satisfactorily be addressed clinically and when the patient refuses or is unable to control problematic conduct. In institutional settings, assistance may be obtained from the institution's security personnel, human resources department, and/or legal counsel. Measures available to private practitioners include involuntary hospitalization, identifying and (if possible) blocking harassing phone calls with the assistance of the telephone company, retaining an attorney, and (depending on the jurisdiction) filing a complaint in court for harassment, threats, or stalking and, as needed, seeking a restraining order. In taking these actions, the clinician must remain mindful of patient confidentiality, communicating only as much information as is necessary to meet the emergency. However, a patient's right to confidentiality is not a legal shield for violating the rights of a clinician.

KEY REMINDERS

- Communications with patients should be carried out in a manner that is professional in tone and content, nonintrusive, appropriate for the type of therapy and the patient's background, and respectful to and understandable by the patient.

- Inadvertent meetings with patients out in the community are inevitable, especially in small or geographically isolated communities or in communities united by interest or affiliation.

- When encountering a patient outside the therapy setting, it is essential to respect the confidentiality of the patient–clinician relationship and to behave in a professionally and socially appropriate manner.

- Unplanned encounters with patients should be documented and processed clinically with the patient.

- Patient-instigated contacts outside the clinical setting should be addressed therapeutically and, if they rise to the level of stalking, by extratherapeutic interventions.

CHAPTER 7

Clothing and Physical Contact

In this chapter, we deal with boundary issues in the realms of clothing and nonsexual physical contact (such as hugs and handshakes). These are relatively straightforward, compared with complexities surrounding therapists' self-disclosures and patient encounters outside the office. Nonetheless, in each of these areas there are context-specific judgments and precautions to be considered.

CLOTHING

Clothing worn or not worn, or clothing put on or taken off, makes a statement. It is a medium through which patient and therapist communicate with each other, and that form of communication can involve boundary crossings or violations. For example, an article of clothing can represent the therapist's body, the therapist's power, or the therapist's love, as we saw in the case of gifts of clothing in Chapter 4.

The Therapist's Attire

As part of establishing the therapeutic frame, therapists should dress consistently according to their own standard of professional attire, a standard appropriate for the context in which they practice. Appropriate professional dress reinforces the message that therapy is work. Even (or especially) in a home office, a therapist should avoid arriving sweaty in a jogging outfit.

Professionalism is conveyed in some situations by a suit and tie, in others by dress shirts and slacks (other than jeans), depending on the standards of the peer culture. Some settings that emphasize informality, such as frontline drug counseling, may support more casual attire. Safety is also a consideration. For example, clinicians on inpatient units ordinarily do not wear ties, since these can be used to choke the wearer.

Formal attire can connote seriousness and professionalism, whereas informal attire may convey accessibility, a nonjudgmental position, and a relaxed attitude. Each of these choices has a downside as well. Formal attire can be seen as cold and distancing; informal attire can be seen as expressing lack of purpose or even seductiveness. If you dress in less than the male or female equivalent of a business suit or sport jacket and tie, be alert to the possibility that patients (especially older ones) will take this as a sign of disrespect. Be prepared to explore this reaction. You may hear, for example, an older European immigrant say, "He didn't even care enough to put on a tie." At the other extreme, some more recent immigrants may not trust anyone wearing a suit, which they associate with oppressive authority figures.

A therapist who dresses provocatively may be sending a message of sexual availability. The therapist may not realize the impact of his or her attire, and the patient may not feel comfortable raising the issue, thinking it out of bounds. If you find yourself becoming very conscious of your appearance in preparation for a session, if you feel you need to wear your most attractive outfit to look good to the patient, as though you were going out on a date, then you may be developing what psychoanalytic therapists call an erotic countertransference. This calls for discussion with a supervisor or consultant.

Caretaking and Role Reversal

Clothing is a common focus of patients' caretaking impulses and the role reversal that can result, as discussed in Chapter 3. Knowingly or not, a therapist may not meet a patient's personal standards. Some therapists deliberately dress unimpressively, either as a persona they adopt (like the absent-minded professor) or as part of a systematic challenge to the patient's magical expectations of the therapist's omniscience and omnipotence. The latter is a considered therapeutic gesture, which is not the same as leaving oneself vulnerable to a patient's reparative interventions.

Many therapists are relatively indifferent to dress. Beyond this, a therapist may unconsciously act so as to invite caretaking on the part of the patient. The therapist may be in a vulnerable position in life, or may simply be acting as he or she has learned to act with a parent or a spouse: "Mom, where's my socks? Where's my underwear?" "Honey, where are my cufflinks?" Not by intent but by personal style, the therapist may trigger the patient's interest. A patient of a certain age (e.g., adolescent) or background (e.g., fashion-conscious) may react in a rejecting way: "How can this schlump help me?" Other patients will offer caregiving, with an explicit or implicit message such as (in the case of a male therapist), "Oh, you poor man. You're wearing these rumpled clothes. That's not good enough for someone in your position. You deserve better. Let me help you." Or perhaps: "Your wife obviously isn't taking care of you; allow me." A female therapist might be told, "I would buy you better jewelry than that." The therapist's task is not to allow conscious or unconscious personal agendas (the patient's or the therapist's) to breach the therapeutic frame. The therapist can stay in role, maintain the frame, and invite exploration by saying, "I notice that you seem to be trying to take care of me."

Provocations by the Patient

In Chapter 1 we described the case of a young woman who took off her clothes above the waist during a session with a male therapist. A patient's disrobing is an extension of the ordinary provocation of overly revealing dress. How might therapists best react to such unforeseen situations? At one extreme, Berne (1972) pointed out that it is an error for a male clinician, facing a patient with her skirt pulled up high, to tell the patient about the sexual fantasies her presentation inspired him to have. This is not appropriate self-disclosure. Nor is it appropriate to put the patient on the defensive by impugning her motives. Rather, the therapist can simply say, "Please pull your skirt down." In one such case, a young woman arrived for an evening session with a male therapist wearing tiny jean shorts, a skimpy halter top, and flip-flops. She proceeded to sit on the couch in a provocative posture. Her therapist responded tactfully but directly by telling her that it was simply not appropriate for her to come to a therapy session dressed as if she were going to the beach. This response established a respectful, professional tone while making clear what therapy is and is not.

In addition to avoiding the extremes of demeaning the patient or being drawn into the patient's seductive behavior, one should resist the impulse to retreat into legalism. We saw this in the Chapter 1 case when the therapist ran into another office in a panicked search for the applicable professional regulations. Had he been practicing in Rhode Island, he might have found a definition of "sexual contact" between therapist and patient that included (in addition to intercourse, sustained kissing, and fondling) the following:

> Exhibition by the MHP [mental health professional] in view of the patient or former patient of the MHP's genital area, groin, inner thigh, buttocks, or breast; voyeurism by the MHP in the form of viewing the patient's or former patient's genital area, groin, inner thigh, buttocks, or breast. (Rhode Island Senate Bill 96-S-2968, 1996)

This law gives the patient a civil cause of action whenever either the patient or therapist crosses legs while wearing shorts or a skirt above the knees. Such ill-advised legislative micromanagement exemplifies what we and our colleagues in the Harvard Medical School Program in Psychiatry and the Law have called "critogenesis"—meaning (by analogy with "iatrogenesis") harm caused to patients by legal provisions and processes (Bursztajn, 1985; Gutheil, Bursztajn, Brodsky, & Strasburger, 2000). Under such statutory restraints, Gutheil and Gabbard (1998) explain:

> Therapists would be forced into maintaining rigid and unswerving eye contact in a way that would totally constrict their free-floating attention and free-floating responsiveness to subtle enactments within the patient–therapist field. For psychodynamic therapy to be effective, therapists must immerse themselves in the experience of the patient without feeling undue restrictions regarding where they may look or how they might feel or think. Patients who characteristically evoke erotic reactions in others because of the way they behave, look, dress, talk, or move will inevitably evoke similar reactions in the therapist. This countertransference identification may lead the therapist to think about the patient in sexual terms. Like any other transference–countertransference interaction, the meaning of this erotic tension must be explored and understood to help the patient in other relationships outside of therapy.
> Freedom of thought is necessary for the therapist's achievement of an optimal state of effectiveness. (p. 413)

In the following case, a therapist is able to stay on task while attending freely to the patient's nonverbal behavior.

> A woman in her 20s diagnosed with histrionic personality disorder regularly wore provocative clothing in sessions with her male psychiatrist, such as a two-part blouse that would alternately open up and fold together. When the psychiatrist presented this case to a supervision group, he was teased about having noticed the patient's

blouse. The psychiatrist understood, however, that the patient was playing out an intensely erotized relationship with her father. When he quoted the patient's reported remarks to her father, such as "Don't you like me better than your tennis buddies?" the group agreed that this naked appeal, coming from a grown woman, expressed an excessive attachment to a parent. The therapist's noticing the blouse was a prelude not to intrusive personal comments but to understanding the direct, usable clinical meaning of the patient's self-display. The therapist could then explore with the patient the sources of her behavior and how she might learn to satisfy her needs more effectively.

For the inexperienced therapist, there may be a conflict about noticing the blouse. What matters, however, is the therapist's unwavering professionalism and clinical focus in the interest of the patient. An experienced therapist can enjoy talking with an attractive person without having the therapy contract sidetracked by personal gratification.

Limit setting is likewise in order if the patient asks or actually begins to take her clothes off. This is one instance, however, in which the appropriate response is, in part, gender-specific. When a male patient takes off his clothes in a session with a female therapist, the patient's behavior is not just provocative (a clinical issue) and compromising (a clinical and risk management issue); it is also a threat of sexual assault (a safety issue). If a male patient starts taking off his clothes, the female therapist's likely first perception (one that is reality-based, whether or not warranted in a given situation) is the danger of rape. Therefore, the therapist needs to decide quickly whether to take self-protective action such as leaving the office or calling for help.

Otherwise, direct limit setting is the first response when a patient begins to disrobe. The therapist calmly says, "This behavior is inappropriate, and it isn't therapy. Please keep your clothes on [put your clothes back on]." For some patients the therapist's words and demeanor will be enough to restore structure and control.

What if the patient does not respond to verbal limit setting? The usual next step is to open the office door. If that fails to restrain the patient's behavior, you can call to someone outside the office (such as a secretary, nurse, or bystander), "This young woman saw fit during her session to take off her clothes. I wonder if I might ask you to step in and chaperone." If necessary, you can leave the office to look for a chaperone; however, leaving the patient alone in the office has risks of its own.

Precautionary Measures

Anticipation and fantasy rehearsal can be helpful in preparing for difficult, tense situations such as this. Be aware that such situations do occasionally arise, and develop protocols for responding in consultation with
colleagues or supervisors. Generally, one cannot expect to know in advance when a patient is susceptible to disruptive or dangerous behavior.
However, as with the precautions taken for high-risk patients in prisons
and inpatient settings, a patient's history or observed behavior may warrant preventive measures.

For example, in the case of a patient who has repeatedly begun to
disrobe in the office (or masturbated or made aggressive sexual advances toward a therapist), the therapist can engage in a risk–benefit
analysis with the patient as to the advisability of leaving the office door
open during their sessions. Such an analysis is based on ensuring three
preconditions for therapeutic work: first, the survival of both parties;
second, the safety of both parties; third, the comfort of both parties.
These threshold criteria can be weighed against the potential compromise of privacy and confidentiality as part of the informed-consent dialogue. The therapist can explain: "We've been under a lot of stress here,
which has been distracting for me, as it must be for you, too. As a result, I'll feel safer and more comfortable with the door open. Then I'll
be better able to give you my full attention. But we'll need to be alert to
pause in our discussion if people pass close by the door." Faced with
this alternative, some patients will choose to restrain their behavior.
Otherwise, the decision to keep the door open can be revisited once the
patient's behavior stabilizes.

Termination and Referral

Having taken action to restore order and decorum, the therapist faces the
question "Can this therapy succeed?" As discussed in Chapter 6, this
question may present itself even in less serious cases in which no deliberate boundary violation has occurred. A patient who has gone so far as to
disrobe in the office appears to be looking for something other than therapy. This behavior calls into question whether there is a basis for continuing to work together. It is generally advisable, therefore, to see the patient
with a consultant to debrief the incident and decide whether to continue
therapy. In some cases it is also advisable for the therapist to consult with
an attorney.

Under some circumstances therapy can recover from such an episode as long as the patient is able to move beyond the interaction. However, if the patient persists in the behavior (as with any other persistent boundary challenge) or continues to dwell on the incident rather than process it therapeutically, termination and referral may be necessary. In such cases, debriefing serves the additional purpose of making the termination as therapeutic as possible.

Termination on grounds of misbehavior does not relieve a therapist of the duty to avoid abandonment by making an appropriate referral (perhaps to a therapist of the patient's gender or to one with relevant expertise). What if the patient does not give you permission to talk to the subsequent therapist about the reasons for termination? Since this behavior does not constitute a sufficient emergency or threat of violence to justify breaking confidentiality, you can simply tell the subsequent therapist, "I'm referring this patient to you because of the patient's behavior. I don't have permission to tell you what that behavior was, but the patient knows this is the reason for termination." The new therapist can then follow up by telling the patient: "I understand this was a behavioral termination. You weren't finished with therapy. What was the behavior?" If the patient declines to talk about it, the therapist can say, "That's a potential problem. Whatever happened, we need to keep it from happening here." The patient makes a choice concerning disclosure, and the therapist decides whether to proceed with therapy.

PHYSICAL CONTACT

In a courageous firsthand account of her own psychotherapy during her residency in psychiatry, Korn (2003) described going to her scheduled session on September 11, 2001, after the destruction of the World Trade Center. Her therapist, "Dr. B," gave her "a brief hug" before she left the office. She found this gesture "odd," but "somewhat comforting and perhaps appropriate" on that tragically disorienting day (p. 70). As Gabbard (2003) explained in his commentary on Korn's personal narrative, therapists around the country acknowledged how "professional roles and boundaries were dropped to a large extent in the wake of the disaster" in response to the mutual shock and grief felt by patient and therapist (p. 71). In Korn's case, "If the departure from the therapeutic frame had stopped there [i.e., with the hug on 9/11], and if they had processed it between them, we might have regarded the incident as a boundary crossing rather than a boundary violation" (Gabbard, 2003, p. 71). Instead, Korn reported, the hug became a regular session-ending ritual on the part of

Dr. B, who from their first meeting had "always greeted me with a handshake, sometimes putting his other hand over mine" (p. 71). Korn observed that Dr. B was "experimenting" with boundaries in ways that she would not do with her own patients, but she accepted these departures on the basis of his greater experience.

During a session that followed the breakup of a romantic relationship, Korn sobbed in the therapist's office. Dr. B "walked across the room, knelt down on one knee and held my hand with both of his for a few minutes until I stopped crying" (p. 71). "While outside of therapy such a gesture may be regarded as supportive and comforting," Gabbard comments, "within psychotherapy this type of overture to the patient may be fraught with meaning and erotically charged" (pp. 71, 74). As the months went on, feeling that she was not progressing in therapy, Korn expressed her intention to decrease the frequency of her sessions. Countering that this would be an unwise move at a time when she was feeling so vulnerable and badly needed someone to trust, Dr. B offered free sessions. Soon after that, the ritual hug led to a brief kiss, which Dr. B rationalized unconvincingly by saying, "You are proud of your kiss" (p. 72). Here, in the guise of building her self-confidence, Dr. B was trying to tell his patient how she felt, whereas the purpose of therapy was for her to discover how she felt. Korn terminated therapy with Dr. B after a fellow resident validated her growing concerns by telling her about similar experiences with this therapist. When she confronted him about his inappropriate behavior, Dr. B replied that he "wish[ed]" they had "talked about it" (p. 73), as if processing boundary crossings (and, by implication, the boundary crossings themselves) were the patient's responsibility. It is, of course, a therapist's responsibility to see that any boundary crossings are appropriately discussed.

Korn's distressing experience exemplifies the so-called slippery slope by which unexamined boundary transgressions, such as Dr. B's two-handed handshake, can escalate to more blatant violations. By no means does this escalation always occur, let alone lead to sexual misconduct. Empirically, therapists who engage in nonsexual physical contact with patients have not been found to be more likely than other therapists to become sexually involved with patients (Pope, Sonne, & Holroyd, 1993). However, gender-specific nonsexual physical contact—that is, touching patients of the opposite sex more than patients of the same sex—is associated with a higher risk of sexual involvement with patients (Holroyd & Brodsky, 1980). Korn's "Dr. B," whose behavior provoked a complaint from a second female patient, fits the profile of male therapists who engage selectively in physical contact with women.

To Touch or Not to Touch?

The belief that all physical contact between therapist and patient (with narrow exceptions) is to be avoided comes primarily from the classical psychoanalytic tradition, from a heightened awareness of the risk of retraumatizing sexually abused patients, and from the practical realities of risk management (Appelbaum & Gutheil, 2007; Gutheil & Gabbard, 1993; Pope et al., 1993). A counterinfluence (now greatly diminished) has been the humanistic psychology movement that flourished in the 1960s and 1970s. As Gutheil (1999a) recalls, "In the 'old days' when everyone wanted to be Leo Buscaglia, PhD, hugs were seen as a form of benign, occasional physical contact punctuating the surrounding therapeutic expanse of talk" (p. 59). Still, a number of developments in recent years have militated against a total prohibition on physical contact with patients.

First, there are well-established nonpsychodynamic therapies that involve physical contact. In Rolfing or massage therapy, the client consents to specified forms of physical contact that are thereby included in the therapeutic contract. Likewise, a cognitive-behavioral therapist might, for example, "with both hands on the patient's shoulders, physically and emotionally support an agoraphobic patient on a crowded street or bus" (Hundert & Appelbaum, 1995, p. 350). As a rule, such supportive, nonintimate contact is limited to public settings. These types of therapy have their own contracts and ethics codes that define appropriate and inappropriate touching in context-sensitive ways.

Second, although few recall today that psychiatrists traditionally performed their own physical examinations, the "remedicalization" of psychiatry, involving a deemphasis on psychodynamic exploration, is bringing some psychiatrists back to their long-discarded role of attending to their patients' medical needs. Physical examinations of newly admitted inpatients by psychiatrists (when no internist is present) are not unknown, since a patient must be examined before medication is prescribed. Thus, the Massachusetts Board of Registration's guidelines for physicians practicing psychotherapy allow for physical contact "appropriate for the purposes of physical examination and medical treatment, consistent with the psychotherapeutic treatment being provided" (Hundert & Appelbaum, 1995, p. 350). A psychiatrist, would, for example, refer a psychotherapeutic patient to a suitable clinician for a pelvic examination. From the opposite direction, the emergence of family practice as a primary care specialty has brought family counseling explicitly within the scope of practice of physicians who, unlike psychiatrists, routinely "lay hands on" patients.

As in the days of the all-purpose "country doctor," the family is being counseled by the same doctor who physically examines every member of the family. Family physicians are bound by the same ethical principles as psychiatrists (including avoidance of sexual, flirtatious, or other exploitative behavior), but the boundaries they observe are different. The differences are accepted because they are congruent with patients' expectations in an informed-consent context. Patients come to the doctor for comprehensive medical care, which can include psychological counseling if the patient chooses.

Third, it is necessary to address the question of touching, like other boundary issues, in a culturally sensitive manner. Individuals raised in European and Latin American societies are more likely than those raised in the United States to expect to shake hands at the beginning and end of each visit (Epstein, 1994, p. 209). Since French Canadians regularly greet each other with a kiss on both cheeks, this greeting is considered acceptable between therapist and patient on appropriate occasions (Smith & Fitzpatrick, 1995). By contrast, some Muslim patients are offended by any physical contact. Cultural expectations also differ with respect to eye contact. Nonetheless, as Gabbard & Nadelson (1995) point out, some clinicians have used their own cultural backgrounds as an excuse to take liberties that patients of different backgrounds find offensive. Clearly, the clinician needs to be sensitive to the patient's culturally derived assumptions and expectations (Gartrell, 1992).

Cultural sensitivity with respect to boundary issues can be fostered by empirical research comparing the attitudes of clinicians in different cultures. In one of the first such cross-cultural studies in this area, the attitudes of clinicians in the United States and Brazil toward a wide range of boundary-related behaviors were compared (Miller et al., 2006). Overall, there was little difference between the two groups in their ratings of how professionally unacceptable and how potentially harmful to patients particular behaviors were. In the relatively few instances where cultural differences were found, the Brazilian therapists usually rated the behavior in question more professionally unacceptable and harmful to patients than did the American therapists. (This was especially true for certain types of self-disclosure.) The main exceptions were two greeting behaviors, shaking hands and kissing on the cheek, which the Brazilian therapists rated less professionally unacceptable and harmful than the Americans did. This greater acceptance by Brazilian therapists of the routine touching that takes place as part of greeting or comforting is consistent with broader cultural differences. Standard greetings in Brazil, even between people who do not know each other well (unlike in the United States), include shaking hands with an arm clasp, kissing on both cheeks, and hugging.

Fourth, touch has a specific supportive function in treating persons with AIDS, who sometimes are made to feel "untouchable," like "lepers." Gutheil (1999a) recommends "that clinicians who work with HIV-positive patients should contrive to touch such patients nonsexually at some point during each therapeutic encounter, e.g., by a handshake, pat on the shoulder or squeeze of the arm, specifically to counter the social ostracism such patients may feel" (p. 59). (Occasionally an immunocompromised patient may prefer not to be touched for fear of disease transmission.)

Finally, animal and infant research demonstrates that touch is a basic form of human communication and emotional support, starting with the earliest mother–infant contacts. A number of writers have questioned whether nonsexual physical contact should or can be kept out of psychotherapy (Hilton, 1997c; Horton, Clance, Sterk-Elitson, & Emshoff, 1995; Kertay & Reviere, 1993; Lichtenberg, Ruderman, Shane, & Shane, 2000; Maroda, 1994; McLaughlin, 1995; Pope, 1994). Simon (1992) outlines appropriate exceptions to the prohibition against physical contact in psychotherapy:

> Occasions may arise in treatment when a handshake or a hug is an appropriate human response. Clinically correct touching often occurs in the course of administering a procedure or treatment. Therapists who work with children, the elderly, and the physically ill frequently touch their patients in an appropriate, clinically supportive manner. An absolute prohibition against touching the patient would preclude such therapeutic human responses and supportive clinical interventions. (p. 279)

The importance of context in interpreting and implementing clinical guidelines is made clear by this poignant story told by Gerald Koocher, president of the American Psychological Association:

> On occasion, I tell my students and professional audiences that I once spent an entire psychotherapy session holding hands with a 26-year-old woman together in a quiet darkened room. That disclosure usually elicits more than a few gasps and grimaces. When I add that I could not bring myself to end the session after 50 minutes and stayed with the young woman holding hands for another half hour, and when I add the fact that I never billed for the extra time, eyes roll. Then I explain that the young woman had cystic fibrosis with severe pulmonary disease and panic-inducing air hunger. She had to struggle through three breaths on an oxygen line before she could speak a sentence. I had come into her room, sat down by her bedside, and asked how I might help her. She grabbed my

hand and said, "Don't let go." When the time came for another appointment, I called a nurse to take my place. By this point in my story, most listeners who had felt critical of or offended by the hand holding have moved from an assumption of sexualized impropriety to one of empathy and compassion. The real message of the anecdote, however, lies in the fact that I never learned this behavior in a classroom. No description of such an intervention exists in any treatment manual or tome on empirically based psychotherapy. (Koocher, 2006, p. xxii)

A patient's age, gender, culture, religion, social status, sexual orientation, physical health and mobility, emotional condition, and presenting problems—as well as how the patient and therapist may differ in some of these respects—are all contextual factors entering into this delicate area of clinical decision making.

Risks of Physical Contact with Patients

In a questionnaire survey of patients' experiences of touch in psychotherapy, a large percentage of those who responded felt that touch fostered greater trust and openness with their therapists. Few patients experienced the touching as negative (Horton et al., 1995). Such self-reports, however, typically express only the conscious level of a patient's reaction. As Twemlow (1997) cautions: "A touch liked by the patient does not mean in the long run that such contact is helpful to the therapy. In fact, unless its meaning is carefully explored such unconsidered physical contact is often unhelpful, if not harmful, to the overall process" (p. 359).

Exceptions notwithstanding, the question of physical contact with patients needs to be approached with considerable caution. The therapist's intentions may be strictly clinical and supportive, but the therapist cannot be sure how the patient will interpret the gesture, or how and when the patient may communicate that reaction. There is the risk that the patient will confuse the therapeutic interchange with other, often dysfunctional, intimate relationships in his or her experience. A male therapist's taking the liberty to touch a female patient may reinforce the patient's feeling of disempowerment (Alyn, 1988). Irrespective of gender, placing the patient "in the therapist's hands" can reinforce the therapist's power and the patient's vulnerability. Moreover, the therapist's touch may tap powerful emotional content, which the therapist must be prepared to help the patient integrate (Kepner, 1987; Smith, 1985).

Although customary practices differ in different treatment settings, patients and therapists are subject to these dynamics in any setting. On inpatient units any physical contact is generally discouraged, because many patients suffer from psychotic disorders and some have been sexually assaulted. At the other end of the scale, although the culture of some residential settings allows and supports more physical contact than others, especially in group meetings and activities, clinical staff members need to be alert to potential problems arising from this practice. The fact that hugging occurs routinely in a group home does not preclude a patient's feeling invaded by a hug.

Several case examples illustrate how readily patients can misinterpret physical contact on the part of a therapist. One woman alleged sexual misconduct on the basis of a therapeutic exercise intended to help her express her anger. The therapist had her get down on her knees and instructed her to push hard against his hands. By the patient's own testimony, both of them were fully clothed, and only their hands touched. Yet, the patient found this "the most overwhelming sexual experience of my life." In presenting this case, Caudill (1997c) comments, "Many people are so overwhelmed by the intensity and intimacy of the therapeutic relationship that they experience an otherwise inconsequential gesture or statement as a full-fledged romance or romantic intrusion" (p. 98). In this case, the therapist might have taken more care to consider such possible reactions with the patient as part of obtaining the patient's informed consent to the exercise.

The following case shows both the clinical and legal risks involved in nonsexual boundary violations that patients (and juries) may interpret as sexual:

> A therapist claimed that her school of practice involved hugging her female patient at the beginning and end of every session, without apparent harm. She eventually had to terminate therapy with the patient for noncompliance with the therapeutic plan. The enraged patient filed a sexual misconduct claim against the therapist. Despite the evidence showing that this claim was probably false (a specious suit triggered by rage at the therapist), the insurer settled because of the likelihood that a jury would not accept the principle of "hug at the start and hug at the end but no hugs in between." (Gutheil & Gabbard, 1993, p. 195)

Despite the apparent absence of sexual misconduct, the legal resolution of this case was damaging to the therapist; nor did the clinical outcome benefit the patient. Instead of supporting the patient in mourning the deprivations of her childhood and thereby working through her resentment and grief, this therapist gave the patient the direct gratification of hugs. In this way, the therapist made herself a physical substitute for the patient's absent or withholding parent(s). When the critical distinction between the symbolic and the concrete is obscured, the patient may come to expect continued gratification of infantile longings, and (as in this case) may react vindictively when that gratification is withdrawn. Short of such a disastrous outcome, the patient's anxiety-fueled energy to confront conflicts may dissipate, causing the therapy to stagnate (Casement, 1990; Gutheil & Gabbard, 1993).

The question of touch in therapy is especially highly charged in the case of survivors of abuse. In their experience, touch may have been a way of expressing dominance as well as affection, a way of inflicting harm as well as of soothing and comforting. Any kind of touch may have sexual connotations for a patient who has been sexually abused. Likewise, a victim of physical assault may react to any hand gesture as a threat. Physical contact is also foreseeably problematic in the treatment of patients diagnosed with personality disorders, who often request special treatment or consideration, as in this kind of exchange:

PATIENT: Your words don't help me. I need something different.

THERAPIST: Words are what we use in therapy.

PATIENT: You're not listening. I'm not like every other patient. I need something different from what you give most patients.

Such appeals have, of course, clinical meanings that need to be understood. Additional complexities arise in the case of patients with dissociative identity disorder. A gesture that one state of mind experiences as entirely benign may appear sinister when the patient is in another state of mind. As Epstein (1994) explains, citing Freud (1913/1958b): "A psychotherapist's work involves a special type of intrusion into the patient's *psychological* space. A treatment situation that combines a crossing of *both mental and physical boundaries* is probably too confusing for many psychologically disturbed individuals and should be segregated into distinct functions" (p. 212; italics in original).

The following vignette shows how easily a patient with borderline personality disorder, abetted by an experienced clinician's poor judgment, can lose the distinction between physical contact with therapeutic intent and acting out sexually:

A patient with very primitive borderline personality disorder was being treated on an inpatient unit. Unit staff had evolved a plan involving giving the patient hugs—a regressive response—as a reward, paradoxically, for mature and realistic behavior, despite the fact that this patient had a known history of major psychotic regressions, confusions of fact and

fantasy and of intimacy and sexuality, sexual abuse by her family in childhood, and, on one occasion, confessing that she had fabricated sexual
accusations for attention. Despite this background, her experienced therapist acknowledged giving her, on various occasions, a large number and
variety of hugs, including social hugs, reassurance hugs, goodbye hugs,
and congratulatory hugs. On one previous occasion in reaction to a
threatened termination of therapy this patient had explicitly accused this
therapist of sexual advances. When confronted she retracted the accusation as false and attributed it to a wish to punish yet keep the therapist.

   On the particular occasion in question, the patient had threatened
to commit suicide in the context of a planned termination of therapy
and was being seen for a second, extra appointment on the same day as
her regular one. During this session the patient showed impulsivity,
loose associations, and serious regression. At the end of the session, the
patient requested a goodbye hug and the therapist acquiesced and attempted a social hug. The patient suddenly began to breathe heavily
and thrust her pelvis, then drew a vibrator from her purse, which led
the therapist to disengage and set a limit. The patient regressed, sobbing and threatening suicide, but refused hospitalization. She then attempted to persuade the therapist to take her home himself rather than
have her face the "unsavory characters" found at the bus station. He de-
layed several times, but then he drove her home from this tumultuous,
out-of-control session. (Gutheil, 1989, pp. 600–601)

Predictably, the patient accused the therapist of having sexual relations with her both in the office and in his car when he drove her home.
Also predictably, she once again retracted the accusations. Her escalation
in response to the therapist's hugs followed from her history of confusion
about boundaries, specifically about what was and was not sex. Her therapist and the unit staff gave her more confusion when she badly needed
clarity. Aside from the overt boundary violations and loss of control, this
patient regularly maneuvered the therapeutic discussions into areas
likely to earn her hugs. This made her therapy as an exchange of talk,
aimed at understanding, essentially useless.

   There are particular considerations and precautions associated with
each of the more common forms of physical contact between patient and
therapist.

Handshakes

A handshake is the one form of physical contact that a therapist generally
can engage in safely with a patient who initiates the gesture. Socially
sanctioned as a nonerotic greeting traditionally associated with men doing business, it "is the least sexualized form of planned, purely volitional

touching that occurs between therapist and patient" (Davidson, 1991, p. 5). Even so, in exploratory individual therapy, Epstein (1994, p. 209) recommends that the therapist not initiate a handshake with a patient after the first session. Usually it is not problematic to accept a patient's handshake, although some patients who are in intensive psychodynamic therapy and/or have poor spatial boundaries may need to be advised that therapy will be more productive without even this form of nonverbal interaction (Szekacs, 1985).

Like a hug, however, a handshake can be used by a patient to pull a therapist into an erotic embrace, as in this incident described by a female psychiatrist.

> A male patient who had seen me some years ago for a relatively brief period (about eight sessions) called for another appointment—basically to discuss a marital problem he had been unable to resolve. As I entered the waiting room, he stood up and came toward me with outstretched hand, verbalizing greetings as he crossed the room. As I shook hands with him, he used the handshake to pull me to him, reeling me in as it were. He clasped me to his chest and put his other arm around my shoulder all in one motion. What had begun as a handshake had developed into an embrace. So there we were, in the middle of my waiting room with the patient's arm around me, holding me quite close. I felt I had given no encouragement for this contact. Yet, obviously this would not have happened had I not been willing to shake hands in the first place. (Davidson, 1991, p. 5)

A more subtle form of undermining occurs when the patient experiences the handshake as part of a relaxation of constraint—and of internal conflict—on the way into or out of the therapist's office. This form of resistance is illustrated by the following example.

> On leaving analytic sessions, a patient always took the analyst's hand for a handshake. This behavior was left unanalyzed until it emerged that this was the patient's way of symbolically undoing any conflict or friction that had arisen during the session. The handshake would make everything magically "all right" so that no affect would carry over to the next session. When this was analyzed, the handshaking was stopped by mutual agreement and the underlying material emerged thereafter. (Gutheil & Simon, 1995, p. 339)

Hugs

Although friends and associates (especially women) commonly exchange nonerotic hugs both in private and in public, it is evident that hugs, unlike handshakes, tend to contain erotic messages. Therefore, there are virtually no circumstances in which it is appropriate for a therapist to initiate a hug with a patient. It is also inadvisable for a therapist to accept a hug from a patient, with two main exceptions. One occurs at moments of profound grief when an immediate, uncomplicated human response is called for and the therapist's failure to return an embrace is likely to harm or even rupture the alliance (Gabbard, 1999a, 2005; Gartrell, 1992). The meaning of such boundary crossings can be explored later. Generally, there is also no need to rebuff a patient's hug at the conclusion of an extended course of therapy, when there is no opportunity for subsequent exploration and it may be too awkward to turn away from the patient at that moment (Davidson, 1991; Gutheil & Gabbard, 1993). However, if the patient returns for additional consultation, it is then advisable to explore the meaning of the hug.

Cases earlier in this chapter demonstrate the risks of arousing the patient's sexual or romantic fantasies with hugs. In a case reported by Gabbard and Nadelson (1995), a patient inexplicably accused a physician of having had "genital contact" with her. Investigation revealed that "during a hug the patient had experienced the pressure of the physician's genitals on her pelvis as 'genital contact,' reawakening old trauma" (p. 1448). As is often the case, a patient's construction of present reality was conditioned by past experience.

Another kind of risk is illustrated by the following case (using pseudonyms). Mrs. Arnold, a middle-aged woman suffering from chronic depression and dissatisfaction associated with marital problems and past traumas, requests a hug from her therapist, Dr. Stevens, at the end of a stressful session. Dr. Stevens's brief hug of reassurance becomes a regular ritual at the end of each session. Occasionally, at her request, the patient sits next to the therapist and puts her arm around him as she talks about her deep longing for the maternal nurturance of which she was deprived. Dr. Stevens sees himself engaged in a therapeutic effort to make restorative contact, at a deeply affective level, with a patient whose attachment to her mother was severely ruptured. He is not sexually stimulated by this contact and is unaware that Mrs. Arnold has come to feel both stimulated and frustrated by it. She becomes increasingly dependent on these moments of physical closeness with the analyst, which foreseeably become the main focus of the sessions for her. As her condition deteriorates into potential suicidality (which Dr. Stevens sees as further justifying his physical nurturance), she seeks the advice of another psychiatrist. This consultant explains to her that Dr. Stevens has lost control of her treatment and that she needs to find another therapist (Dewald & Clark, 2001, pp. 82–85).

Awareness of dynamics such as these has persuaded many therapists to adopt Gartrell's (1992) policy of "no hugs" except in extraordinary circumstances—for example (in the case of a female therapist) when a patient had been raped the night before a session. This policy should be carried out with sensitivity to cultural differences and (where appropriate) exploration of the feelings associated with the desire to be hugged or held. As Gartrell notes, many patients appreciate clear limit setting at the outset, and the explanations and explorations can contribute to forming a strong therapeutic alliance.

Kissing

Kissing a patient has such clearly erotic connotations that clinicians surveyed predominantly disapprove of it and associate it with sexual misconduct (Herman et al., 1987; Stake & Oliver, 1991). In a major survey in which 94% of therapists considered handshakes unquestionably or often ethical and 44% had the same opinion of hugging (although only 12% hugged patients often), 85% deemed kissing a patient unethical in all, or all but rare, circumstances. Nearly all respondents never (71%) or rarely (24%) kissed a patient (Pope et al., 1987). There is, then, a consensus that kissing between therapist and patient, as in the introductory case of "Dr. B" above, typically is part of a pattern of sexual misconduct rather than a defensible therapeutic technique. This consensus, however, is not equally strong in all cultures, as shown by the study of Brazilian and American therapists discussed above (Miller et al., 2006).

Responding to Patients' Requests for Physical Contact

A therapist's response to patients' requested or enacted physical contact needs to be carefully considered, not impulsive or defensive. Some patients start out feeling that they can't make it without the reassurance of a hug at the end of each session. This form of support may feel soothing and therapeutic to both the patient and therapist. Then, one day it may suddenly feel like an intrusion, an impending assault, or an unhealthy enmeshment. These potential reactions need to be anticipated.

When a patient says, "I would like a hug at the end of a session," as with "I would like to meet for longer sessions" or "I would like to meet twice a week instead of once," the therapist needs to take into account the feelings and motives behind these demands rather than fall into either of two extreme reactions. A therapist who finds these demands intrusive and reacts defensively may appear arbitrary, rigid, distancing, and rejecting. At the other extreme, a patient in deep pain and emotional crisis can lead some therapists to express their human sympathy at the expense of their professional judgment (and, ultimately, the patient's well-being). In exploratory therapy, a therapist avoids these extremes by replying "Let's talk about that." This models a mature way of satisfying one's needs without acting impulsively.

Many patients with a history of victimization and trauma have never experienced clearly defined boundaries. Their tendency to push a therapist's limits reflects their inability to set and protect their own limits. A therapist who calmly but firmly sets clear boundaries is modeling how to say "No" with respect and consideration for another person. In appropriate cases it can be helpful to remind the patient that his or her demands are part of a pattern being explored in therapy, and that part of the therapist's responsibility to the patient is not to allow any chance of repeating the dysfunctional pattern.

In almost all cases it is best to empathize with the patient's wish to be treated as "special" and to explain that acting on that wish is not likely to help the patient. The therapist can initiate a mourning process with words like the following:

> "I know it makes you sad that I can't hug you and hold you, and I know it makes you angry. I hope we can talk about those feelings, because what we're doing here is recognizing the limits of therapy. I can't ever provide you with the perfect parenting that you missed, and there's something poignant and sad about that. You can't go back and make everything right in the past. What we can do is talk about how that makes you feel and help you grieve the losses of childhood."

Casement (1985) described a case in which he successfully conveyed this distinction between the concrete and the symbolic to an initially resistant patient. The patient wanted him to hold her hand to make up for her mother's having been unable to do so during childhood surgery. After considering her request, Casement explained to the patient that she needed to experience the trauma as it had occurred in order to work through it. At first enraged, the patient became receptive when Casement told her that he felt he could help her only by tolerating the despair that she felt and was making him feel. Reflecting on this statement, the patient said that for the first time she felt she could trust him and that she was amazed that he could bear such painful feelings as she was experiencing.

Even without this level of interpretation, patients value and appreciate clear limit setting. One patient who had been sexually involved with a

previous therapist told her subsequent therapist that she could not tolerate any physical contact, even a handshake. During her third year of therapy she began to beg to be held and comforted by her therapist. The therapist responded to the patient's sobbing and pleading by empathizing
with her pain but reminding her of the way they had contracted to work
together. After the patient had worked through her feelings about wanting to be held and comforted, she confided that even when she had most
longed for physical contact with her therapist, she was terrified that the
therapist would break their initial agreement by acquiescing to her demands (Pope, 1994, pp. 75–76).

When the patient, instead of requesting to be hugged or held, makes
a direct physical advance, the therapist can discourage the patient by
words and/or physical positioning. If the patient repeatedly attempts to
throw his or her arms around the therapist, an appropriate response is

> to step back, catch both wrists in your hands, cross the patient's wrists in
> front of you, so that the crossed arms form a barrier between bodies, and
> say firmly, "Therapy is a talking relationship; please sit down so we can
> discuss your not doing this any more." (Gutheil & Gabbard, 1993, p. 195)

The patient may feel hurt, but that reaction needs to be risked and explored. If the physical contact threatens to escalate to the equivalent of a
wrestling match and perhaps to violence, the therapist can open the door
and, if necessary, leave the office. If the patient persists in trying to force
physical contact, termination and referral may need to be considered.

The following dramatic example shows how a therapist can simultaneously repel a determined physical advance and further therapeutic understanding. The patient was a married woman enacting her tendency to
sexualize relationships:

> At the end of a session in which she had been unusually stiff and silent,
> she suddenly got up from the couch and threw her arms around [the male
> therapist] tightly. She pushed her hips against his but her eyes were fran-
> tic and angry. When he looked at her with concern, she turned her face,
> pressed her head into his neck and began to make aggressive, rigid pelvic
> thrusts against him. His response was to place his hands gently on her
> taut and twisted neck, asking, "What is this bad and painful feeling up
> here when you also are asking for closeness?" She loosened her grasp on
> him and collapsed to the floor, heaving with sobs, her face contorted. . . .
> She guessed that she had always used sex for "a little bit of body close-
> ness." (Shor & Sanville, 1974, p. 91)

Suddenly confronted with an angry, aggressive sexual advance, this therapist remained calm and stayed engaged verbally, keeping the focus on

exploring the patient's feelings even at a very tense moment. By so doing, he brought the patient back into the therapeutic dialogue, with productive results. As therapy proceeded, this physical aggression was not repeated.

Still, accepting physical contact initiated by the patient proves on occasion to have been a helpful response, even in psychodynamic therapy, as in a case reported by McLaughlin (1995). An impulsive patient grabbed and held her male therapist's hand as she sobbed for several minutes. The clinician found this incident to have been a crucial breakthrough, in that it showed the patient that the therapist did not regard her as untouchable. Buoyed by a sense of increased trust and security, she was able to communicate more openly with him than she had previously. The therapist also accepted occasional hugs from this patient without apparent damage to her therapy.

Reparative Measures

When inappropriate physical contact occurs, whether because of the therapist's error of judgment or other circumstances, it is usually possible to repair the situation and perhaps advance the therapy by going over what happened with the patient and exploring how the patient has experienced it. Even accidental (or seemingly accidental) contact can be a stimulus to understanding. In one reported case, a male patient's hand brushed against a female psychiatrist's clothed elbow in the hallway on their way to the consulting room. Although his touch lasted no more than a second, the psychiatrist's surprisingly intense erotic reaction alerted her to explore the patient's preoccupation with his attractiveness to women (Davidson, 1991).

Likewise, when physical contact occurs in an emergency—for example, when a therapist must perform mouth-to-mouth resuscitation on a patient who has collapsed or had a cardiac arrest in the office—the patient may be uncomfortable with the quasi-intimate contact even though the boundary crossing involved no unethical conduct. At another level, if the patient has had a fantasy of the therapist as a "life saver," the concrete realization of this fantasy can also raise uncomfortable, albeit illuminating, issues. Exploration (with consultation as needed) can determine whether the incident has been sufficiently disturbing to the patient to warrant termination and referral. At the same time, the possibility of the inadvertent contact's leading to a therapeutic breakthrough should not be reflexively ruled out.

A change in setting or circumstances may precipitate an escalation of a patient's needs, leading the patient to cross physical boundaries. In one such case, a female therapist visited a female psychotherapy patient in the hospital where the patient was awaiting major surgery. The patient jumped out of bed and threw her arms around the therapist, drawing her into an extended embrace. When the patient returned to psychotherapy, she insisted that the therapist had initiated the embrace. The therapist and patient explored the significance of this encounter in the months that followed, including their different perceptions of what had happened. It emerged that, under the stress of impending surgery that further threatened her already weak sense of bodily integrity and self-esteem, the patient had taken advantage of the "intimate" hospital setting to embrace the therapist. By persuading herself that the therapist had embraced her, she could believe that she was not as unattractive as she feared. Discussing these underlying meanings brought into focus an important emotional conflict for this patient (Davidson, 1991).

Whatever the origin of a boundary crossing, it is the therapist's responsibility to discuss it with the patient, assess its impact on the therapy and, if possible, use it as an impetus for therapeutic progress. This is all the more true when the therapist realizes that, in initiating or accepting the physical contact, he or she either made a clinical error or unconsciously acted on his or her own needs. The following case example, adapted from Gabbard (1999a), shows how a therapist can undertake reparative explanation and exploration:

> A divorced female therapist in her 40s was treating a male patient of about the same age who told her that he loved her. Near the end of one therapy session he leaned forward and grasped her hand in an expression of gratitude. The therapist clasped the patient's hand with her other hand as well, a gesture by which the patient appeared deeply moved. Reviewing this session, the therapist realized that she was losing her therapeutic stance with this patient. She then consulted a colleague. She explained that, having no one to go home to at night, she welcomed the patient's protestations of love. She realized, however, that it was not helpful to encourage the patient, even passively, to act out his feelings.
>
> On the consultant's advice, the therapist began the patient's next session by opening up discussion of what had happened the preceding time. Although the patient had initiated the handclasp, he expressed concern that the therapist might have been losing control when she returned the gesture. Encouraged to explore this concern further, he went on to say that the incident reminded him of his mother's emotional dependence on him. The therapist indicated that, from that point on, it would be best to avoid physical contact such as handholding in favor of discussing the feelings that moti-

vated such enactments. Ongoing discussion brought out other ways in which the patient's relationship with his mother was reflected in the dynamics of the therapeutic interchange.

This vignette can serve as a model for correcting therapeutic error and responding effectively to boundary crossings. The therapist monitored her own actions and explored their motivations. She sought consultation and then discussed the boundary crossing promptly with the patient. Appropriate limits were reestablished so that the incident would not be repeated. The therapist did not burden the patient with her self-exploration, but focused instead on the patient's feelings and experiences. In this way, an act that could have compromised therapy became instead a springboard for productive investigation.

Some Further Guidelines

Reviews of literature on physical contact with patients acknowledge that there is little quantitative empirical research on the effects of non-sexual touch in therapy (Goodman & Teicher, 1988; Holub & Lee, 1990; Kertay & Reviere, 1993; Kupfermann & Smaldino, 1987; Willison & Masson, 1986). Nonetheless, these and other commentators do offer guidelines for distinguishing cases of unexplored wishes that require limit setting from instances of massive regression or acute grief for which words alone fail and touch is clinically indicated. The guidelines generally offered are consistent with those developed in this chapter, although some are more permissive. There is a consensus that, given the pervasive risk of rationalization, consultation and caution in the use of touch are advised. The following precautions are also especially useful to keep in mind:

1. "Theoretical considerations must never override concern for the individual patient, the therapeutic relationship, and ethical issues" (Kertay & Reviere, 1993, p. 39).
2. In this as in other areas, informed consent is critical. The contract with the patient spells out what is permitted and what is not. The contract can be used later to set limits if necessary (Pope, 1994, pp. 75–77).
3. The therapist needs to maintain awareness of his or her feelings toward the patient, questioning any possible use of therapeutic touch to satisfy the therapist's own needs for sexual excitement, control, a place of importance in the patient's life (e.g., ideal parent, savior), personal closeness, intimacy, emotional comfort, or

protection from the patient's disturbing feelings and expressions (consensus).

4. Touch that makes the patient uncomfortable is not therapeutic, and touch that creates discomfort in the therapist is also to be avoided (Willison & Masson, 1986, p. 499).

5. "Because touch may have multiple meanings in treatment, therapists must listen carefully to their patients' associations about the wish to touch rather than assuming they understand the meaning based on their interpretation of the wishes" (Davidson, 1991, p. 6).

6. "The guideline that I use in determining when to provide physical comfort is whether it seems inhuman not to. And I have met with good results" (Maroda, 1994, p. 153).

KEY REMINDERS

- The clothing worn by both the therapist and patient makes statements and conveys meanings that can affect the clinical interchange.

- Therapists should dress consistently according to their own standard of professional attire, a standard appropriate for the context in which they practice.

- Clothing-related boundary challenges and provocations on the part of a patient, such as inappropriate dress or disrobing during sessions, need to be addressed clinically with limit setting and exploration.

- Although a total prohibition on physical contact with patients is unrealistic, the question of touch in therapy must be approached with caution and clinical understanding.

- Decisions concerning touch in therapy, including how to respond to patients' requests for physical contact, require consideration of numerous contextual factors.

- In many instances of inappropriate physical contact (such as those resulting from errors in clinical judgment), reparative measures can restore the alliance and advance the therapy.

- Persistent or serious boundary ruptures involving either clothing or physical contact may necessitate termination and referral.

CHAPTER 8

Sexual Misconduct

Sexual misconduct by psychotherapists is fundamentally different from the kinds of boundary crossings and violations considered up to this point. Here there are no questions of degree. There is no need to determine whether a boundary violation in one context may be a benign crossing or useful therapeutic technique in another. Context is important for understanding the transgression of sexual boundaries in psychotherapy, but this behavior is unethical in any context. (For the historical development of this ethical position, see Eth, 1990; Freud, 1915/1958c; Greenson, 1967; Saul, 1962.) By now there is a unanimity of reputable opinion that having sexual relations with a patient is incompatible with any form of professional mental health treatment. This consensus includes those who believe that the current preoccupation with boundary violations has gone too far (see the "backlash" discussed in Chapter 11). Therefore, the term "sexual misconduct" is used generically to refer to any and all instances of such behavior. In the following chapter we will outline various ways in which patients can be harmed by therapists' sexual misconduct (see Simon, 1994).

In a cogent summary, Smolar and Akhtar (2002) explain why therapist–patient sex always lies outside the boundaries of appropriate therapy. They state that "elements of the therapist's role must remain constant amidst the patient's fluctuating needs, wishes, and vulnerabilities in order for the relationship to remain therapeutic." Smolar and Akhtar then list three characteristics of sexual interaction that fatally compromise a therapeutic relationship. First, sexual intimacy necessarily involves a weakening or suspension of reality testing as well as indulgence in fantasy and regressive thinking. In such a state of mind, the therapist cannot remain grounded in the therapeutic role. Second, since sexual intimacy gratifies both parties' emotional needs, it does not permit the therapist to fulfill the ethical duty to attend only to the patient's psychic needs. Third, sexual intimacy breaks down the essential asymmetry of the therapeutic relationship by creating a situation of equality inimical to maintaining the therapist's authority.

Notwithstanding the clear ethical imperative to abstain from sex with patients, overheated rhetoric denouncing therapist sexual misconduct can be counterproductive. Historically, sexual issues have been most difficult to discuss with cool rationality even in the mental health professions. In an atmosphere of anxiety and fear, highly implausible and even bizarre accusations can be accepted as fact. Decision makers, including regulatory boards that act defensively for fear of unfavorable publicity, cannot be counted on to make reasoned determinations based on the evidence. The following case exemplifies the sensationalism associated with some claims of therapist sexual misconduct, as well as the difficulty in disentangling fact from fiction.

Twin brothers Dennis and Charles Momah, both physicians in Washington State, were the subject of allegations of sexual misconduct by female patients. These allegations resulted in Charles Momah's being sentenced to 20 years in prison for sexual crimes (he has appealed his conviction). One patient, Perla Saldivar, sued Dennis Momah in 2004 for sexually assaulting her during an examination. Subsequently she added Charles Momah to the lawsuit, claiming that Dennis Momah allowed his brother to impersonate him so that he, too, could assault her. In 2006 Pierce County Judge Katherine Stoltz dismissed Saldivar's case. In a counterclaim filed by Dennis Momah, who attributed a stroke he suffered in 2004 (ending his medical practice) to Saldivar's "false accusations," Judge Stoltz ruled that Saldivar's allegations had been contradictory, "contrary to common sense," and inconsistent with medical evidence. Finding Saldivar's allegations against both brothers to have been "knowingly and intentionally fabricated," Judge Stoltz ordered Saldivar to pay $2.8 million plus attorneys' fees to Dennis Momah for the resulting damage to his reputation. She also ruled that Saldivar's lawyer, Harish Bharti, was an "active and knowing participant in the fabrication of Perla Saldivar's ever-changing accusations against Dennis Momah." The judge ordered Bharti, who represented most of the former patients who sued the Momahs, to pay Dennis Momah $250,000 and the court $50,000 in sanctions, as well as to post the judge's ruling on his website for at least a year. Saldivar and Bharti announced that they would appeal the judge's rulings, while Momah appealed the dismissal of a defamation suit he had filed against Bharti in 2004. (summarized from Ostrom, 2006)

The challenge for the practicing clinician is not deciding when to do what, but how to avoid being caught unawares by patients' wishes or threats or by one's own vulnerabilities. It is unlikely that anyone reading this book is a predator. Yet, some readers may identify with therapists who found that they had committed serious boundary violations, in some cases sexual, after believing that "this couldn't happen to me" (Norris et al., 2003).

Clinicians prepare for such challenges by maintaining a practical (and, ideally, theoretical) awareness of boundary issues and by being alert for signs of personal vulnerability or lapses in therapeutic professionalism. Epstein and Simon's (1990) "Exploitation Index," a list of "early warning indicators" of boundary violations (outlined in Chapter 13), is a useful tool for monitoring one's relationships with patients. Pope et al. (2006) explore various clues that sexual or other personal feelings about a patient may be affecting the therapy—clues such as "Interesting Slips and Meaningful Mistakes" (pp. 72–74) and "Fantasies, Dreams, Daydreams, and Other Imaginings" (pp. 74–76). By attending to the questions and guidelines outlined for other areas of boundary concern in this and the previous chapters, one keeps up a level of clinical and ethical vigilance that makes the mere suspicion, let alone the reality, of sexual misconduct all the more remote.

Still, even the most ethical, prudent clinician can be severely tested by manipulative, sometimes threatening, behavior on the part of patients who have not learned more constructive ways to resolve conflicts and satisfy their needs. The last part of this chapter will provide guidelines for recognizing and responding to such behavior, which can escalate to false accusations of sexual misconduct.

COMMON DYNAMICS OF THERAPIST–PATIENT SEX

The vignettes in this section illustrate some commonly observed dynamics in cases of therapist–patient sex. This is not a systematic taxonomy of characteristics of therapists or patients that predispose to sexual exploitation; such causal factors, or "vulnerabilities," are discussed in Chapter 10. Rather, the cases that follow show some typical variations on a disturbing theme, common patterns of interaction to watch for in patients, colleagues, trainees, or supervisees.

Exploitation

A sexual relationship between a therapist and patient is exploitative in the sense that the therapist (consciously or not) places his or her interests, wishes, or desires ahead of the patient's therapy and well-being. Such relationships are always exploitative. However, this dimension of therapist sexual misconduct is more apparent in some cases than others—cases such as the following:

> A woman who had obtained the street drug "Ecstasy" wanted to experience it under controlled circumstances. She arranged with her male psychotherapist to take the drug in his presence. While she was in this drugged state, the therapist prevailed upon her to have sex with him. Civil and criminal actions against the therapist followed.

This case is an example of outright coercion. Hypnosis is also used for this purpose, as in the case of a lay hypnotist who was found to have abused nine women (Hoencamp, 1990). Another sign of a predatory therapist is multiple victims, as in the following case:

> A male psychiatrist in the armed services was accused of taking sexual liberties, including fellatio, with young male patients. The psychiatrist was found to be regularly performing physical examinations—in particular, prostate examinations, which, by his own testimony (incredibly), he did without using gloves. Such examinations normally are not within the scope of outpatient psychiatry, but the psychiatrist claimed falsely that military medical protocols required him to perform them. The young forensic expert retained by the defense based his opinion on an assessment that the defendant's character was inconsistent with the allegations against him. Indeed, this married psychiatrist was outwardly a pillar of the community. Yet, credible allegations of similar behavior years earlier at another military base supported the inference that he was living a secret life at the expense of his patients. His claim to being an upstanding family man was further damaged by his having been arrested for solicitation in a rest-stop sting. This pattern of corroborative behavior outweighed any character evidence. Although evidence of past behavior may or may not be admissible at trial, it is an important principle of clinical and forensic assessment that predatory behavior repeats itself.

Some of the patients exploited by this psychotherapist had been victims of childhood sexual abuse. One patient said, "I came to you with a plate of problems. Now I have two plates." That is a statement that could be made by many, if not most, victims of therapists' sexual misconduct.

Role Reversal and/or a Misplaced Desire to Help

Violations of the sexual boundary between therapist and patient often are an expression not of a psychopath's predatory urges but of normal human needs inappropriately acted out. Role reversal may occur when a helping professional is made vulnerable by age, illness, bereavement, divorce, or other personal losses. It often begins when the therapist confides in the patient about personal matters and sometimes ends in sexual misconduct.

The therapist's vulnerability may be reinforced or intensified by the patient's vulnerability, displayed so openly in the therapeutic setting. Whereas a predator opportunistically exploits this vulnerability, the empathic therapist, seeing the world through the patient's troubled eyes, may rush to heal the patient's wounds. As noted in Chapter 2, empathy exerts a powerful gravitational pull, and grief can be seductive—*especially if you yourself feel a reciprocal need for nurturance and intimacy.* Some therapists become sexually involved with a patient because they believed this was the only way they could prevent the patient from descending into suicidal despair (a dilemma discussed later in this chapter). At least consciously, these therapists were trying to achieve the broadly therapeutic goal of keeping the patient alive. The most reliable restraints on this misdirected "helping" impulse are training, supervision, and consultation at the professional level, together with personal therapy or counseling when needed.

Rationalization

Therapists who engage in sexual misconduct often come up with expedient rationalizations for their conduct. One form of rationalization is illustrated by a case (using pseudonyms) from Dewald and Clark (2001, pp. 99–100).

> After 2 years of therapy, Dr. Bayer becomes increasingly attracted to his patient, an attractive, talented young woman who has difficulty feeling accepted by men. Dr. Bayer begins to make direct, detailed comments about how attractive this woman is and how a man might make love to her. When the patient tells the therapist how she is simultaneously excited and frustrated by these verbal overtures, he

replies that he is merely trying to build her self-confidence and give her an idea of the kind of romantic relationship that could be available to her. Whenever she speaks of an actual opportunity for a relationship with a man, Dr. Bayer responds in a discouraging, disparaging manner.

In this case there is no "slippery slope," since Dr. Bayer makes no physical overtures and does not transgress or loosen any other boundaries in the analytic setting. His rationalization of unprofessional conduct thus seems akin to that of teenagers who claim to be sexually virtuous because they have done "everything but." Yet, his intrusive verbal behavior clearly violates the patient's intimate personal space, effectively destroying her therapy. Dr. Bayer is not a serial predator or systematic boundary violator, but he would have done much better to seek consultation when he found himself becoming attracted to his patient.

Therapists who do "go all the way" with a patient are ready with their own rationalizations, as in the following case:

> A male psychologist who practiced time-limited supportive therapy at a health maintenance organization treated a female patient. The HMO's protocols reflected an expectation that patients might return to their therapist when they faced new practical problems or intensified stresses in their lives. In this case, the psychologist foreclosed the possibility of such a return to treatment by initiating a social and then sexual relationship with the patient as soon as the first course of treatment was concluded. As he explained to the patient, he had been only "like an adviser or coach" for her, since he "didn't do deep Freudian analysis" and had no ongoing responsibility for her care. If she needed help later, he told her, she could "just as easily come back and see somebody else." However, he did not specifically refer her to any other clinician. Months later, the patient came to question this explanation and to see the situation differently. Feeling deprived of the professional support her former therapist could have offered her, she reexamined the reasons she had become intimately involved with him, wondering to what extent it was a real personal attraction and to what extent it had developed out of his special role in her life. What especially concerned those who reviewed the case was that the patient appeared to blame herself, questioning both her criteria for choosing men and her "gullibility," even as she filed a complaint against the psychologist with his professional regulatory board.
>
> In the board hearing, the psychologist based his defense on the claim that the kind of short-term practical therapy he offered did not entail the development of transference. He did not take into account

that, whether or not the technical term "transference" applies, the structure of clinical work creates certain dependencies and vulnerabilities. The patient still feels involved and connected with the therapist. These dynamics need to be acknowledged and respected and their consequences provided for.

The psychologist also cited the First Amendment right to freedom of association and claimed that this patient was competent to make her own decisions. While conceding that in legal terms he might be right on both counts, the board refocused the issue as a clinical and ethical one. In those contexts the potential for undue influence on the therapist's part weighed heavily. Whether or not it is permissible in any circumstances for a therapist to become intimately involved with a former patient, this psychologist's having begun a personal relationship with a patient immediately at the conclusion of therapy created an overwhelming presumption of undue influence. Moreover, the psychologist's failure to make a timely referral made it reasonable for the patient to assume that he was still her therapist. The board suspended the psychologist's license pending his completion of a rehabilitation program, and his employment at the HMO was terminated.

The practice of having intimate personal relationships with former clients is rife with rationalization. The ethical and legal complexities of this situation will be discussed in Chapter 9.

Patient Vulnerability to Sexual Exploitation

The following presents a few brief descriptions of how patient vulnerability to sexual exploitation is commonly manifested. These examples should not be understood as representing all patients sexually exploited by therapists. Plainly, some motivating factors are specific to gender, age, diagnosis, or individual characteristics. What is known about the psychological dynamics, life histories, and circumstances that predispose patients to be vulnerable to therapists' sexual misconduct is outlined in Chapter 10.

One patient used the following words to describe her response to a therapist's sexual overture: "He led me to the bedroom and I followed like a little duckling" (Gutheil, 1991, p. 665). This language, which calls to mind Konrad Lorenz's experiments on imprinting with newly hatched birds, expresses a combination of powerlessness, dependency, fragile self-esteem, and idealization of the therapist. Rutter (1989a) quotes two patients along the same lines: "The opportunity to have such a special relationship with this man who meant so much to me was something I absolutely could not turn down" (p. 122). "So of course I couldn't say no. . . . By now I had become so totally dependent on him for any chance of expressing myself" (p. 126).

Underlying this mechanistic compliance in many cases is a history of sexual abuse. When this history emerges in therapy, the therapist exploits rather than explores the emotional vulnerability that is revealed. From early in life, the patient may have been conditioned to submit: "You'd better go along with your father's demands for sex, if you know what's good for you." The therapist, meanwhile, may rationalize the unethical conduct as a benign boundary crossing: "Unlike the patient's father, I have only the purest intentions." Emotionally deprived, traumatized patients are often so vulnerable to the slimmest reawakening of hope, the slightest promise of nurturance, that they feel they cannot turn away from any intimate connection, however compromised (Pope & Bouhoutsos, 1986; Rutter, 1989a). Thus, the presence of so many previously abused individuals among the victims of sexual abuse by therapists makes the latter form of abuse especially tragic and destructive.

A different sort of motivation was expressed by another patient who later filed suit against the offending therapist: "I knew it was wrong; I knew I was being abused and taken advantage of. But to me it was a chance of a lifetime. I was afraid I would never have such an exciting relationship again." Here the very illicitness of the relationship gave it a special allure, as if this woman felt that no suitable "real-life" partner could give her such an exotic and colorful experience. As in the Tom Rush song "Ladies Love Outlaws," there are cases in which the patient sees herself as civilizing a wild creature (Gabbard, 1994a). Therapists' behavior is sometimes driven by similar personal motivations. In one case a female therapist treating a female patient found the patient's husband (as he appeared in the patient's narratives) such an intriguing and challenging character that she decided to "tame" him by treating him as well. Subsequently she became romantically involved with him. The couple's divorce foreseeably was followed by a lawsuit brought by the female patient against the therapist.

The following case demonstrates how a patient's suggestibility can interact with a therapist's psychopathology to produce an unintended escalation of sexual excitement (a process which, of course, it is the therapist's responsibility to restrain and redirect):

During her first therapy session, a female patient asked her male therapist, "May I smoke in your office?" The therapist answered sarcastically, "No, but you can suck my thumb if you want." His inappropriate remark had the unexpected impact of stimulating the patient's sexual fantasies. Sexual misconduct and subsequent litigation followed.

The therapist's failure to set limits on his sexual behavior with a patient was consistent with his having made such an unprofessional, provocative remark to a patient (let alone a new patient) in the first place. Directed to receive rehabilitative therapy, the therapist was diagnosed with bipolar disorder with paranoid features.

Sexual dynamics between a patient and therapist can be catalyzed in various ways (Gutheil, 1991). The patient's disclosure of past sexual abuse may sexualize the therapeutic relationship from the perspective of the patient, the therapist, or both. In reaction to such disclosure, the therapist may perceive the patient as an active sexual being or as a passive sexual object; either of these images can stimulate the therapist to violate sexual boundaries. Secrecy and guilt not only can add to the erotic excitement, but also can create a bond (fragile as it may prove to be) between the two conspirators. At the same time, aggression commonly plays a role on either or both sides. Some therapists act out fear or contempt for the damaged but alluring victim, while some patients turn the sexual relationship into a source of power over the therapist's personal and professional life—a power struggle that may have its ultimate resolution in court.

The ethical and legal responsibility to prevent the enactment of any of these dynamics belongs solely to the therapist, as is made clear by the three axioms presented in Chapter 1. As Hoencamp (1990) notes: "It is the right of the patient to bring his/her weaknesses to a therapeutic relationship. The therapist has no right to abuse the patient's weaknesses or the situation into which he/she has placed the patient" (p. 294).

FEELINGS OF ATTRACTION TO PATIENTS

Being responsible not to act out feelings of attraction to a patient does not mean being exempt from such feelings. It is only normal for practitioners to feel attracted to (or repelled by) their patients or clients. In a major national survey of 585 psychologists, 87% reported that they had been sexually attracted to patients, and 63% felt guilty, anxious, or confused about those feelings (Pope et al., 1986). As Edelwich and Brodsky (1991) observe, "What frees the clinician to act with clear ethical purpose is an acceptance of and comfort with the normal human feelings that are incidental to the clinical interaction" (p. 120). National surveys have found that most therapists have had sexual fantasies about a patient, and a substantial minority report having had such fantasies while having sex with another person (Bernsen et al., 1994; Pope, 2001; Pope et al., 1986; Pope et al., 1987). In one survey, nearly half (46%) of respondents reported occasionally having a sexual fantasy about a patient, while an additional one-fourth (26%) had such fantasies more frequently (Pope et al., 1987). Although psychologists have been surveyed most often, surveys of other disciplines such as social workers (Bernsen et al., 1994) have had comparable results.

These figures are in contrast to surveys regularly finding the percentage of therapists who actually have had sex with a patient to be in the single digits (e.g., Pope et al., 1986; Williams, 1992). Pooling the data from national studies, Pope (2001) estimated that perpetrators make up about 4.4% of therapists (7% of male therapists, 1.5% of female therapists). Surveys of physicians (summarized in Gabbard & Nadelson, 1995) have yielded similar figures. Although self-report studies of actual sexual relations with patients may involve greater underreporting than self-reports of sexual fantasies, it is safe to say that far more therapists feel attracted to patients than act on that attraction.

A survey of psychologists licensed in Missouri provides insight into how therapists refrain from acting on feelings of attraction to patients (Stake & Oliver, 1991). Whereas only 1.3% of respondents reported that they acted on feelings of sexual attraction to patients, 17.1% acknowledged disclosing their feelings to the patient without acting on them. (Male therapists were significantly more likely to do so than female therapists.) Half of the respondents (49.3%) discussed the feelings with their supervisor, 18.8% with their own therapist. At the same time, 69.5% reported that they worked through their feelings by themselves. (Subjects were instructed to check all applicable responses.) Finally, 22.1% referred the patient to another therapist—a last resort to be considered when it is determined, with the help of supervision and consultation, that a therapist cannot safely and effectively continue to treat a particular patient (see Edelwich & Brodsky, 1991). Overall, the psychologists surveyed were appropriately inclined to seek help from others in dealing with feelings of attraction to patients.

Feelings of attraction between patient and therapist occur naturally even in therapies in which those feelings are not, as a matter of course, deeply explored. The emotional reactions and dynamic processes that analytically oriented therapists refer to as erotic transference and countertransference are found in many other kinds of therapy. You may not intend to stand in for a significant figure in a patient's life, but the patient may still cast you in that role. Moreover, you may react by casting the patient in the role of a significant figure in your life.

A guiding principle for coping effectively with a patient's feelings of sexual attraction to a therapist, and vice versa, is to recognize that these attractions often occur together, in interaction with each other. Each can stimulate the other, and each can shed light on the other. Mental health professionals across disciplines and theoretical approaches can benefit from some exposure to analytic literature on the management of erotic transference and countertransference (Bridges, 1994; Celenza, 1991; Elise, 1991; Folman, 1991; Gabbard, 1990; Gorkin, 1987; Jaffe, 1986; May, 1986; Person, 1985, 2003). Insights and principles derived from analytically oriented therapy have been adapted (without analytic terminology) to provide practical guidelines for physicians (Golden & Brennan, 1995) as well as for non-analytic clinicians and counselors of any discipline (Edelwich & Brodsky, 1991).

Inexperienced therapists often experience sexual feelings as a threat and therefore respond with avoidance, denial, cold aloofness, or premature, punitive limit setting. These responses can shut off valuable clinical material and drive the patient away (Bridges, 1994; Gabbard, 1990). The therapist may also prematurely refer the patient to another clinician (Edelwich & Brodsky, 1991). Too often the patient is left feeling rejected and abandoned, or else therapy becomes an impasse between a shamed, frustrated patient and an angry, self-protective therapist. At the other extreme, a therapist may encourage the patient's expression of sexual fantasies for the voyeuristic pleasure of listening to them and the sadistic pleasure of frustrating them. Another common error is to project one's own sexual arousal onto the patient, in effect blaming the "seductive" patient for one's own unconscious conflicts (Gabbard, 1990). As Bridges (1994) cautions, "The sexual dimensions of clinical practice and relationships are dangerous when they are denied, projected, or otherwise disowned" (p. 427).

A therapist's nondefensive recognition and examination of his or her own sexual feelings toward a patient facilitates nonexploitative acceptance and exploration of the patient's sexual feelings toward the therapist (Edelwich & Brodsky, 1991; Havens, 1993; Pope et al., 1993; Pope et al., 2006). An analytic therapist needs to reassure the patient that the whole range of human emotions, including love, anger, hate, fear, anxiety, resentment, and sexual desire, can be part of the therapeutic experience

(Gabbard, 1990). Sometimes the patient needs to express those feelings to learn about the conflicts he or she has experienced in other relationships. In this exploration, a therapist who is comfortable with his or her sexual feelings has an additional source of clinical data to draw upon. Bridges (1994) illustrates these principles with a case in which a female therapist felt intense sexual attraction to a male patient. The patient's sexualizing the relationship was a defense against his feelings of dependence and powerlessness in relation to his mother. The therapist colluded in this defensive posture until she regained her clinical perspective by analyzing experiences in her own past that paralleled the patient's. In other case illustrations involving female patients and female therapists, sexualized countertransference developed from a therapist's initially unacknowledged identification with a patient's feelings of loneliness, loss, or extreme vulnerability (Bridges, 1994).

With training and experience, therapists can develop the mental and emotional resources to incorporate into therapy those distracting, disturbing feelings that appear as unwelcome intrusions on therapy. For example, one therapist makes a practice of responding to a patient's declarations of love for him by saying, "That's wonderful! Now, you'll take those feelings out into the world with you" (Bridges, 1994, p. 430). These words convey caring, encouraging feedback while reaffirming the boundary between therapy and the rest of the patient's life.

At the same time, experienced therapists know that it is difficult, and unnecessary, to deal with such conflicts and tensions alone. As Bridges's (1994) case studies demonstrate, even ethical, highly trained clinicians often need supervision and consultation to work through the deep emotional and experiential currents that otherwise might lead to unwise enactments or therapeutic impasse. Clinicians of all disciplines can benefit from Gabbard's (1990) advice:

> When therapists find themselves sexually aroused by their patients, or are the object of a patient's intense sexual desire, consultation with a colleague is advised. Poets have known for centuries that desire may cloud judgment. A colleague's objective feedback may help a therapist steer a truer course through the turbulent seas of erotic feelings in therapeutic relationships. (p. 7)

A supervisor or consultant can serve as a "prosthetic superego," supporting the therapist in maintaining or recovering a professional (i.e., clinical and ethical) perspective. In addition, personal therapy can provide deeper exploration as well as a safe place to disclose feelings that are difficult to discuss with a supervisor.

RESPONDING TO PATIENTS' SEXUAL DEMANDS

It is well recognized that a patient's protestations of love for a therapist can mask intense hostility and aggression, even sadism (Gabbard, 1990; Kumin, 1985–1986)—feelings that therapists may knowingly or unknowingly reciprocate (Maltsberger & Buie, 1974; Pope & Tabachnick, 1993; Winnicott, 1949). When therapy runs aground in the face of the patient's insistent demands for sexual gratification, the therapist may come to feel like an object used to fulfill the patient's needs (Frayn & Silberfeld, 1986).

With some patients, straightforward, compassionate limit setting can set the therapy back on course. For example, the therapist might say, "There are many people out there who are available to sleep with you, but as a therapist I'm trying to make a different contribution to your life. I'd like to be your therapist, and what you're asking is not what a therapist does." In some cases the following variation can be appropriate: "I understand that you want to feel sure of our relationship, and that it's hard for you to be sure that you do have a relationship with someone unless the relationship is sexual. But this room here is meant to be a safe space for you to learn what it's like to have a caring relationship without sex, so that you can confront the problems for which you came to get help."

If the patient persists in making sexual demands, the therapist might say, "I've made clear that I'm not going to sleep with you because that's not therapy. Moreover, reducing your therapy to this one question makes any reasonable exploration of the problems you brought to therapy impossible. We need to look seriously at whether therapy can be of use to you or can even continue at all if you insist on staying on this one track that isn't going anywhere. We can go on with therapy, but to do so, we'll have to get off that subject."

COERCION AND BLACKMAIL

In the absence of, or in spite of, such preventive limit setting and redirection, some patients escalate to blackmail, threatening suicide, self-mutilation, disrobing, sabotage of therapy, or false accusations of sexual misconduct if the therapist does not agree to violate boundaries to satisfy the patient's immediate needs (Gutheil, 2005a). Therapists can meet this threat more effectively if they disabuse themselves of the notion that boundary violations actually help prevent suicide. On the contrary, assuming the omnipotent role of "rescuer" may cause a truly suicidal patient to deteriorate further, either by exacerbating the present crisis or by making a recurrence more likely (Eyman & Gabbard, 1991; Gabbard & Wilkinson, 1994, pp. 59–67). As with any other threat, the proper response is a clinical one, such as "If you really are suicidal, you should be in the hospital. If the risk is not imminent, then we should meet more often and follow that symptom."

When a clinician is threatened by a patient, the appropriate response generally is to reaffirm boundaries and make every effort to refocus the patient on the clinical agenda. Take apart the illegitimate "if–then" statement by disconnecting the premise from the conclusion of the blackmail. Thus, the therapist might say, "Let it be on the record that I'm not going to sleep with you. Now, let's deal with what that feels like, what you plan to do about it, and how we should respond." If the patient says, "I'm going to have an anxiety attack," the therapist replies, "Let's treat your anxiety." If the patient "threatens" to sink into a deep depression, a similar response is called for: "Let's explore it." Blackmail is a quid pro quo: "If you will do X for me, then I won't do Y to myself/you." A contract, on the other hand, is a plan for achieving a shared goal: "I agree to do X, and, in conjunction with that, you agree to do Y." In place of the illicit bargain of blackmail, the therapist attempts to reestablish the therapeutic contract: "I will agree to see you more often. Will you agree to work to stave off suicidality, and to let me know if it's getting worse so that you can go back into the hospital?"

Another regrettably common threat takes the form of "If you don't have sex with me, I'll go to the state licensing board and say that you did." In that case, the therapist should confront the patient with the practical consequences of this blackmail while maintaining a therapeutic focus: "I hope you won't do that, because it would doom our therapy, but we should explore why you feel you need to do it." At the same time, the therapist writes a note: "Patient said she would accuse me of having sex with her if in fact I did not sleep with her. Patient was reminded I would not sleep with her and was asked to explain why she would jeopardize therapy in this manner. Explored issue." In addition to sharing this note with a supervisor or consultant, the therapist can obtain an "anonymous advisory" from the state licensing board. Without naming the patient, the therapist reports the threat and requests the board's advice. In this way, the therapist has put the incident on record and documented his or her efforts to repair the situation in case the patient later files a claim of sexual misconduct or of abandonment, the latter in the event that therapy has been terminated as unsalvageable. Termination may be required if the patient's persistent threats and coercive behavior create a hostile relationship, making it impossible for therapy to progress.

Coercion and blackmail on the part of patients do not necessarily take the form of a single, easily recognizable "quid pro quo" demand. The following case, a complex and challenging one, shows how a conscientious, reasonably well-trained therapist can be overwhelmed and held hostage by a pattern of boundary-eroding patient behaviors (Gutheil, 2005a). The length of this case presentation is a function of the central importance of the various interactions between therapist and patient and the various pressures exerted on the therapist to an understanding of the clinical dynamics and ethical implications of what transpired. In effect, this case can serve as a composite of numerous situations in which therapists feel trapped into boundary excursions.

A married female therapist with a master's degree in counseling psychology was treating a married female patient diagnosed with borderline personality disorder and possible dissociative identity disorder. The patient was a severe self-mutilator with considerable exposure to various therapies. The therapist, who had attended training seminars and studied standard texts on this patient's disorders, was well prepared clinically, but not for the dynamics of patient–therapist interaction in this case. These dynamics grew out of the patient's abuse history, which had left her feeling deeply shamed and cut off from her bodily sensations. As a result of the traumas she had suffered, this patient had an intense need for privacy. Her extreme sensitivity to intrusion and exposure, which had made hospitalization problematic, also was manifested as a phobic resistance to supervision or consultation, as well as to having particular facts written down in her chart. To allay her fear and anxiety, the patient was allowed to read most of the therapist's notes and to impose on the therapist a generic, euphemistic form of expression that weakened the documentation of the case (see Gutheil & Hilliard, 2001).

Over a few years of treatment, the patient's condition improved. This was accomplished, however, at the cost of numerous boundary crossings undertaken to navigate this patient's minefield of traumatic associations. These included frequent after-hours phone calls and the exchange of personal cards and letters. By pressing her therapist to depart from usual practices in order to circumvent her special dynamics and sensitivities, the patient was, in effect, holding the therapist hostage over a boundary question. On one occasion the therapist, in consultation with her supervisor, made a home visit. She was asked to stay at night to help desensitize the patient to a time of day associated with her past abuse. The therapist slept on the sofa, not in the patient's bed, as falsely portrayed in the patient's subsequent complaint.

Ironically, as the patient improved to the point of beginning to feel her body as a genuine presence, she initiated serious challenges to physical boundaries. At one point she took the therapist's hand and attempted to place it on her own breast. The therapist withdrew her hand and documented the behavior—which did not prevent the patient from claiming later that the therapist "touched my breast."

Her body numbness alleviated by treatment, the patient began to feel physical sensations in the office. During one session, in a seeming attempt to confirm this progress, she began to masturbate in the therapist's presence. The therapist told her that if she persisted in doing so, the therapist would have to leave the room. The patient pleaded with her to stay, claiming that in the therapist's absence, the erotic stimulation would evoke memories of past abuse, and the patient would be driven to cut herself. Held hostage by the threat of self-mutilation (and by her fear of being held liable for it), the therapist chose to stay in the room for a time, and before long the patient stopped masturbating. However, the therapist had left herself open to the charge that she had observed the patient in this act for her own voyeuristic gratification.

This episode epitomized the double bind in which this patient placed her therapist. For the therapist to stay in the room would be to participate passively in a boundary violation. To leave, to get consultation, or to bring someone else into the room would risk provoking severe self-mutilation, as in previous instances of symbolic repetition of past abuse. Even when this threat was not made explicit, the patient's history presented an implicit threat of self-destructive behavior if the therapist did not accede to the patient's boundary-crossing requests. Moreover, since hospitalization had been a very traumatic experience for this patient, the therapist hesitated to set firm limits for fear the patient might decompensate and would need to be hospitalized.

In retrospect, the therapist realized that when the patient started masturbating the appropriate response would simply have been to tell the patient to stop doing it. If the patient did not desist, the next step would have been to open the door and ask someone else to come in. Undoubtedly the patient would have taken this as a serious rejection, possibly precipitating a crisis, but it would seem to have been a necessary intervention and a necessary risk to take. At the time, however, the therapist felt too trapped and intimidated by the threat of immediate consequences to take the long view. This patient's history and her way of relating to the therapist set land mines blocking most of the reasonable paths that a therapist would ordinarily take in dealing with boundary challenges, including documentation, consultation, limit setting, and hospitalization.

> Finally, when the patient requested that the therapist stay overnight with her a second time, the therapist, after speaking with her supervisor, refused to do so. The patient then called the clinic that employed the therapist and brought a complaint against her. The patient had second thoughts about this retaliatory act when the clinic, as a way of investigating the matter, had someone sit in on the therapy for the patient's safety. Falling back on her presentation of dissociative identity disorder, the patient disavowed her complaint as having been made by a disavowed/disappointed "alter" and complained bitterly about the measures taken to protect her from the alleged misconduct, which she characterized as invasions of her privacy in therapy. Although her retraction of specific charges was accepted, she could not undo what she had started. Therapy continued with observers sitting in, ostensibly for the patient's protection but, in all likelihood, for the clinic's protection as well. The patient experienced this monitoring of her therapy as yet another violation.
>
> The patient later filed a complaint with the counselor's professional licensing board. In the board complaint, all of the boundary crossings that the patient had, in effect, extorted from the therapist were presented as though they had been initiated by the therapist to gratify the therapist's own needs. The patient's role in bringing about these crossings was ignored or minimized. The patient also alleged extensive perverse sexual behavior on the therapist's part, much of it implausible. It is quite possible that these scenarios represented relivings of actual abuse by someone else at another time in the patient's life. However, when the board began to look into the complaint, the euphemisms and vagaries to which the therapist had felt she was limited in documenting the patient's treatment were not sufficient to refute the patient's claims (Gutheil & Hilliard, 2001; see also Chapter 12).
>
> At the board hearing, through strenuous effort on the part of her counsel, the therapist was cleared of the allegations of sexual misconduct. However, the board faulted her and the clinic for inadequate supervision and consultation. Were it not for those deficiencies, the board reasoned, she would not have felt so helpless to set limits and would not have allowed herself to be held hostage to the extent that she did. Some board members said that they found especially helpful the distinction the defense-retained expert drew between boundary crossings and violations. However, the board held that consultation before the fact could have helped the therapist estimate the risk of misperception by the patient—for example, the risk that a home visit

would be perceived as a sexual overture. In her understandable fear of retraumatizing the patient, the therapist failed to weigh the countervailing risk that this badly damaged patient would "get it wrong." In light of the sheer number of boundary crossings and the ease with which this patient could misinterpret them as violations, the board sanctioned the therapist in some of the areas charged, and the risk of a civil lawsuit remained.

Everything this therapist did in working with a very difficult, complicated patient had a good clinical intention. Therapists who stretch normal boundaries for regressed, dependent patients often do so for good therapeutic reasons such as the following:

- "I'm doing it in an attempt to individualize therapy by meeting the patient at his or her own level."
- "I just want to give this victimized, traumatized patient what he or she needs."
- "I don't want to be cruel or sadistic."

It is important to be alert to such rationalizations, as they may arise. Likewise, it is essential to be alert to less defensible reasons for acquiescing to emotional blackmail by patients, including rescue fantasies and the wish to play the role of an idealized parent or lover. Whatever the governing motivations, a case such as the one just described teaches the following lessons for dealing with difficult patients, those who pose serious challenges to the maintenance of the therapeutic frame (Gutheil, 2005a).

First, good intentions are not enough. The impact on the patient must also be considered. Moreover, there may be a gap between what the therapist intends and how it is interpreted and understood, first by the patient and then by a finder of fact.

Second, although boundary crossings are distinguishable from violations, subsequent reviewers and evaluators will not necessarily appreciate the difference. Even when they do, a series of benign boundary crossings may leave the impression that "something's wrong." In the words of an old Scottish saying, "Many a mickle maks a muckle" [many littles make a big].

Third, you sacrifice full, clear documentation at your peril. If you take the risk of departing from standard procedures, you need to record in the chart the clinical rationale. There are reasonable concessions that can be made to patient preferences, but compromising professionalism in this critical area is not one of them (Gutheil & Hilliard, 2001). Instead, you can explain to the patient, "Documentation is essential for your care. For example, if I get hit by a car, somebody else has to be able to take over."

Fourth, consultation and supervision are of critical importance. Together with documentation, they provide a protective structure of professional disclosure and accountability, not to mention the benefit of having more than one mind applied to the clinical problem. A patient who attempts to keep a therapist from obtaining an anonymous consultation should be told that this is not acceptable.

Fifth, the clinician is responsible for setting and maintaining boundaries, even if the patient threatens self-harm or flight from therapy. One of a therapist's fundamental tasks is to refrain from reinforcing a patient's primitive strivings and instead to foster and encourage adult strivings. This cannot be accomplished by giving in to blackmail. In the foregoing case of a blackmailing patient, the therapist likely would have done better at some point to tell the patient that her latest demand was a deal breaker. A therapist concerned about the costs of resisting blackmail should also consider the costs of paying the blackmailer. No therapy can proceed and progress if its only goal is to prevent self-harm. Furthermore, a therapist must accept that therapy may fail or be rejected because the patient does not find it immediately gratifying. Tolerating these uncertainties and risks, while making every reasonable effort to engage the patient in exploring his or her choices and behavior, is part of the therapist's burden.

KEY REMINDERS

- A sexual relationship with a patient is incompatible with any form of professional mental health treatment and therefore is always unethical.

- By recognizing and examining his or her own sexual feelings toward a patient, a therapist is better able to accept and explore the patient's sexual feelings in a way that is neither exploitative nor punitive.

- A therapist can respond to a patient's sexual demands most effectively with straightforward, compassionate limit setting—followed, if necessary, by reminding the patient that acting out a sexual fixation on the therapist is antithetical to the purpose of therapy.

- Even when a patient escalates to threats and blackmail, the therapist remains responsible for setting and maintaining boundaries.

PART III

Implications

CHAPTER 9

What Harms Are Caused?

Serious boundary violations are destructive to therapy and cause foreseeable (although not universal) harms to patients. This chapter briefly outlines these harmful consequences as a reminder of why the prevention of boundary violations is an important priority. The primary emphasis here is on the harms caused by therapists' sexual misconduct, which have been most systematically studied. However, as detailed in the clinical and legal case examples throughout this book, many of the same psychological harms can be caused by other boundary violations that precede, or occur in the absence of, therapist–patient sex (Simon, 1991b).

It should also be noted that actual and alleged boundary violations cause substantial harm to clinicians through disciplinary and legal sanctions (see Chapter 12) and to the credibility and effectiveness of the mental health professions (see Chapter 11).

SURVEY AND CLINICAL RESEARCH

Investigation of the harmful consequences of sexual relationships between patients and therapists began when this practice became a matter of public concern in the 1970s (Collins, Mebed, & Mortimer, 1978; Masters & Johnson, 1976; Taylor & Wagner, 1976). In Bouhoutsos et al.'s (Bouhoutsos, Holroyd, Lerman, Forer, & Greenberg, 1983) survey of California psychologists, 90% of their patients who had had sex with a previous therapist reportedly had suffered ill effects. In an early controlled study of female patients, those who had had sexual contact with a male therapist or other health care practitioner experienced greater mistrust and anger toward men and more psychological and psychosomatic symptoms than those who had not. The severity of psychological impacts was significantly related to prior vulnerability (severity of symptoms or history of sexual victimization) and the marital status of the practitioner (Feldman-Summers & Jones, 1984). Pope and Vetter (1991) extended Bouhoutsos et al.'s survey findings to a national sample with a higher return rate. In the judgment of their subsequent therapists, female patients more regularly experienced some degree of harm if the intimate relationship was initiated before termination of therapy (95%) than after termination (80%)—a finding that did not hold for male patients.

Other researchers supplemented these survey findings with in-depth psychodynamic exploration. In a group therapy project for women who had been sexually involved with therapists, Sonne et al. (Sonne, Meyer, Borys, & Marshall, 1985) identified three major clinical issues that repeatedly emerged: difficulties with trust, poor self-concept, and difficulty expressing anger. Group participants struggled with their inability to trust not only others but themselves as well, since they tended to blame themselves for the sexual boundary violations. They also felt shamed and demoralized by the loss of the "special" status they felt they had enjoyed until the therapist terminated their intimacy or was revealed to be sexually involved with other patients (see discussion of "cessation trauma" later).

Apfel and Simon (1985a) constructed a psychodynamic typology of harmful effects on patients, which included the following:

1. Ambivalence toward therapy and mistrust of subsequent therapists.
2. Questioning of one's sense of reality and sanity.
3. Repetition instead of exploration of childhood traumas.
4. Bondage to the offending therapist.
5. Exacerbation of original symptoms.
6. Constricted intimacy with others.
7. Rage and desire for revenge.
8. Excesses of guilt and shame.
9. Impaired imagination and inhibited exploration of fantasies.
10. Crisis and disorganization brought about by the abrupt ending of a relationship.

These effects occurred despite the fact that, in the cases studied, the sexual relations typically did not include intercourse. Indeed, the guilt, shame, and humiliation felt by the patient often was associated with the sexual inadequacies or perversities of the therapist.

METHODOLOGICAL QUESTIONS

As a body of research on the harmful effects of therapist–patient sex developed, the researchers themselves raised questions about the validity of their findings (Pope, 1990a, 1990b; Pope & Vetter, 1991). For example, the surveys excluded victims of such misconduct who did not seek subsequent therapy. The surveys also relied on the perceptions and judgment of the respondents. Furthermore, caution was required in attributing the observed harms to the sexual misconduct as opposed to the patient's preexisting problems, including past traumatic events as well as personality disorders.

Clinical reports are useful in establishing that certain symptom patterns do in fact occur in association with particular life experiences and in allowing for in-depth analysis of those patterns. For several reasons, however, it is difficult to make valid inferences about causation of harm from clinical reports (Williams, 1995). In any particular case, causal attributions may simply reflect the therapist's beliefs or uncritical acceptance of the patient's reports. The inference that a patient's symptoms resulted from a therapist's sexual misconduct is based on speculation about what the patient's condition would have been had the misconduct not occurred. Moreover, even if it is accepted that the harm suffered by a patient was caused by sexual involvement with a therapist, the question arises whether the same symptoms might have been precipitated (as they commonly are) by the unhappy ending of some other intimate relationship. Finally, even a large number of clinical reports cannot establish the rate of occurrence of such harm in the general population.

These uncertainties, compounded by various sampling biases, raise questions about the validity of survey results based on self-reports of patients or their subsequent therapists (Williams, 1992). Patients who believe they have been harmed by sexual involvement with a therapist tend to be more motivated to participate in a survey than those who do not feel they have been harmed. This self-selection bias also affects surveys of therapists about their patients' experiences of sexual boundary violations on the part of previous therapists. Therapists' responses to such surveys (indeed, their motivation to respond at all) may vary with the types of patients in their caseloads, what their patients do or do not tell them, and their own theoretical orientations and interpretive methods.

Subsequent research has benefited from methodological questions such as those raised by Williams. For example, Luepker (1999) attempted to distinguish between preexisting problems and those caused by sexual boundary violations by giving respondents the following response items:

> (1) has not been a problem; (2) existed previously but remained the same during and after the misconduct; (3) existed previously but became worse during and after the misconduct; and (4) emerged as a *new* problem during and after the misconduct. (p. 53)

Among the symptoms and impairments reported to be increased during and after the misconduct were posttraumatic stress disorder, major depressive disorder, suicidal ideation and suicide attempts, use of prescription drugs, concern about alcohol and non-prescription drug use, disruptions in relationships and daily functioning, negative effects on sexual feelings and functioning, and reduced earning capacity. Luepker's study design took a significant step toward remedying a major deficiency of previous research. However, it was still subject to the limitations of self-report surveys of a particular clinic population. Respondents who identified themselves as victims of therapists' sexual misconduct would be biased toward reporting increased impairments whether or not such exacerbations could be corroborated by objective means.

IS THERE A "THERAPIST–PATIENT SEX SYNDROME"?

Difficulties in assessing harms and attributing causation bear upon the validity of the "therapist–patient sex syndrome" proposed by Pope and Bouhoutsos (1986). This syndrome has been defined by the following symptoms:

1. Ambivalence
2. Guilt
3. Feelings of isolation
4. Emptiness
5. Cognitive dysfunction
6. Identity disturbance
7. Inability to trust
8. Sexual confusion
9. Mood lability
10. Suppressed rage
11. Increased suicidal risk

As Pope and Bouhoutsos acknowledge, patients vary in the degree of harm they subjectively experience. One may undergo the trauma without having some or all of the symptoms, and one may manifest similar symptoms as a result of other causes. Consistent with Williams's (1992) critique, Pope and Bouhoutsos describe the central problem in linking observed or reported damage to a particular cause:

> For many patients there may be no data deriving from formal testing and assessments performed prior to the sexual involvement with the therapist. Without such baseline data, the assessment of the damage that was due to the sexual involvement becomes more complex and difficult. (p. 64)

Clinical experience has taught that victims of sexual exploitation by therapists often manifest the symptoms identified by Pope and Bouhoutsos (and other symptoms as well), as do patients with major depression or schizophrenia. The main difficulty with using the purported syndrome to attribute causality is the considerable overlap among patients involved in sex with therapists, patients who were previously sexually abused (especially in childhood), and patients diagnosed with borderline personality disorder. Pope and Bouhoutsos themselves observe that the therapist–patient sex syndrome "bears similarities to aspects of the borderline (and histrionic) personality disorder" (p. 64). Disentangling causes from effects in this cluster is problematic. Previous sexual abuse is commonly found in the histories of individuals diagnosed with borderline personality disorder, and both previous sexual abuse and borderline personality disorder are known to predispose patients to being vulnerable to sexual misconduct by therapists. On the other hand, a therapist's sexual misconduct may produce symptoms consistent with borderline personality disorder in a patient who previously has not shown such traits. Thus, in a given case, recognition of the comorbidity of past sexual abuse, borderline personality disorder, and sexual abuse by therapists is only the beginning, not the end, of clinical or forensic investigation (Gutheil, 1992c).

Although the idea of a "therapist–patient sex syndrome" has been found useful for educational purposes (Pope, 1994, pp. 117–121), the attempt to substitute such an a priori construct for case-by-case analysis leads to several practical difficulties. For patients, it can be a self-fulfilling prophecy, predisposing them to assume a victim role. In this way, it can shut off open-ended therapeutic exploration of other potential causal dynamics. In cases where therapist–patient sex syndrome is a false diagnosis, the treatment, too, is likely to be misdirected. In the forensic arena, "therapist–patient sex syndrome," unlike most other descriptive entities, includes assumptions about history and causation as part of the diagnostic formulation. As a result, when a plaintiff's expert witness testifies that the plaintiff exhibits this syndrome, the jury may take the diagnosis both as proof of the disputed factual claim that the misconduct occurred and as a statement about causation, an essential question in establishing liability (Gutheil, 1992c; Gutheil & Gabbard, 1992).

ARE THERE CASES IN WHICH NO HARM OCCURS?

Cases in which patients suffer no apparent harm from sexual boundary violations have been documented clinically, although they are relatively rare and tend to have an unusual flavor, like the following example:

> A young woman with schizoid and paranoid tendencies had difficulty forming a therapeutic alliance for any length of time. After several unsuccessful attempts at treatment, she became sexually involved with a resident in psychiatry who was treating her. By then her diverse (if fragmentary) experiences in psychotherapy had given her a grasp of basic terminology and analytical thinking, which she deployed with such confidence that she saw herself as teaching the resident. Following this experience, she found that she was better able to form a therapeutic alliance. Eventually she undertook graduate studies and became a psychiatric social worker.
>
> Exploring these events in subsequent therapy, the woman came to understand that her grandiose self-confidence had protected her from injury to her self-esteem resulting from the sexual boundary violation. To her, in fact, the resident's involvement with her had more the feeling of transference than countertransference! A role reversal that usually is damaging to patients constituted, for this patient, a process of discovery and rehearsal of her desire to help people.

The (probably small) minority of patients who are not harmed by therapists' sexual misconduct typically show some combination of ego strength and lack of emotional involvement in the sexual relationship with the therapist. However, we cannot uncritically accept assurances that a patient has suffered no harm, just as self-reports of harmful consequences cannot be taken solely at face value. Whereas some patients magnify the harms they have suffered in order to assume the victim role, others fail to report actual harms for a variety of reasons, including a desire to protect the offending therapist and feelings of guilt and shame about the involvement.

In cases of apparent improvement, the patient's mental stability, self-esteem, and sense of well-being may be propped up for a time by the illusion of a nurturing relationship. In some cases the price of the appearance of progress is continued bondage to the therapist in place of understanding, autonomy, and growth (Apfel & Simon, 1985a; Langs, 1984–1985). The benefit is almost always gained at a price and therefore is transient and ultimately illusory, like the good feeling that comes from taking an addictive drug (Simon, 1994).

CESSATION TRAUMA

The shallow, illusory nature of the gratification obtained from a sexual relationship with a therapist commonly is revealed when the relationship ends. The triggering event may take the form of the therapist's abruptly breaking off the relationship, refusing to leave his or her spouse, terminating therapy, or otherwise appearing to abandon the patient. A mere brusque response to a telephone call has been known to lead to bitter disillusionment after a 20-year relationship. Traumatic endings also occur when the patient finds out (from rumors, talking with a fellow patient, or media accounts of litigation brought by other patients) that the therapist has been sexually involved with another patient or patients as well.

The sudden shattering of the patient's feeling of being "special" can lead the patient to reinterpret every aspect of the relationship as exploitative rather than gratifying. This devastating experience has been termed "cessation trauma" (Gutheil, 1999b; Gutheil & Gabbard, 1992; Simon, 1994). It may lead to intense feelings of embarrassment and humiliation, severe disorganization, major depression, and suicidal crises. A diagnosis of posttraumatic stress disorder may be warranted. Litigation often is initiated under these circumstances, as in the following case:

> A woman in her late 30s with a childhood history of physical and emotional abuse had been treated for depression, anxiety, and drug and alcohol abuse. When she came under the care of a female psychologist who was in her 50s, the psychologist diagnosed multiple personality disorder. In addition to other unorthodox methods of treatment, the psychologist engaged in breast feeding with a 5-year-old alter and sexual contact with 13- and 16-year-old alters. When other patients confronted her about the attention she gave this patient during group therapy sessions, the psychologist established more definite boundaries in the therapeutic relationship. Feeling abandoned, the patient tried in vain to restore the intimate relation-

ship. Eventually she saw another therapist and sued the psychologist, claiming that as a result of the defendant's negligent care she could no longer practice her vocation of making jewelry and had to work as a house and office cleaner. The jury awarded the plaintiff $205,000 in compensatory damages and $120,000 in punitive damages (*Meek v. Holmes*, 1995).

In such cases, "The seeds of the trauma were latent in the pathologic relationship from the outset, but the trauma stands revealed only at its end" (Gutheil, 1999b, p. 9).

A question that sometimes arises is whether any reparative actions can reduce cessation trauma. Although the impact of the misconduct can in some cases be diminished, the fact remains that the mental health practitioner has gone over the line by having a sexual relationship with a patient. That cannot be undone, and therapy (if it has continued to that point) cannot continue. Normal procedures for termination and referral should be followed to maintain continuity of care and minimize feelings of abandonment (in a clinical, if not personal, sense). It may also be possible to reduce the emotional harm to the patient by candid acknowledgment of the wrongdoing, regret for the ill effects, and a promise that the unethical conduct will not be repeated. Such an assurance can be meaningful, since some patients file complaints and legal actions to protect future patients from exploitation. Moreover, a good-faith effort to mitigate the damages one has caused can benefit the therapist in a civil action and in a licensing board's evaluation of the therapist's potential for rehabilitation and fitness to practice.

INTRINSIC AND EXTRINSIC HARMS

It is useful to distinguish between *intrinsic harms*—that is, harms that occur regardless of individual variations in the dynamics of the experience—and *extrinsic harms*, which can vary with the individual and the circumstances (Gutheil & Gabbard, 1992). Intrinsic harm is the inevitable, and fatal, damage done to therapy by therapist–patient sex. For the reasons outlined by Smolar and Akhtar (2002), two people cannot have both a sexual relationship and a therapeutic relationship (see Chapter 8). Thus, the intrinsic harms caused by therapists' sexual misconduct include the failure to provide appropriate therapy, the provision of substandard therapy with a substantial risk of harm to the patient, and the lost window of opportunity for the patient to progress both in therapy and in life.

A pathologic relationship with a clinician can represent a detour not only from appropriate beneficial therapy but also from normal experience, growth, and development. In the words of one patient who sued her therapist for sexual misconduct, "I gave up my adolescence for this guy"; that is, she had never learned normal dating and formation of relationships while engaged in a longstanding relationship with her therapist. Other female litigants have asserted that their opportunity for childbearing had passed during the years when they were intimately involved with their therapists. It should be noted that many individuals lose years of their lives in unproductive dysfunctional relationships—with partners who are not their therapists—and suffer lost opportunities as a result. Nonetheless, mental health professionals have a clear responsibility not to create, replicate, or perpetuate problems for their patients.

Extrinsic harms are those, beyond the irreparable damage to therapy, that patients foreseeably, although not invariably, suffer as a result of therapists' sexual misconduct. These must be assessed on a case-by-case basis. The consequences outlined above, with reference to sources such as Apfel and Simon (1985a), Luepker (1999), Pope and Bouhoutsos (1986), and Simon (1994), constitute extrinsic harms (see Pope, 1994, ch. 5, for a detailed discussion of consequences and interventions). In particular, there is a consensus among clinicians that revictimization of those who have a history of sexual abuse at the hands of family members or others is a major tragedy and clinical challenge (Kluft, 1990; see Chapter 10). In the area of loss of trust in therapists and resistance to subsequent therapy, the undoing of therapeutic gains that may have been made before the boundary violations began must also be considered. The following case shows how difficult it can be for a patient, once victimized, to extend the trust needed to benefit from therapy.

> A young woman consulted a cognitive-behavioral therapist for treatment of well-documented social anxiety disorder. Subsequently the therapist told the patient that he should accompany her on *in vivo* exposure exercises such as ordering food in a restaurant. Although therapist-accompanied exposure treatment is legitimate, this therapist expanded the treatment to include, successively, walking around the block with the patient, going out to eat with her, and inviting her to his apartment. These activities led to a sexual relationship, followed by a successful lawsuit brought by the patient. The patient required several years of intensive psychodynamic therapy to undo the damage.
>
> After 5 years, still suffering from the social anxiety disorder for which she had not been properly treated, the patient again requested

CBT. Her new therapist, also male, prescribed relaxation training as the first step in a very gradual desensitization hierarchy. In an unusual variant of the technique, the patient practiced the relaxation response in the therapist's presence only with her eyes open. After 3 months she finally felt safe enough to close her eyes while she was with the therapist, who regarded this development as a marker of progress in therapy.

Harmful consequences can extend to many areas of a person's life, including work and the ability to earn a living (Luepker, 1999), as in the following case:

A female singer went to a male psychiatrist for treatment of performance anxiety. Several years into the treatment, the psychiatrist allegedly persuaded her to have a sexual relationship with him in the guise of therapy. Finding that her condition was deteriorating, the patient attempted to free herself from the relationship by moving from the Midwest to the West Coast. Even there (showing continued dependency along with recognition of exploitation and harm) she maintained continued telephone contact with the psychiatrist until 9 years after she had begun treatment with him.

Unable to resume the career that previously had earned her $70,000–150,000 per year, the singer sued the psychiatrist for undue familiarity, resulting in posttraumatic stress disorder and occupational paralysis. Although the psychiatrist denied the allegations, a jury found for the plaintiff, awarding $1.5 million in damages (*Holladay v. Boyd*, 1995).

Also not to be overlooked are the harms suffered by "secondary" (also referred to as "indirect" or "associate") victims of therapists' sexual misconduct–namely, spouses, intimate partners, children, and other family members and friends of the patients involved (Luepker, 1995, 1999; Milgrom, 1989). Children, for example, may experience anxiety, impaired school performance and peer relationships, and other effects of parental stress and conflict. Likewise, other patients of the offending (or falsely accused) therapist may suffer from the disruption of therapy or loss of trust in their therapist. Marital conflict and divorce are major precipitants of litigation against sexually exploitative therapists, as in the following example:

A married couple and their two adult children each entered into individual therapy with a female social worker (already a potential boundary violation). A few years later, the husband separated from his wife. A month after that, the social worker told the wife that she could no longer treat her because of conflicting loyalties to her and her husband. She did, however, continue to treat the adult children. After another month, the wife learned that the social worker had begun dating her husband. Confronted by the wife and children, the social worker allegedly insisted that the relationship was not improper. The couple subsequently divorced, and the husband married the social worker.

The wife and children sought psychological intervention for severe depression, sleeplessness, difficulty with concentration, and loss of trust in others. They sued the social worker for allegedly violating the National Association of Social Workers' code of ethics by (1) abandoning and failing to refer a patient in need of treatment and (2) initiating a personal relationship with the relative of a patient to the patient's detriment. The parties settled for $475,000, shared equally by the plaintiffs (*Jackenthal v. Kirsch*, 1995).

POSTTERMINATION RELATIONSHIPS

The clinical professions have continued to struggle with the ramifications of relationships, sexual and otherwise, between clinicians and former clients (see, e.g., Anderson & Kitchener, 1998; Friedman & Boumil, 1995, ch. 9; Gabbard & Pope, 1989). The need to maintain boundaries after termination of therapy has been most clearly articulated in the psychoanalytic context. Gabbard and Lester (2002), citing research showing the persistence of transference after termination, assert the orthodox position that "posttermination sexual relationships should be regarded as unethical and clinically ill-advised in virtually every situation" (p. 149). If a posttermination relationship were held out as a permissible option, the patient might be distracted from the work of analysis by a desire to win the analyst's favor. Both patient and analyst might be inhibited from confronting and exploring difficult issues. Moreover, from the perspective of analytic theory, the wish to cling to a relationship with the analyst as a "real person" can be a form of resistance to the mourning process necessary to completing the analysis.

> Many patients, particularly those in the mental health professions, approach analysis with a secret agenda of paving the way for a post-analytic relationship—sometimes sexual, sometimes not—that will allow the analyst to be a "real person." Interpretation of this fantasy paves the way for the necessary grief process. Any hint of collusion with it, either through avoidance or subtle encouragement of it, may leave a crucial sector of the personality unanalyzed. (Gabbard & Lester, 2002, pp. 153–154)

Finally, in a study of 71 successfully analyzed patients, Hartlaub, Martin, and Rhine (1986) found that two-thirds had returned to their analysts for additional work within 3 years of termination. An analyst who has become a friend or lover is no longer available to provide the needed services.

The analytic position of urging abstinence from nontherapeutic relationships with ex-patients has not been the consensus among the mental health professions, although opinion has moved in that direction. In Borys and Pope's (1989) survey of 4,800 psychiatrists, psychologists, and social workers, whereas respondents were virtually unanimous in their disapproval of sexual relations with a current patient/client, only 68% favored absolute prohibition of such intimacies after termination. In an early national survey of 395 psychologists practicing psychotherapy, 11% acknowledged having had intimate relationships with former clients, as opposed to 3.1% with clients during the course of therapy. Respondents expressed divergent views about the propriety of posttermination intimacies. The largest group (44.7%) regarded such relationships as highly unethical. Another 23.9% judged such relationships only somewhat unethical, while 31.3% believed them to be neither ethical nor unethical, or even ethical to some degree. Among the factors to be taken into account in assessing the ethics of intimate posttherapy relationships, time since termination was by far the most frequently cited—a rather simple benchmark for making a complex determination (Akamatsu, 1988). Similar findings were obtained in other surveys around the same time (Conte, Plutchik, Picard, & Karasu, 1989; Herman et al., 1987).

By contrast, a survey of psychologists practicing psychotherapy found that 7% believed it to be ethical (unquestionably or under many circumstances) to become sexually involved with a former client (Pope et al., 1987). This relatively modest percentage reflects the changing cultural climate of the late 1980s and early 1990s, when public exposure of seemingly rampant sexual abuse by psychotherapists cast a disturbing light on a wide range of boundary transgressions. During this period the foreseeable harms caused by posttermination sex were brought under the same ethical scrutiny as those caused by sex during therapy. Nonetheless, training programs in clinical psychology have not consistently succeeded in making trainees aware of this and other complex boundary issues (Housman & Stake, 1999).

As early as 1982, Edelwich and Brodsky (1982, 1991) identified three foreseeable (if not universal) negative consequences of allowing sexual relationships after termination: compromising of the therapeutic process by the anticipation of a possible love affair; denial of future safety and support in a therapeutic alliance that both parties have worked to create; and corruption of the subsequent personal relationship by the unequal power and privileged knowledge inherent in a therapist–patient relationship. Brown (1988) outlined dynamics by which serious harm could befall the patients involved, other patients, and the community. Concerns such as these led to recommendations that prohibition of sexual intimacies with former clients be written into professional ethics codes (Sell, Gottlieb, & Schoenfeld, 1986; Vasquez, 1991). Shopland and VandeCreek (1991) developed rationales for prohibition from the perspectives of psychodynamic theory, feminist/sexual abuse theory, and family systems theory. Like Edelwich and Brodsky, they hypothesized that when sexual relations occur after termination it is likely that the therapeutic role (objectivity, professional judgment, and concern for client welfare) was in some sense abandoned before termination; moreover, the illusion that termination means freedom from ethical constraints can only encourage such relationships.

As professional organizations took up this question in revising their ethics codes, Appelbaum and Jorgenson (1991) made a proposal intended to "balance the goals of protecting former patients and avoiding unnecessary interventions into consensual relationships" (p. 1466). In place of an absolute ban on posttermination relationships, they recommended a 1-year waiting period during which even social contact would be prohibited. Beyond 1 year after termination, a therapist would not be sanctioned for entering into an intimate relationship with a former patient, except in the case of defined categories of patients likely to remain highly vulnerable to undue influence. Those categories might include former patients in long-term dynamic psychotherapy, psychotic patients, and victims of past sexual abuse (Gonsiorek & Brown, 1989; Schoener, 1992).

In formulating this proposal, Appelbaum and Jorgenson took into account the wide range of patient populations with different diagnoses, vulnerabilities, and prognoses, together with the shift to short-term, non-transference-based therapies with a time-limited sense of fiduciary responsibility. Empirically, they questioned the reliability and validity of research purporting to demonstrate the persistence of transference over time. Moreover, they noted that, both in their own extensive forensic and legal experience and in that of the Minneapolis Walk-In Counseling Center (see Schoener, 1992), only about 1% of cases of sexual contact with a former patient begin more than a year after termination. Thus, a rule prohibiting contact for at least 1 year would address the predominant modus operandi of predatory therapists while protecting patients from acting out their idealizing fantasies and dependency needs in the immediacy of the therapeutic exchange, with its potent dynamics and potentially coercive pressures.

A major concern raised by Appelbaum and Jorgenson was that a permanent ban on intimate relationships between therapists and former patients might not be legally sustainable in light of the constitutional guarantee of freedom of association. A time-limited ban, while admittedly an oversimplified response to complex dynamic processes, would keep the regulatory and enforcement process manageable by avoiding the need for intrusive investigations of personal relationships while still catching the worst and most frequent offenders.

Appelbaum and Jorgenson's position is supported by Schoener's (1992) report, based on consultation in several thousand cases of alleged therapist–patient sex, that "the vast majority of complaints of post-termination exploitation come in situations where there has not really been a termination or in which there was a 'quickie termination' to justify sex" (p. 981). From another perspective, Malmquist and Notman (2001) have questioned whether the use of the concept of transference (itself continually debated and revised within psychoanalysis) meets current standards of scientific acceptance in the legal arena. Transference inevitably occurs in a wide range of human relationships. Intimate personal relationships are regularly compromised by undue influence, coercion, and various dysfunctional circumstances even in the absence of a prior therapeutic relationship. Therefore, the corruption of a subsequent personal relationship by the emotional residue of a therapeutic relationship may not be as appropriate a basis for professional and legal restrictions as the corruption of the therapeutic relationship itself. Malmquist and Notman cite the international perspective provided by Coleman (1988), who found that other countries limited regulation of posttermination sex to the ethical as opposed to the legal arena and generally declined to regulate such consensual behavior except in cases where the sexual relationship arose directly out of the therapeutic relationship.

These considerations notwithstanding, Appelbaum and Jorgenson's (1991) article in the *American Journal of Psychiatry* was answered by numerous letters, most of them in vigorous dissent to their proposal. In 1993 the American Psychiatric Association moved in the opposite direction from that favored by Appelbaum and Jorgenson. Its ethical guidelines previously had stated that sexual involvement with a former patient "almost always is unethical." Those words were revised to read "Sexual activity with a current or former patient is unethical" (American Psychiatric Association, 2006). The American Psychological Association (2002) and the American Association for Marriage and Family Therapy (2001)

provide for a 2-year waiting period but strongly discourage sexual relations with former patients even after that interval, thereby placing the
burden on a psychologist to show (if a case comes under scrutiny) that his
or her conduct was not injurious and exploitative. The National Association of Social Workers (1999) places the same burden of proof on a social
worker, but without specifying a waiting period. Clinicians should also
be aware of restrictions imposed by state licensing laws, which may differ
from those of professional organizations.

Since 1991 the American Medical Association has prohibited sexual
contact between physicians and former patients, with no time limitation,
"if the physician uses or exploits the trust, knowledge, emotions, or influence derived from the previous professional relationship." This rule takes
into account the widely varying contexts of patient–physician relationships, ranging from the impersonal to the emotionally involving. However, it may place too much faith in the capacity of physicians to discrimi-
nate among those contexts. Most physicians are not trained to evaluate
the ongoing potential for undue influence in a relationship. It is all too
easy to rationalize "Oh, no, that's not me" when even a straightforward
surgical procedure can create, on the patient's part, a feeling of attachment to the physician who "saved my life." The AMA rule necessitates, in
effect, a retrospective investigation of the dynamics of every relationship
between a physician and a former patient that becomes a matter of dispute (see Appelbaum, Jorgenson, & Sutherland, 1994).

The *reductio ad absurdum* of termination of therapy with sex in mind
is the facetious example in which the therapist looks down at his watch
and says, "Let's see, we're terminating at one o'clock; see you for dinner
at seven" (Edelwich & Brodsky, 1991, p. 96). Unfortunately, numerous actual cases fit Schoener's (1992) description of no real termination or "a
'quickie termination' to justify sex." In one such case, a Pennsylvania
court affirmed a licensing board's revocation of a psychologist's license
for sexual misconduct even though the last billed therapy session took
place 2 months prior to the first act of sexual intercourse with the patient.
The court found no evidence that formal termination of therapy had been
discussed before the sexual relationship began. Moreover, during the last
paid therapy session the therapist sat next to the patient, held her hand,
and told her he loved her (*Morris v. State Board of Psychology*, 1997). In another variation on this theme, the Supreme Court of Washington upheld
severe disciplinary sanctions against a social worker who began a 2-year
sexual relationship with a patient the day after therapy was concluded.
Prior to termination, the social worker had suggested to the patient that
the two might become friends after therapy ended. During the final ses-

sion, their conversation became intimate and sexually suggestive. The court agreed with lower courts that the social worker had engaged in unprofessional conduct that rendered her unfit to practice (*Heinmiller v. Dept. of Health*, 1995).

The idea of a "waiting period" after which intimate relationships with former patients become permissible is itself not impervious to being lampooned. In an actual case in the authors' consultative experience, the therapist looked up at the calendar at the time of termination and informed the patient, "We can start having sex 1 year from today." Yet, an absolute ban on posttermination intimacy can likewise be reduced to absurdity at the limits of its application, as in the following example:

> You are a psychiatrist providing weekend coverage for a colleague. A patient of your colleague's who has run out of medications comes to the emergency room, and you write a refill prescription to enable the patient to get through the weekend. As you realize, seeing and prescribing for this patient establishes a treatment relationship between the two of you. She is "your patient," if only until her regular doctor returns. For one thing, you can be held liable for any harmful effects of the medications you have prescribed.
>
> Ten years later you meet the same woman at a party and begin a dating relationship. What's the problem? You may not even remember seeing this person in the emergency room, and she may not remember you. But if the situation comes to light, you are "having sex with a former patient."

The policies of some human service agencies take into account that transference and undue influence are unlikely to develop when a staff member gives a client practical assistance on a single occasion. Until 1993, as noted above, the American Psychiatric Association's ethics code allowed for obvious exceptions such as the one in the instant case by specifying that sexual activity with a former patient "almost always is unethical." The revised code, by declaring sex with current and former patients alike to be unethical, raises the specter of indiscriminate enforcement. Most likely, in the hypothetical situation described here, an ethics committee would issue a warning letter without such lasting consequences as an entry in the National Practitioner Data Bank. Still, you cannot count on an ethics committee or licensing board to respond reasonably. Just as a flexible rule invites manipulation and exploitation, an absolute rule risks abusive enforcement.

If the harmful consequences even of sexual relations with current patients can vary, it is hardly surprising that those of posttermination intimacy can also be unpredictable. Spindler (1992) reported the case of a woman who was traumatized by having sex with her ex-therapist 15 years after an apparently successful termination of therapy. In subsequent therapy the patient came to understand that her previous therapy had ended with a transient transference "cure" based on her wish to repeat a childhood sexual experience of which both she and her therapist had been unaware.

Yet, there have also been posttermination relationships with long-term outcomes such as the following:

> In the 1970s a male therapist who was treating a female patient was advised by his supervisor that he appeared to have romantic issues about the patient. While the therapist was considering whether to work through the issues or refer the patient to another clinician, the patient told him that she wanted to terminate in order to start "seeing" him socially. The therapist agreed to terminate but informed the patient about the "1-year rule" then in effect at his agency. Several months later the patient called the therapist and announced, "I don't play by anybody else's rules." The two began dating. As their relationship developed, they spent much time processing (with each other, though not with a supervisor or consultant) questions about unequal disclosure and undue influence that arose from their therapist–patient relationship.
>
> The couple married and raised a family. Twenty years after giving up their therapeutic relationship in favor of a personal one, they were afraid to tell people how they had met because of the hypercritical climate of opinion that had since arisen.

It was with such cases in mind that Schoener (1992) wrote: "Regarding marriage to former patients, do we denigrate or declare such relationships as a priori exploitive? If so, what about the children who result, some of whom also enter our field as therapists?" (p. 981).

Although some professional organizations as well as some laws and regulations do provide for time-limited prohibitions, "once a patient, always a patient" remains the consensus in the mental health professions (Edelwich & Brodsky, 1991, pp. 93–112; Epstein, 1994, pp. 218–220; Gabbard, 2005; Simon, 1992). Inhibition, avoidance of issues, selective self-presentation, or overt or subtle bribes (on either side) motivated by the prospect of future personal gratification can undermine any form of therapy. As Gabbard (2005) has written:

> Neither party can speak freely about their observations if they want to preserve a positive image in the eyes of the other. It is only by virtue of the

fact that the therapist–patient relationship will never be anything but professional that patients can speak freely about all of their problems. (p. 31)

Other concerns, not involving intentional manipulation, apply specifically to psychodynamic therapy. For instance, in the absence of a structure that precludes acting on romantic fantasies, a therapist may repress feelings which, if safely acknowledged and explored, might contribute to understanding the patient (Sonnenberg, 1992).

Epstein (1994) summarizes the prevailing viewpoint as follows:

> In my opinion, legalistic arguments about permissible waiting periods ignore the fundamental purpose of the therapeutic frame. I do not believe it possible for a therapist to conduct coherent psychotherapy unless he or she can *permanently* relinquish the prospect of *ever* obtaining gratification from the patient for *anything* besides the contracted compensation. The treatment frame is a reflection of the therapist's ego boundaries. If a therapist *seriously* entertains an actual plan for sex with a patient after termination, it suggests that he or she suffers from impaired ego boundaries. (p. 219)

An appropriate termination, in which therapist and patient reflect on the progress that has been made, does not imply that therapy is "over." On the contrary, the patient needs to be free to come back to resume the process of reflection when called for. Often the patient does come back, even years later, to undertake a piece of work that builds on the work previously done. Not only in psychodynamic therapy, but in cognitive-behavioral therapy as well, patients confronting new problems or variations of old problems regularly benefit from the continued availability of a therapist whose guidance has been helpful before. Once professional boundaries have been crossed and the patient and therapist have become lovers, business partners, or even friends who meet to gossip over lunch, that guidance is no longer available.

Even if the patient does not return to the therapist's office, it is valuable (some would say essential) for the therapist to retain a special place in the patient's consciousness as a remembered guide and mentor. This process of internalization ("What would Dr. So-and-So say?") is analogous to the assimilation of parental values, standards, and behavioral maxims. Such ongoing consultation with one's "inner therapist" (psychodynamic, cognitive-behavioral, or whatever) is also sacrificed when professional boundaries are breached.

For the practicing clinician, then, the dilemmas posed by the

Appelbaum–Jorgenson proposal are best resolved by recognizing that there are different spheres of regulation, each with its own valid application, including civil law, criminal law, regulation by licensing boards and professional associations, and voluntary self-restraint. Although an outright prohibition of intimate relationships with former clients may not be sustainable constitutionally or advisable from policy and administrative standpoints, the clinician can and should simply choose to forgo such problematic relationships. As Simon (1992) concludes:

> Suffice it to say that the most credible clinical position for a therapist is to stay out of the patient's life after treatment ends. The patient should be allowed to go forward with his or her life, unencumbered by the therapist and the inevitable psychological baggage carried over from treatment. (p. 280)

Nonsexual Relationships after Termination

Nonsexual posttherapy contacts (both accidental and deliberate) have been subjected to a scrutiny parallel to that accorded sexual contacts but with a greater range of both opinions and actual incidence reported. In a survey of 327 psychologists (52% male, 99% with doctoral degrees) who had been practicing psychotherapists for an average of 14 years, 29% reported that they had engaged in business relationships with former patients, compared with 6.5% reporting sexual relationships (Lamb et al., 1994). Male respondents were four times as likely to report sexual relationships and significantly more likely to report business relationships than female respondents. Respondents (on average) regarded sexual relationships with former clients as very inappropriate within the first year after termination and somewhat inappropriate even after 3 years. Business relationships, on the other hand, were viewed as less inappropriate than sexual relationships at any time, and ratings of inappropriateness decreased at a steeper rate with the passage of time for business than sexual relationships. Respondents varied more widely in their ratings of business than sexual relationships, in part because some respondents took into account the lack of business alternatives in isolated communities, and considered some types of business relationships (e.g., patronizing a store owned by a former patient) more acceptable than others (e.g., employing a former patient).

In an exploratory study of psychologists' nonsexual, nonromantic relationships with former patients, 63 respondents reported on 91 incidents of intentional as well as circumstantial contacts (Anderson & Kitchener,

1996). These included friendships and other personal relationships, social interactions and events, business or financial relationships, collegial or professional relationships, supervisory or evaluative relationships, work-place relationships, and combinations of the foregoing (e.g., collegial or professional plus social). Predictably, this wide range of situations yielded a full spectrum of attitudes about the ethical propriety of such contacts. Of particular interest is the finding that none of the participants who described friendships with ex-patients saw them as ethically problematic. By contrast, a majority of those who described less deliberate forms of repeated, mutually revealing contact found those relationships ethically problematic. Examples include the therapist's becoming a neighbor of a former client, a former client's dating a child of the therapist, or a former client's marrying a friend of the therapist's spouse.

Overall, a majority of respondents in Anderson and Kitchener's study considered the posttermination relationships they had participated in or observed to be ethically appropriate. This finding differs from those of surveys (e.g., Borys & Pope, 1989) in which clinicians, asked to evaluate such dual relationships in the abstract, have responded in a more judgmental way. It is likely that clinicians who have actually experienced or witnessed posttherapy contacts with patients have formed a deeper appreciation of the complexities of those situations and have been in a position to assess potential harms on an individualized basis. Nonetheless, respondents expressed considerable unease about the complications those relationships could create. Typical of their concerns was a comment made by one of the participants who judged the business or financial relationships they described to be ethically problematic:

> My relationship with the former client as the former therapist causes me to cut this person slack [in two business or financial arrangements]. . . . The former client thrives and appears to benefit greatly, but I'm not always so sure it is good for me. Also it could cause too much dependency on me (Anderson & Kitchener, 1996, p. 62).

A useful finding of this study was that the harmful consequences of posttherapy contacts can often be minimized by anticipating problems that may cause discomfort, discussing them before termination, and agreeing on clear boundaries. Some respondents also found that when they did choose to form some kind of relationship with a former patient, it was helpful to process the therapeutic and personal implications of the situation and to maintain two-way communication as needed.

Gartrell (1992) examined the dilemmas of managing relationships with former clients in a lesbian community. Among the considerations she cited for avoiding friendships with former clients (besides those already outlined in this chapter) were the following:

> When clients state a desire to establish a friendship with me after termination, they typically anticipate that I will continue to be as caring, supportive and available as I have been as a therapist. Such clients do not desire a true friendship, but rather an extension of the therapeutic relationship in a more informal way. Rarely has the expectation that the friendship would involve *mutual* care-taking and support been expressed. And when that desire has been expressed, clients have only a one-dimensional picture of me, which has not included any opportunity to judge my potential as a friend (p. 46).

In addition, Gartrell noted, she could not possibly have the time or inclination to offer friendship to all former clients, nor could she elevate some ex-clients to the special status of friend while leaving others to feel rejected (which could undo gains made in therapy). These considerations are especially relevant in a community bound together by interest, lifestyle, and personal identification, where clients and former clients are especially likely to have ongoing contacts with the therapist and with one another. In such an environment, Gartrell chose to cultivate "a style that allows *friendliness, but not friendship*" (p. 46).

Gartrell's resolution of this issue is essentially similar to Borenstein and Fintzy's (1980–1981) advice to psychoanalysts who come into contact with former patients. They recommended a friendly, cordial response, neither excessively aloof nor excessively intimate, as best serving the ex-patient's growth and development (cf. Schachter, 1990, 1992). These seasoned observers point the way for mental health clinicians of any profession or background to cope sensibly with what might seem limitless permutations and combinations of contacts with former patients. It may take a long time for professional organizations to sort out the relevant distinctions and set workable standards in this area, especially with respect to nonsexual relationships. That is not to mention the wildly inconsistent disposition of cases by courts and licensing boards. (See Chapter 11 for the case of a senior clinician who suffered serious consequences for hiring two former patients as housepainters.) In any event, no professional standards or regulations are likely to capture all the nuances and wrinkles that can appear in the world outside the consulting room. Nonetheless, for the clinician who stays focused on clinical, ethical, and legal responsibilities, a little common sense can go a long way.

The position that has been developed in this chapter is that a clinician can best serve patients by maintaining an ongoing sense of ethical and fiduciary responsibility, at least to the extent of avoiding undue influence or intrusion into the patient's life, thereby allowing the patient the prerogative of resuming therapy if and when needed. In other words, one's ethical stance is no different and one's conduct little different whether one is dealing with a current or a former patient. It follows from that axiom that the guidelines presented in Chapter 6 for responding to inadvertent out-of-office contacts with patients apply to former patients as well.

Judgment is called for, of course, in navigating circumstances such as isolated communities (e.g., geographic, religious, or gay and lesbian), unavoidable collegial contacts with ex-patients who are involved in the mental health professions, and regular personal contacts brought about by, say, children or mutual friends. Other kinds of judgments are called for as well, such as whether shopping at a store owned or operated by an ex-patient will necessitate direct personal contact with the patient. Obviously, there is a difference between paying a standard price for a product off the shelf and entering into business deals with a former patient. The latter raises the same questions of undue influence, endangering the gains made in therapy, and precluding future therapy that call for avoidance of sexual relationships with former clients.

KEY REMINDERS

- Sexual misconduct and other serious boundary violations are destructive to therapy and have been documented to cause foreseeable (although not universal) harm to patients.

- In addition to potential harms that need to be evaluated on a case-by-case basis, sexual misconduct by psychotherapists results in a failure to provide appropriate therapy, the provision of substandard therapy, and a lost window of opportunity for the patient to progress both in therapy and in life.

- In a phenomenon that has been termed "cessation trauma," the damage done by a sexual relationship with a therapist often becomes devastatingly evident to the patient when the relationship ends.

- Sexual relationships with former patients are prohibited or strongly discouraged by the major mental health professional organizations, both because questions of undue influence remain and because of the value of preserving the availability of the therapist (as well as the internalized persona of the therapist) for consultation.

CHAPTER 10

Vulnerabilities

W hat makes a therapist more likely to engage in serious boundary violations? Are some types of patients especially vulnerable to boundary violations? Recurring patterns in the case vignettes in Part II suggest that it is possible to identify risk factors that make boundary challenges and transgressions more likely. This chapter briefly summarizes those risk factors, or vulnerabilities, both in therapists and in patients, followed by some issues specifically related to the therapist's and patient's gender. Knowing these danger signs is useful for prevention— whether for an individual, agency, institution, or profession—as outlined in Chapter 13.

It is worth reemphasizing that to analyze the patient's contribution to the dynamic interaction is not to blame the patient for conduct for which the therapist bears sole ethical responsibility. The three axioms presented in Chapter 1 apply here, as does the discussion in Chapter 2 on the inherent vulnerability of the therapeutic dyad. Repeated one-to-one encounters in a setting deliberately isolated for privacy, with highly personal information disclosed and feelings expressed, provoke challenges to the very boundaries they necessitate. Add to this setup a patient's need to idealize, a therapist's wish to be idealized, and the rescue fantasies of both parties, and you have what Robert Hilton (1997b) has called "the perils of the intimacy of the therapeutic relationship." Hilton describes these perils as follows:

> In summary, effective psychotherapy involves an intimate relationship in
> which both client and therapist are in peril. The peril is in being open

authentically to each other to the degree that each faces potential re-traumatization at the other's hands. The client must challenge the "role" of the therapist in order to feel safe, chosen, and back in control of his life. The therapist needs his role challenged in order to recover his true self, to affirm his self-esteem as a person, and to accept his limits as a good parent. This is not an easy task, and often the therapist, while unconsciously wanting and needing the confrontation when it comes, responds defensively by moving away, against, or toward the client. The "role" of the therapist functions as a form of self-organization and beneath this role lie all of the unmet needs and emotions of a frightened and disorganized child. Yet the therapist is responsible for having worked enough with these unmet needs to be able to invite the client where he needs to go. (p. 85)

Acknowledgment of this mutual vulnerability, while maintaining protective limits and responsibility for the client's well-being, is part of the foundation of the relational model of therapy developed by feminist therapists (Jordan, 1995; Miller & Stiver, 1997). This and other theoretical frameworks are represented in the sources cited here in order to indicate both the different terms in which therapists' vulnerabilities can be conceived and the universality of the underlying concerns.

The sealed-off environment in which therapy often takes place can turn into a "magic bubble," a collusion of mutual admiration and/or mutual need that becomes impervious to the restraining influences of consultation, supervision, good judgment, and common sense (Gutheil, 1989). This potential pitfall is there in any therapeutic dyad but is especially hazardous for therapists and patients with the characteristics identified in the following sections.

In the brief profile descriptions that follow, you may recognize yourself, a colleague, a supervisee, a patient, or someone concerning whom you are consulted. Some of these profiles have been constructed with specific reference to sexual boundary violations. Nonsexual boundary violations do not necessarily lead to sexual misconduct; however, therapist sexual misconduct tends to occur in the context of a progression of boundary violations. Therefore, the sexual misconduct profiles in this chapter may also apply, in substantial degree, to therapists and patients involved in the full range of boundary violations, such as financial exploitation, inappropriate self-disclosure, and inappropriate social or physical contact.

Of course, there are variations within this picture. A lonely therapist in a midlife crisis who "falls in love" with a patient is more likely to be taken advantage of financially by the patient than to profit illegitimately from the relationship. Conversely, a therapist who engages in "insider trading" on the basis of financial information unwittingly disclosed by a patient may not commit any boundary violations—least of all sexual—of which the patient is aware. Then there is the psychopath or sociopath who can be characterized as a polyexploiter, victimizing patients socially, sexually, financially, spiritually, and morally.

VULNERABLE THERAPISTS

New Yorker writer Janet Malcolm's book title, *Psychoanalysis: The Impossible Profession* (Malcolm, 1994), reflects a common perception. Psychotherapy is indeed a difficult occupation (Coale, 1998; Hedges, Hilton, Hilton, & Caudill, 1997; Sussman, 1995a). In numerous ways therapists put themselves on the line—personally, emotionally, professionally, and legally. Vulnerability to boundary violations is not limited to antisocial or severely impaired individuals. Thus, typologies of therapists susceptible to boundary challenges and excursions should not be taken to obscure the risk that this could happen to anyone (Norris et al., 2003). Indeed, one's vulnerability may arise from the very motivation that brought one into the profession—to help others. Sussman (1995b) lists some of the unconscious motives that can lead a person to the practice of psychotherapy (cf. Sussman, 1992):

- The wish for magical powers
- The hope of being admired and idolized
- The hope of making up for the damage one believes one inflicted on one's family as a child
- The hope of transcending one's own aggression and destructiveness
- The hope of escaping one's own problems by focusing on those of other people
- The hope of holding on to or becoming like one's own therapist
- The hope of achieving a deep level of intimacy within a safe context
- The hope of meeting one's own dependency needs vicariously by attending to those of one's patients
- The hope of transcending ordinary limitations and frustrations by achieving breakthroughs in understanding and interpersonal connection

These observations are consistent with the characterization of psycho-therapists as "wounded healers" who choose this line of work to heal themselves vicariously (Eber & Kunz, 1984; Groesbeck & Taylor, 1977). Miller (1981) has elaborated the theory that many psychotherapists were compelled as children to satisfy their parents' unconscious expectations at the expense of their own emotional and developmental needs. As a re-sult, they are at risk for acting out unresolved narcissistic conflicts at the expense of dependent, vulnerable patients.

Genova (2001) analyzes the impact of these personal dynamics from a cultural and evolutionary perspective. In this analysis, the therapeutic dyad developed as a makeshift, not very workable, substitute for the emotional reciprocity with which people met one another's needs and re-sponded to one another's suffering in traditional communities. Accord-ing to Genova:

> As isolated and anonymous individuals encounter each other, having lit-tle past or future together, two things happen. The first is that, without the support of a true community, the limits of an individual helper's re-sources are reached sooner and more often. There are not enough helpers to go around. The second is that the help seeker often brings a greater backlog or depth of unmet need, as well as depth of frustration if current needs are not met, to each encounter. In this context—on purely Darwin-ian grounds—altruism ceases to be so attractive. Competing and more immediate self-preservation instincts gain a stronger position. The helper often shifts, under their influence, to strategies that are sure, in the near term, to conserve resources: ways of obtaining immediate gratification or discharging uncomfortable affect at the help seeker's expense. It is in this perverse sense that the helper is trying to make his originally altruistic in-volvement deliver some reciprocal benefit, or at least stop being a drain. (p. 64)

Mental health professionals have resorted to sanctioned ways of in-sulating themselves from the onrush of human need that would otherwise engulf them. Some do it by relying heavily on prescribing medications; oth-ers retreat into research, administration, or private practice with a selected clientele. Boundary violators, Genova believes, are often those who, unable to resort successfully to these distancing mechanisms, are left to practice (in Malcolm's words) an impossible profession. The absence of a nurturing community creates a substantial risk that the therapist will join the patient in "a regressive longing for the world of the perfectly nurtured child" (p. 66). This is an inherent vulnerability of the therapeutic dyad. Readers who wish to explore psychoanalytic interpretations of boundary transgres-sions can consult numerous sources (e.g., Apfel & Simon, 1985a; Celenza,

1991, 1998; Claman, 1987; Epstein, 1994, pp. 248–254; Gabbard, 1994a, 1995b; Gabbard & Lester, 2002; Gorkin, 1985; Kohut & Wolf, 1977; Marmor, 1976; Person, 1985, 2003; Shackelford, 1989; Twemlow, 1997).

Profiles of therapists at high risk for boundary violation have been found useful for a number of practical purposes. These include timely recognition and intervention in problematic situations, evaluation of patients' claims, assessment and rehabilitation of offenders, and self-help for clinicians. Typologies of therapists who become involved sexually with patients grew out of early studies of such therapists (Averill et al., 1989; Belote, 1974; Butler & Zelen, 1977; D'Addario, 1977; Dahlberg, 1970; Holroyd & Brodsky, 1977; Stone, 1975, 1976; Zelen, 1985). By now these classification schemes are based on clinical and forensic caseloads numbering in the hundreds or even thousands. The fact that authors with different clinical and theoretical perspectives identify similar themes provides a form of corroboration, pointing to a common reality under disparate vocabularies.

Schoener and Gonsiorek's Classification

The most comprehensive, widely used typology of offenders is based on the experience of the Walk-In Counseling Center of Minneapolis (Gonsiorek, 1995a; Schoener, 1995a; Schoener & Gonsiorek, 1989). It consists primarily of clinical diagnostic categories (some of them in language now outdated but easily translated into current nomenclature) and assessments of their potential for rehabilitation.

1. *Naïve.* This group consists of inadequately trained and/or inexperienced mental health professionals as well as non-mental health professionals (e.g., family physicians and clergy) who provide counseling services. They have an inadequate understanding of professional ethics and of the boundary between professional and personal relationships. These individuals usually respond well to appropriate retraining unless their psychological and interpersonal naiveté is characterological rather than situational.

2. *Normal and/or mildly neurotic.* This large group of boundary violators consists of situational offenders who, at a bad moment in their lives, let down their guard and "fall in love" with a patient. Whether the "slippery slope" of boundary violations progresses to sexual misconduct depends on the strength of internal and external restraints. These individuals almost always have only one victim, show remorse for their unethical conduct, and are good prospects for rehabilitation.

3. *Severely neurotic and/or socially isolated.* These therapists tend to have chronic problems with depression, feelings of inadequacy, low self-esteem, and social isolation. They often appear as overworked clinicians dedicated to their patients, but at the cost of meeting personal needs through their clinical work. Their boundary violations may progress to sexual intimacy in the same inadvertent way as occurs with situational offenders, but those transgressions tend to be repeated, albeit years apart, as long as the underlying deficits are not remedied. Therapists in this group vary in their potential for rehabilitation because of their longstanding intrapsychic and life problems.

4. *Impulse control disorders.* These individuals exhibit severe behavioral dyscontrol in a number of areas, such as financial crimes, sexual assaults or harassment, and a range of paraphilias. They act without sufficient appreciation of the consequences of their behavior. Although their relative lack of calculation leaves them open to exposure, they may still be found to have exploited many victims by the time they are caught. Clinical experience indicates that these individuals cannot be rehabilitated and therefore should be removed from positions where they can harm others.

5. *Sociopathic or narcissistic personality disorders.* Like the previous group, this one consists of repeat offenders. However, since their exploitation of patients is deliberate and calculated, they are better able to avoid detection. Usually highly skilled at manipulation, they may select vulnerable clients with little capacity to defend themselves and then stage-manage the therapeutic situation to facilitate inappropriate intimacies. Unlike those with impulse disorders, they are capable of behavioral control, which they employ as needed to give an appearance of propriety and maintain their professional reputation. Their manipulativeness extends to appearing remorseful when caught and making a show of participation in a rehabilitation program. In fact, they are almost always impervious to character change and should be removed from positions of clinical responsibility.

6. *Psychotic and severe borderline disorders.* This is a small group characterized by significantly impaired reality testing and general functioning. Because of their severe, chronic impairments, the future behavior of these individuals tends to be unpredictable, and therefore they are not considered amenable to rehabilitation and reinstatement as clinical professionals.

7. *Sex offenders.* These are pedophiles and other aggressive sex offenders, including sexual sadists and frotteurs, who may also suffer from mental disorders or character traits associated with the groups listed

above (see Simon, 1999). They commit offenses that would be criminal even outside the context of therapy. Although sex offenders' potential for rehabilitation in general society remains a matter of debate, the health care and clerical professions offer such a temptation to reoffend that these are generally not considered appropriate work settings for such individuals.

8. *Medically disabled individuals.* These are therapists whose inappropriate behavior is caused not by disorders or deficiencies of character but by medical conditions, most commonly neurological impairments or bipolar mood disorder. In the latter case, a therapist during a manic episode may engage in out-of-character impulsive acts, such as sexual behavior contrary to one's usual sexual orientation (behavior otherwise uncommon among therapists who violate sexual boundaries). In the absence of an underlying character disorder, the rehabilitation potential of medically impaired therapists depends on the treatability of their medical condition (e.g., brain damage or mood disorder).

9. *Masochistic/self-defeating individuals.* This category, added by Schoener and Gonsiorek after it was first proposed by Gabbard (1994a; Gabbard & Lester, 2002, pp. 113–114), resembles that of overworked, chronically depressed, socially isolated clinicians, with an added risk factor. These therapists find themselves unable to resist (as it is their responsibility to do) the insistent boundary-breaking demands of patients, typically those with personality disorders. As the patient demands extended sessions, hand holding and hugging during sessions, frequent off-hours telephone calls, reduced or no fees, and eventually a sexual relationship, the therapist feels increasingly tormented and helpless. According to Gabbard (1994a), such therapists have internal conflicts about setting limits, which they feel is sadistic. In some cases acting out their own childhood abuse as well as the patient's, they turn their aggression inward, choosing to suffer instead of making the patient suffer. Some therapists who have exhibited this pattern have described having sexual relations with the patient as an out-of-body experience characterized by numbing, dissociation, and depersonalization, much like a rape or incest victim—or a patient seduced by a therapist. (This analogy does not, of course, diminish the therapist's ethical responsibility for the boundary violation.) Afterward, they often acknowledge their unethical conduct, seek help, and throw themselves on the mercy of the authorities. Although therapists in this group do not act in a deliberately exploitative way, their deeply dysfunctional personality structure makes their prognosis for rehabilitation guarded.

Variations and Elaborations

Psychiatric Disorders

To supplement Schoener and Gonsiorek's (1989) classification scheme, which is not based strictly on standard diagnostic terminology, a brief discussion using current diagnostic categories may be helpful. Therapists with Axis I psychiatric disorders represent a relatively small proportion of boundary violators. The mentally ill therapist who engages in boundary violations typically suffers from a psychotic disorder of the affective type. Mania or hypomania and substance abuse are found with some frequency (Gutheil, 1999b). However, the most common diagnoses are personality disorders (Axis II) (Gutheil, 2005b, 2005c). Narcissistic, antisocial, borderline, histrionic, dependent, and schizoid personality traits are all associated with a heightened risk of sexual and other boundary violations. For evident reasons, the risk is especially high with patients who have similar traits or other vulnerabilities. Although paraphilias or perversions are also a risk factor, clinicians who act on such impulses with patients usually are found to have a personality disorder on the narcissistic-to-antisocial continuum (Gabbard & Lester, 2002).

Claman (1987), Epstein and Simon (1990), Gabbard and Lester (2002, pp. 117–121), Gutheil (1999b, 2005c), and Strean (1993) emphasize the preponderance of narcissistic traits and issues among boundary violators. Predatory repeat offenders, as opposed to those who are vulnerable and needy for love, tend to have severe narcissistic personality disorders with prominent antisocial features. Gabbard and Lester (2002, pp. 117–121) identify six common (though far from universal) themes in the narcissistic struggles of therapists who violate sexual boundaries with patients:

1. Grandiosity
2. Sadomasochistic conflicts
3. A tendency toward action over reflection
4. Superego disturbance
5. Perception of a deficit in the patient that requires an enactment to be filled
6. Overvaluation of the power of love to heal both therapist and patient

The "Lovesick" Therapist

Gabbard (1994a; Gabbard & Lester, 2002, pp. 96–113) has analyzed the dynamics underlying various situations in which a therapist "falls in love" with a patient. "Lovesick" therapists generally correspond to the second or third of Schoener and Gonsiorek's types. They differ from sociopathic predators in that they tend to become involved with one particular patient rather than a succession of patients. Although they may exhibit various psychopathologies that were outlined above, their narcissistic conflicts typically are less severe than those of habitual offenders. Often they practice competently and ethically until, at a vulnerable moment, they encounter a "special" patient who, for whatever reasons, engages their neediness. In the presence of this patient the therapist seems to enter an altered state of consciousness in which normal judgment and restraint are suspended. This impairment usually does not carry over to the clinician's dealings with other patients. Twemlow and Gabbard (1989) estimated that half of all therapists who become sexually involved with patients can be characterized as lovesick rather than psychotic or psychopathic. There continues to be general agreement that this is the most common category of sexual boundary violator among both male and female therapists (Celenza, 1998; Celenza & Hilsenroth, 1997; Gutheil, 1999b).

The archetypal lovesick therapist is an aging man who, when experiencing a crisis of illness, bereavement, marital problems, career setbacks and disappointments, or fears of mortality, seeks reassurance and validation in an emotional attachment to a younger female patient (Epstein & Simon, 1990; Gutheil, 1999b). In some of these cases, attainment of high professional or institutional standing creates a form of narcissistic vulnerability, an illusion of being beyond accountability. How can you seek consultation when no one is as wise and as experienced as you are (Norris et al., 2003)?

Therapists who have difficulty tolerating loss and mourning may seek to avoid terminating with patients by forming personal relationships with them (Gutheil & Simon, 2002). The writer David Evanier (2002) described how his psychiatrist, a distinguished older man, took him into his home and family and asked him to be "my Boswell." After the psychiatrist's wife became ill with lymphoma, he became increasingly dependent on his young patient's companionship. As Evanier tells it:

> "My patients become my rescuers," he told me out of the blue one day on the way to the synagogue. I didn't know what to make of it until a colleague of his confided to me, "He's known for never letting go of his patients." And he added: "There was a time before you knew him when his capacities seemed unlimited. He had cancer when he was 40. He was not the same man after that."

After his wife died, this psychiatrist, then in his 70s, started dating his female patients.

Female therapists who are vulnerable to "lovesickness" include those for whom being a therapist provides a chance to bond intimately with other women. When the patient is male—typically a young man with behavioral problems, including impulsiveness and substance abuse— the therapist may be vicariously enjoying the patient's risk-taking lifestyle. Or she may be caught up in the common fantasy of rescuing and reforming a wayward, rowdy young man (Gabbard, 1994a; Gutheil, 1999b).

Common Fantasies

The "rowdy man" fantasy mentioned above is one example of the *rescue fantasy*. It often leads therapists—especially the less experienced and the "lovesick"—to become sexually involved with a patient. Indeed, the therapist's and patient's needs to rescue or be rescued may mesh into toxic reenactments of their respective pasts (Apfel & Simon, 1985a). This pathway to danger begins in a relatively benign way; it may be said that most successful therapeutic careers have their origins in rescue fantasies. It is when such fantasies are naively maintained and misdirected that they can turn into a belief that the therapist can save the patient singlehandedly rather than help the patient save himself or herself under therapeutic guidance.

Therapists who fail to monitor their attitudes toward patients also readily rationalize their way into the *exception fantasy*, in which they view themselves, the patient, or their relationship as uniquely exempt from ethical codes and boundaries (Gabbard, 1994a; Norris et al., 2003). One may set oneself apart from other therapists, explaining: "I can get away with doing things others can't. I realize that if someone else did this, it would be a problem, but I know what I'm doing. I'm kind of unorthodox; I like to do things my own way; but I'm very careful and I know what I'm doing." Likewise, one may see a particular patient as "special" because of beauty, youth, intellect, creativity, accomplishment, tragic victimization, or a heroic response to life's challenges. This perception may lead one to believe that "I have to be more flexible in my boundaries. I have to give this patient the love she did not get as a child." A tipoff to this loss of professional perspective is the admission that "I don't *usually* do this with my patients, but in this case. . . . " Contrary to all that is known about the dynamics of therapeutic interaction, the romantic relationship may be conceived of as pure and pristine, one made in heaven rather than in a highly specialized setting that is known and even designed to generate intense emotions. "You don't understand," the therapist will protest. "This has nothing to do with therapy. We're truly in love. We are soulmates who just happened to meet as therapist and patient. If we had found each other in any other circumstances, we'd have gotten married."

Finally, sexual boundary violations often involve the *fantasy of exclusivity*, wherein the therapist believes that "I am the only man or woman for this patient." Usually the patient is glad to agree until the fantasy is disproved on one side or the other. It can be traumatizing and demoralizing for a patient to learn that a therapist has "loved" other patients as well. Likewise, it is sobering and humbling, but only realistic, to understand that the patient—who has fallen in love with you as a therapist, not as a person—will likely fall in love with other therapists as well. Finding out that you're not "the one and only" is like learning that the universe does not revolve around the earth.

Clinicians would do well never to underestimate their potential for self-deception. Many therapists who engage in boundary violations insist, and believe, that they are acting in the patient's interest rather than their own. Evasion, externalization, and rationalization are used to deny the reality of boundary problems and their harmful consequences. As discussed in Chapter 13, consultation is the best protection against this failure of reality testing and loss of behavioral control; yet, the need for consultation is itself easily rationalized away in the service of unconscious motives and unexamined behavior (Gabbard, 2001; Norris et al., 2003). Thus, insulation from supervisory oversight and peer support is a common denominator of clinicians' vulnerability to boundary violation.

VULNERABLE PATIENTS

For patients, vulnerability comes with the territory. Anyone who brings deeply personal problems to the intimate setting of therapy is potentially susceptible to boundary challenges. In varying degrees, patients tend to be predisposed to cooperate with, love, or feel completely dependent on or compliant with a therapist. Simon (1999) has identified a number of magical themes in the therapeutic interchange. These take the form of images of the therapist *as perceived by the patient*, whether or not the therapist encourages such perceptions. A patient may see the therapist in one or more of the following ways:

- *Dr. Perfect*—the flawless representation of an ideal.
- *Dr. Prince*—the romantic idol who will rescue the patient.
- *Dr. Good Parent*—the nurturing parent substitute for whom the patient has longed.
- *Dr. Magical Healer*—the patient's savior.
- *Dr. Beneficent*—the devoted caretaker, like a nanny or baby doctor.
- *Dr. Indispensable*—the only clinician who can cure the patient.
- *Dr. Omniscient*—the one who knows and understands all.

The "Special" Patient

As outlined below, patients with certain specific vulnerabilities typically experience these magical hopes, expectations, and fantasies with heightened intensity and, for this and other reasons, will be more likely to act on them. Nonetheless, victims of serious boundary violations also include patients who appear to bring considerable strengths and attractive qualities to therapy. In Belote's (1974) sample of women who had been sexually involved with therapists, patients averaged 16.5 years younger than therapists, a finding consistent with other data (Gutheil, 1991). A patient's youth can contribute to vulnerability by causing the patient to be relatively naive and to submit more readily to the therapist as a respected authority figure. Youth, along with physical attractiveness (a related risk factor in this context), can also make a patient a more appealing victim, playing into the therapist's needs and fantasies. Intellectual capacities and attainments can likewise arouse a therapist's personal interest, feeding a shared or projected narcissism: "I'm special; you're special" (Gutheil, 2005a, p. 479). Thus, although youth, physical attractiveness, and intellectual accomplishment are not (strictly speaking) personal vulnerabilities, they can be precipitating factors, making patients with those characteristics more susceptible to exploitation. Clinical professionals, as patients, have been found to be disproportionately represented in samples of patients sexually involved with therapists (Quadrio, 1996). Recall, for example, the case of inappropriate touching of a female patient by a male psychiatrist discussed in Chapter 7. That patient had been a resident in psychiatry at the time of the events she described (Korn, 2003). The ethics case book of the American Psychoanalytic Association also contains illustrative examples (Dewald & Clark, 2001). Helping professionals are overrepresented in the known victim population in part because they are disproportionately likely to seek therapy (Scott & Hawk, 1986), including subsequent therapy after being sexually exploited by a therapist. They are especially visible to and readily accessed by those conducting clinical research surveys. At the same time, when the patient is also a clinician, a sense of commonality and mutual identification between patient and therapist may be fostered. A patient who is a clinical trainee may look up to a senior clinician as a teacher and model, and one who is a psychiatric nurse or social worker may defer to a therapist with an MD or PhD degree. From the other side, a therapist's potential for overidentification may be heightened by seeing a reflection of oneself (perhaps at an earlier stage of development) in the patient (Bridges, 1995b).

Korn's (2003) account of a knowledgeable patient's uncertainty and drift in the face of a progression of boundary violations is hardly unique. Another courageous patient, Carolyn Bates, contributed a detailed book-length account of how a rational and intelligent young woman could be drawn into sex with a therapist (Bates & Brodsky, 1989). Bates was admittedly naive. Naiveté, misplaced loyalty and trust, and disabling emotional conflicts are commonly experienced by educated, accomplished people in the therapy hour. Vulnerability can appear in selective forms; it can be context-dependent or relationship-dependent. More specifically, in the therapeutic relationship some articulate, high-functioning patients reveal primitive strivings and conflicts masked by their "normal" self-presentation, leading to unexpected boundary challenges (Gutheil, 2005a).

The double-edged character of patients' vulnerability to boundary violation is exemplified and illuminated by R. Hilton's (1997c) observations of therapists who misuse touch in therapy. These therapists tend to have trouble with two types of patients. The first is the "understanding" patient who offers the therapist the loving parental handclasp or hug that the therapist may not have received as a child. The second is the "innocent" patient whose childlike, defenseless manner calls forth the therapist's quasi-parental nurturance. In one case the patient is playing the role of the adult caretaker, outwardly composed and in control; in the other case the therapist assumes that role. Either way, however, both parties are acting out their respective vulnerabilities (see Butler & Zelen, 1977; Zelen, 1985).

A Common Thread of Vulnerability

Wohlberg (1990) found no single profile of patients involved in sexual relations with therapists. All gender and age combinations and a range of diagnostic categories were involved. However, she did find "commonalities," that is, recurring patterns, in the lives of the patient victims. She grouped these vulnerabilities into the categories of current loss, "marker events," and significant developmental turmoil. Loneliness, social isolation, divorce or other relationship loss, and serious medical illness are significant situational risk factors, since a deficit in the relational sphere feeds a longing to replace what has been lost. Among the members of a support group for victims of therapist sexual misconduct, Wohlberg found that approximately one-third were victims of previous incest, one-quarter to one-third were recovering alcoholics, and one-half to three-quarters were victims of other forms of abuse. These findings are consistent with other sources (Averill et al., 1989; Belote, 1974; D'Addario, 1977; Gutheil, 1991). It is possible, however, that individuals who have experience with support groups for substance abusers or victims of rape or incest may be especially predisposed to join similar groups for victims of therapists' misconduct and therefore may be overrepresented in such groups.

Gutheil (1992c, 1999b) has found a pattern of comorbidity among three overlapping conditions: past (typically childhood) sexual abuse, borderline personality disorder (and/or eating disorder or multiple personality disorder), and sexual abuse by therapists. As noted in the preceding chapter, identifying cause-and-effect relationships in this cluster is difficult, since (among other confounding factors) childhood sexual abuse is highly correlated with and may contribute to causing borderline personality disorder (Gabbard & Wilkinson, 1994, pp. 47–51; Gartner, 1996; Herman et al., 1989). Nonetheless, there are clearly identifiable dynamics by which both previous abuse and borderline personality disorder lead to increased vulnerability to therapeutic boundary violations.

A History of Abuse

In an Australian sample of 40 women who experienced sexual abuse in therapy, 68% had a history of either sexual or physical abuse in childhood, while only 10% reported no significant pathology in their families of origin. "Overall," Quadrio (1996) concluded, "the picture is one of gross family pathology" (p. 125). What distinguished these women, according to Quadrio, was "the intensity of their need to feel special, usually in proportion to the amount of abuse and/or neglect they had experienced in childhood." As a result, when their therapists responded to them in a positive, affirming way, "many responded with intense idealization. One may suggest that it is this reflected image of an idealized omnipotent and benevolent personage that is experienced as 'seductive' by offenders" (p. 126).

The prevalence of victims of previous abuse among patients sexually exploited by therapists has been regularly observed (DeYoung, 1981; Kluft, 1990; Luepker, 1989, 1999; Pope & Bouhoutsos, 1986). This relationship is so well established that it has been referred to as "sitting duck syndrome," conveying the vulnerability of the previously abused (Kluft, 1990). In some cases, the abuse victim may be engaged in a "repetition compulsion," an unconscious drive to repeat a trauma in order to master it. In the survivor of sexual trauma, the compulsive repetition of past abuse can take the form of sexualizing subsequent relationships, including the relationship with a therapist. Many incest victims cannot separate caring from sexuality. They have been conditioned to submit to the demands of an abusive authority figure in order to get any kind of attention and relatedness (Apfel & Simon, 1985a; Gorkin, 1985). A person conditioned to depend on an abusive relationship for emotional and even physical sustenance may lose, or fail to develop, the capacity to determine when boundaries are being violated and a relationship is becoming exploitative (Kluft, 1990). Indeed, early childhood abuse can create the expectation that the only "normal" relationship is an abusive one. It has been hypothesized that abuse victims can develop a kind of chemical dependence on the high-intensity, endorphin-releasing experiences produced by abusive interactions, which alone feel emotionally "real" to them (Herman et al., 1989; Van der Kolk, 1989).

Traumatized patients, made anxious by unaccustomed professional distance, may push against boundaries. They are processing the interaction through a historical, experiential filter in which hurt is anticipated, one in which the therapist becomes someone who must be feared, placated, and propitiated for them to get what they want or even to survive at all. Therapy, then, provides a documentary snapshot of a patient's characteristic pattern of relating to others. What the snapshot reveals can then be explored so that the patient no longer will need to reenact that pattern unconsciously and compulsively. Sometimes, though, instead of observing, exploring, and understanding, the therapist rushes in to play the part of the perfect parent, the idealized rescuer—or, worse, that of the actual, exploiting parent. As a result of the therapist's inappropriate, unethical actions, the patient risks being retraumatized.

Borderline Personality Disorder

Patients with borderline personality disorder are prominently represented among litigants in sexual misconduct cases, especially in the small percentage of cases in which the accusation is false (Gutheil, 1989). The neediness and self-dramatization associated with dependent and histrionic personality disorders and the manipulativeness characteristic of antisocial personality disorder also figure in the dynamics of boundary excursions (Gutheil, 2005b, 2005c). Even with actual offenses, both the disinhibition and the vengefulness characteristic of borderline patients make them more likely than other patients to bring legal or regulatory action against a therapist (Gutheil, 1999b). At the same time, there are compelling clinical reasons why borderline patients are especially susceptible to boundary violations and sexual exploitation (Averill et al., 1989; Gabbard, 1991, 1993; Gabbard & Wilkinson, 1994). The following dynamic factors in borderline personality disorder account at least in part for the tendency of these patients to evoke boundary violations of various kinds, including sexual acting out (Gutheil, 1989).

Rage

Borderline rage can intimidate even experienced clinicians into failing to set limits out of fear of the consequences of denying the patient's demands, whether for inappropriate social interaction, personal self-disclosures, or sex. Outwardly, the therapist fears the patient's volcanic response to being thwarted or confronted. Inwardly, the therapist may experience conflicts over his or her feelings of anger and aggression, which patients with borderline personality disorder are particularly likely to evoke. Thus, it is therapists in the "masochistic" category (discussed above) who are most vulnerable to this kind of coercion.

Borderline rage also fuels vengeful action such as the filing of specious legal claims and ethics complaints. False accusations of boundary violations often come about as an expression of rage that the patient feels so strongly as to justify a disregard for truth. Indeed, pathological lying, arising from a number of primitive dynamics, is characteristic of borderline patients (Snyder, 1986).

Neediness and/or Dependency

The neediness and dependency that patients with borderline personality disorder can project call forth the therapist's nurturance, sometimes to the point of overinvolvement. Implicitly and explicitly, the patient entreats and challenges the therapist, on pain of disappointing or appearing to abandon the patient, to become the idealized parent/rescuer who may, in fact, lurk within the therapist's narcissistic fantasies.

Boundary Confusion

Under stress, patients with borderline personality disorder may lose touch with the boundary between "I" and "you" and (through mechanisms such as fusion and projective identification) play on a therapist's weak boundaries to induce similar confusion in the therapist. If the therapist colludes in this boundary confusion, any perception of the real identities of both therapist and patient may be lost in the patient's intense affects, longings, and wishes.

Manipulativeness and Entitlement

Along with their ability to bend reality in the ways described above, patients with borderline personality disorder are known to exercise powerful skills of interpersonal manipulation. They are expert at persuading vulnerable therapists to override their own awareness of professional standards and limits—a transgression therapists often unwittingly acknowledge by explaining to a supervisor or consultant, "Although I don't usually do this with patients . . ." or even "Although I really don't think I should be doing this . . ." Such boundary compromises typically occur when a borderline patient invites a therapist to share in his or her narcissistic entitlement.

Another level of manipulativeness is employed by suicidal borderline patients, who, when their demands for deviation from normal practice are not met, may escalate by threatening suicide (Eyman & Gabbard, 1991). Finally, a patient's manipulations may reach into the legal or regulatory system when the patient (in a characteristically borderline maneuver) turns on the previously idealized therapist. High-functioning borderline patients have presented highly effective cases (however specious) once they move from the conflictual setting of therapy to official forums that reward their articulate, organized self-advocacy (Gutheil, 2005a).

In sum, patients with borderline personality disorder can present a bewildering and intimidating mix of impulsivity, dependency, narcissistic entitlement, boundary confusion, impaired reality testing, pansexuality, splitting, and manipulative mobilization of rescue fantasies. When other personality disorders (narcissistic, dependent, histrionic, antisocial) are also present, the dynamics can be all the more intense. Nonetheless, in keeping with the axioms reviewed at the beginning of this book, these dynamics and the provocations they generate do not justify any deviation from ethical, responsible practice. The therapist needs to be aware of these challenging dynamics and address them clinically and creatively in the patient's interest from within the professional role. Unfortunately, it is when the therapist as well as the patient manifests a personality disorder that the risk of boundary confusion—indeed, chaos—is greatest.

THE QUESTION OF GENDER

Clinical and forensic experience confirm the findings of survey research that the great majority of cases of sexual misconduct occur between a male therapist and a female patient. At the same time, about 20% of cases involve a female therapist (with either a male or female patient), and 20% involve same-sex pairings (Gabbard, 2005; Pope, 1994, pp. 14–20; Schoener et al., 1989). Cases involving a female therapist and a female patient considerably outnumber either the female therapist–male patient or male–male dyads. In a study of sexual misconduct complaints to the ethics committee of the American Psychiatric Association over a 5-year period, only 2 of 85 complaints against male psychiatrists alleged homosexual involvement, as opposed to 6 of 8 complaints against female psychiatrists (Mogul, 1992). To the extent that non-sexual boundary violations are fueled by a romantic dynamic potentially leading to sexual involvement, the same patterns would be expected to hold. However, the overall gender disparities are not as high as with sexual misconduct, since many boundary violations take place outside the nexus of romantic attraction. In particular, serious financial improprieties (except when linked with a sexual power dynamic) are not necessarily gender-driven. Gender and sexual orientation are not underlying causes of boundary violations, as are the personality, life-history, and situational factors discussed earlier in this chapter. However, people experience life as men or women, as straight or gay, and those identities are among the contexts in which boundary violations occur.

In one study of 40 women who had experienced sexual abuse in therapy, 90% of the offending therapists were male—a typical finding (Quadrio, 1996). Psychoanalytically oriented therapists analyze the sexualization of therapeutic relationships in all four possible dyads as arising from various forms of erotic transference (Gorkin, 1985; Person, 1985, 2003). At the same time, the larger social and historical context that shapes therapeutic relationships makes female patients vulnerable to sexual exploitation by male therapists. Quadrio (1996) reviews sociological, sociobiological, and feminist psychological theories that explicate pervasive, deeply ingrained patterns of dominance and submission, with patients and therapists acting out gender roles scripted for them by society or by their genes (cf. Belote, 1974).

In a courageous self-disclosure, Rutter (1989b) gives a personal face to such theories with an account of how he came close to a sexual relationship with "Mia," a 25-year-old patient with severe chronic depression growing out of a history of deprivation and loss. When Mia offered herself to him, Rutter reports, he "was overcome by an intoxicating mixture of the timeless freedom, and the timeless danger, that men feel when a forbidden woman's sexuality becomes available to them. I also sensed that if I went ahead with this sexual encounter, I would be able to count on Mia, as a well-trained victim, to keep our illicit secret" (p. 36). It was extremely unlikely, Rutter calculated, that he would have to answer to anyone if he took advantage of this patient's vulnerability. At that moment Rutter realized that the responsibility to keep Mia's therapy on track rested with him. He asked Mia, who had been kneeling at his feet like a supplicant, to return to her chair and began to explore how she was repeating a pattern of quickly giving herself away to men in order to hold their attention and interest. "To steer her toward the healthy side," he reflected, "I had to fight off some typically masculine components of my sexuality that were all too ready to accept Mia's self-destructive offering" (p. 36). The intense hopes, wishes, fantasies, and dependencies that some women bring to therapy as patients find an all too ready response in some men who are their therapists (Rutter, 1989a, 1989b; cf. Apfel & Simon, 1985a).

In the second most common pairing, that of female clinicians with female patients, the therapists tend to be lesbian, while the patients are a mixed group in terms of their usual sexual orientation. On the one hand, gay and lesbian therapists who are active in those communities face special challenges in maintaining appropriate boundaries between their personal and professional lives in what is often a "small world" (Brown, 1985; Davies & Gabriel, 2000; Gartrell, 1992; Gonsiorek, 1989, 1995b; Kessler & Waehler, 2005; Lyn, 1995; Moon, 2005). On the other hand, female therapists have been known to prey on vulnerable women just as their male counterparts do (Benowitz, 1995). As Gartrell (1992) has noted, "Exploitation of women by women is a serious concern in the lesbian therapy community, and the consequences can be devastating to involved clients" (p. 48). The following vignette exemplifies this opportunistic, self-gratifying behavior:

> A lesbian therapist had "forbidden" her female patient to stay with her long-term boyfriend on supposedly clinical grounds, citing him as the central problem. After the patient had broken up with him (and was consequently vulnerable by being both depressed and sexually deprived) the therapist shared her own personal fantasy of having intense sexual relations with the patient. This repeated boundary-violating self-disclosure and other seductive/coercive maneuvers moved the patient to participate in a prolonged sexual relationship with the therapist, which was poorly differentiated from therapy; for example, the dyad might be lying

entwined in the therapist's bed together, analyzing the patient's dreams. (Gutheil, 1991, p. 664)

Sexual relationships between female therapists and female patients may give more of an appearance of mutual participation and power equality than male–female dyads. In a study of female patients sexually exploited by female therapists, those couples socialized more openly than male–female dyads in similar studies, possibly because two women can more easily socialize together without being suspected of having a sexual relationship. Moreover, community norms may be more permissive of social relationships between female therapists and female patients (Benowitz, 1995). Yet, the female therapists in this study were more consistently the initiators of sexual contact—and did so earlier in therapy—than male therapists in other studies. The latter findings contradict the image of female therapist–patient dyads as expressions of spontaneous mutual affection. That image, a reflection of the belief that women generally are not abusive, may, in fact, inhibit victims from recognizing and calling attention to the exploitation.

Male victims of either male or female therapists have been relatively difficult to study, in part because sex-role stereotyping inhibits men from identifying themselves as victims (Gonsiorek, 1989, 1995b). Indeed, since men are stereotypically viewed as active initiators of sexual encounters, they are not readily perceived as victims. In a study of clinician–patient sex in an inpatient setting, staff members generally blamed the male patient rather than the female clinician who became sexually involved with him (Averill et al., 1989). Male patients often have difficulty seeing themselves as victims; instead, they may feel triumphant about their "conquest" of a female therapist (Gabbard, 1994a, 1994b; Gutheil & Gabbard, 1992). In Mogul's (1992) study of ethics complaints, the two complaints against female psychiatrists for alleged sexual contact with male patients did not come from the patients. On the contrary, both men defended the therapists against the charge of unethical behavior. In such cases, notwithstanding the patients' acceptance of what has occurred, the purposes of therapy have not been accomplished.

In the case of male patients and male therapists, a pattern has been observed in which the patient, isolated and somewhat schizoid, is made vulnerable by the lack of a charismatic paternal figure with whom to identify. The therapist offers such identification as an inducement to intimacy. One such patient tearfully recalled the therapist's calling him "my little blue-eyed beach boy"—terminology expressing possessiveness and relegation of the patient to the role of a child (Gutheil, 1991). (For an in-depth study of gay male clients sexually exploited by male therapists, see Robinson, 1993.)

Forensic experience indicates that, as a rule, therapists who have sexual relations with patients stay within their usual sexual orientation. Typically, they do not become involved with patients of both genders unless they already identify themselves as bisexual. However, some commentators have identified sexual identity confusion as a risk factor for therapist sexual misconduct. In this model, therapists may use their access to patients to experiment with sexual feelings with which they are uncomfortable (Benowitz, 1995; Gabbard, 1994a; Gonsiorek, 1989, 1995b; Quadrio, 1996). In some cases, therapists who are acting out a despised self-image may become sadistic toward patients in whom they see a reflection of that image.

While important, questions of gender can distract attention from basic clinical and ethical principles. A therapist and patient who are both homosexual may form a pseudopersonal, pseudocommunal bond that calls them away from the task of therapy. Likewise, a male patient may believe he "got lucky" when he was able to seduce a female therapist. These diversions, however, only perpetuate and often exacerbate the problems the patient brought to therapy. Sexual misconduct by therapists, regardless of the genders involved, always has the potential to cause serious harm.

POINTERS TO PREVENTION

Recognition of common risk factors for boundary violations contributes to informed vigilance about your own vulnerabilities, those of your patients, and those of the clinical settings in which you practice. Moreover, awareness of such risk factors makes clear the value of the protective and preventive factors, both work-related and personal, outlined in Chapter 13.

KEY REMINDERS

- Vulnerability to boundary violations is rooted in the dynamics of the therapeutic relationship as well as in the personalities and life histories that the therapist and patient bring to the interchange.
- Therapists involved in serious boundary violations range from situational offenders who are emotionally vulnerable at times of

personal loss, illness, or other life stress to habitual offenders with sociopathic or narcissistic personality disorders.

- Patients subjected to serious boundary violations commonly have been made vulnerable by a cluster of factors including social isolation, relationship loss, a history of sexual abuse, and borderline or other personality disorder.
- Gender and sexual orientation, although not underlying causes of boundary violations, are significant contextual factors determining how and with whom boundary violations occur.

CHAPTER 11

Understandings
and Misunderstandings

Concern with therapeutic boundaries has undergone a number of pendulum swings. As noted earlier in this volume, "boundary violation" originally meant only sexual intercourse with someone who was currently a patient. As understanding and sophistication increased about the spectrum of boundary problems (Edelwich & Brodsky, 1991; Epstein, 1994; Gabbard & Lester, 2002; Gutheil and Gabbard, 1993; Reamer, 2001; Simon, 1992), so did the potential for misconstruing the underlying psychological issues and practical dimensions (Gutheil & Gabbard, 1992, 1998; Martinez, 2000; Samuel & Gorton, 2001). Readers of some recent literature may feel pressured to steer a perilous course between the Scylla of total license ("Anything goes as long as you can talk about it") and the Charybdis of a list of absolute prohibitions.

This chapter examines the misunderstandings and pendulum swings of boundary theory that have developed during the past two decades. As we will see, those swings can be summarized in simple terms as "Boundary theory is too loose" (a variant of "bad apple" reasoning) and "Boundary theory is too tight" (the "backlash" response). Both of these extremes, it will be seen, ignore both flexibility and context. Our desired goal is to encourage a dynamically informed exploration of boundary issues while always respecting the axioms listed in Chapter 1. Nonetheless, a careful study of the misunderstandings can lead to a deeper understanding of the principles underlying boundary theory.

OBSTACLES TO DYNAMIC UNDERSTANDING
OF BOUNDARY ISSUES

Three obstacles that have made nuanced discussion of boundary issues difficult are the lure of reductionism, gender bias, and political correctness (Gutheil & Gabbard, 1992).

The Lure of Reductionism

Considering a dynamic interaction between two parties in a context-dependent way is difficult. Rather than as a map of possible pitfalls, it is much easier to view boundary questions as a simple list of forbidden acts. Among other errors, the reductionist view of boundary problems is of simple predator–prey interactions; the predator therapist is the metaphorical "bad apple." The authors' consultative experience reveals that boards of registration and licensing unfortunately succumb to the "list of forbidden acts" model, applying it mechanistically without regard for context. This error leads to false conclusions about boundaries and inappropriate penalties for therapists.

Gender Bias

Gender bias may also enter into reasoning here. Some audiences do not wish to hear about female therapists violating boundaries; it confounds the comfortable assumption that sexual misconduct always involves male therapists who abuse women. In an example witnessed by the authors, at a continuing education conference on sexual misconduct a speaker used a female therapist–male patient example to emphasize a point; two audience members complained that this was offensive since "everyone knew" that all sexual misconduct was instigated by men. In reality, of course, all four gender pairings have been identified in sexual misconduct episodes, although male therapist–female patient is the most common.

Political Correctness

Political correctness also may enter into the discussion in two main ways. First, as discussed earlier, some patients involved in boundary problems with therapists seem to be able to walk away with relatively little psychic damage. This is a politically incorrect assertion since transgressions by therapists must be seen as so horrendous that allowing for the possibility of "little or no damage" is itself offensive. The second dimension of political correctness is the failure to understand that the legal system is adversarial. Thus, if a patient brings a civil suit against a therapist, a defense must be mounted. This fact does not mean that the opposing attorney or the expert witnesses retained for the defense are in favor of sexual misconduct or wish to promote it; rather, fundamental legal principles mandate that every case have a defense.

These conceptual obstacles must be surmounted to permit a clear view of boundary issues and a calm, objective exploration of them.

"BOUNDARIES ARE TOO LOOSE": THE "BAD APPLE" MODEL

This model draws from the predator–prey image noted above. From this viewpoint, bad therapists—the "bad apples" that spoil the barrel—are entirely at fault, while the patients are neutral or passive or ciphers in the equation (Beal, 1989). Besides being simplistic and unrealistic, this view strikes the authors as demeaning and disempowering to women. This misunderstanding takes several forms.

"Blaming the Victim"

This misunderstanding of boundary theory rests on the following claim: if you examine boundary issues as complex, context-dependent two-person interactions, then you *inherently* blame the victim. The victim, such claims assert, should have no "dynamics"; rather, she or he is simply the target of a predator in the form of a bad therapist whose dynamics also do not matter. Clearly, such a view precludes careful examination of "the possible roots of misconduct in terms of a failed treatment alliance" (Schultz-Ross et al., 1992, p. 512) and provides nothing useful to learn, especially about prevention.

To illustrate this point, an article by Gutheil (1989) attempted to show how the dynamics of patients with borderline personality disorder made those patients vulnerable to boundary transgressions by therapists even as they struggled with boundaries of their own. The intent of the article was to provide both a clinical caution and a risk management model, that is, in the service of prevention. A letter to the editor in response to the article (Jordan, Kaplan, Miller, Stiver, & Surrey, 1990) claimed that to diagnose or analyze the dynamics of these patients inherently blamed them:

> We are appalled at the implications of this article; there is a history in the field of psychiatry of this kind of verbal and *diagnostic abuse* of women patients, beginning with labeling patients' early attempts to speak of

sexual misconduct by therapists as "psychotic transference." (p. 129; emphasis added)

Even more important, the "bad apple" model misses the susceptibility of even well-intentioned therapists to being caught in a boundary dilemma. As explained in previous chapters, contrary to the illusion that "This couldn't happen to me," any therapist, under particular circumstances, may face a boundary dilemma (Norris et al., 2003; Samuel & Gorton, 2001). Fortunately, the better one's training and the more consistently one maintains a stance of professionalism, the better the odds of avoiding trouble.

Ignoring Context

In a short story, a narrator described a man grabbing a woman, throwing her forcibly to the ground, and beating her all over her body with his hand. Listeners' horror at this scene melted away when the narrator belatedly included the detail that the woman was on fire at the time.

A middle-aged man described how he grabbed a three-year old girl, took off her clothes with great resistance on her part, and touched her all over her body. He was not reported to child protection authorities—because he was her father, giving her a bath. However, the vignette omitted the tub, the water, and the soap.

Context is critical in understanding events. All valid discussions of boundary issues (e.g., Edelwich & Brodsky, 1991; Epstein, 1994; Epstein & Simon, 1990; Gutheil & Gabbard, 1993; Hundert & Appelbaum, 1995; Martinez, 2000; Reamer, 2001; Simon, 1992; Waldinger, 1994) include context. However, certain settings—particularly adversarial ones, such as courts and boards of registration—see fit at times to ignore this essential criterion. In the absence of context, attorneys or regulatory boards may find their respective tasks simplified to showing that the therapist in question was guilty of acts on the "forbidden list," such as happened in the following example.

A patient gave a therapist a book for Christmas in gratitude. The board of registration, acting on a later complaint from the giver, attempted to show that this was a violation since gift giving, under some circumstances, is a boundary problem (see Chapter 4). What they failed to demonstrate was how the therapist's fitness to practice, or to treat this patient, had been compromised merely by acceptance of a minor gift.

For courts or regulators, testimony in the subjunctive mood—indicating mere possibility—has occasionally been used to disregard context. In this next example a patient, newly arrived in the community, asked a psychiatrist for information on local churches. The psychiatrist supplied a list, including the church he attended. In a later board complaint, the board's expert, a nationally known ethicist, gave this testimony (Gutheil & Gabbard, 1998, pp. 412–413). We have highlighted use of the subjunctive mood throughout:

> Q (board prosecutor): In your opinion, [Doctor,] as a psychiatrist, if a psychiatrist provided a list of four or five churches to a patient and that patient was having idealizing transference with that psychiatrist, one of these churches was the psychiatrist's and the patient knew that, in your opinion, which church *would* the patient choose?
>
> A (expert): In my opinion it *would be likely* that the patient *would be influenced* to go to the church that the psychiatrist recommended—that the psychiatrist was going to. [Emphasis denoting these and all subsequent subjunctive usages added.]
>
> Q: And why *would* the patient do that?
>
> A: Because the patient *would trust* in the psychiatrist's judgment, *would want* to be close to the psychiatrist, *would want* to do what the psychiatrist does or recommends. . . .
>
> A: I don't think that the psychiatrist's job or duty is to recommend churches to patients. There are others who can do that. [Note here that the situation is one where the patient asked and the doctor responded—rather than positing whether recommending churches is a doctor's duty, as this witness's testimony implies.] Second of all, it *would increase the likelihood* that the patient *would* be in a social interaction with the psychiatrist and *would provide* an opportunity that *would be ripe* for all kinds of boundary problems, boundary blurrings, and boundary violations.
>
> Q: Can you describe some of these boundary blurrings that *occur*? [Note the absence of the subjunctive mood (indicating hypothetical circumstances) when the board prosecutor states it; in the board's eyes, it is already fact.]
>
> A: They *could be* sitting next to each other in the church. They *could be* involved in church activities together. The psychiatrist and his own family *might be involved* with the patient and his family. There *would just be an increase in the likelihood* of significant social interaction between them.

Note how all the testimony relates to the *possibility* of problems, although one can equally well imagine the patient's *avoiding* the doctor's church out of a wish for privacy and for other motives. But, although the testimony is given in terms of what *might* happen, the regulatory board, based on the dialogue described above, is ready to assume it *will* do so.

As noted in previous chapters, what might be judged a boundary violation in one type of therapy may be well within the standard of care in another. For example, following the theory of behavioral activation (Beck, 1991; Linehan, 1993), a therapist might take a severely depressed patient (one who has been resistant to medication trials and electroconvulsive therapy) on walks around the hospital grounds in an effort to achieve mood alleviation through psychomotor activity. This intervention would be undertaken after consultation (e.g., a team meeting) with full documentation. Beyond such accepted practice, boundary crossings that take unusual forms may be made with a therapeutic rationale, as in the following example:

> A therapist was unable to have a coherent conversation with a severely psychotic inpatient he was treating until they started playing ping-pong on the inpatient unit. With the diversion of attention onto the game, the patient was able to converse with the therapist and give a history for the first time.

Here, again, context is paramount. Is the therapist wasting the patient's time by playing ping-pong "instead of" doing therapy, as in Pope et al.'s (2006) case of a therapist who played tennis with a patient? Can or should the therapist be reimbursed for this time? Again, the answers in context would involve an analysis of harm or exploitation versus benefit over time (in a civil case) and fitness to practice (in a regulatory board complaint). Of course, the use of play to engage the patient in an alliance, as exemplified successfully by this case, is more common and generally more readily accepted with children and adolescents.

The cost of misunderstanding or disregarding context is also captured in the following consultation:

> A chief of psychiatry in a city hospital, who does only evaluations and psychopharmacology, wrote: "In the midst of divorce my estranged physician-wife filed a complaint against me which was presented to the state board. Over the past few years I renovated a country farmhouse. During this time I ran into two former patients who needed work and hired them to do incidental labor at a competitive wage. My wife's initial contention was that I had an inappropriate relationship with one of the former patients (she based this contention on the fact that she [the ex-wife] saw her [the patient] painting the

deck of the farmhouse while I was at work). I have undergone extensive board evaluations, polygraphs, etc. Conclusion: 'I find no evidence the doctor has had sexual contact with any patient. However, his behavior with Ms. X did show progressive boundary violations [crossings?].' "

The board charged this psychiatrist with unethical practice harmful or detrimental to the public by employing two former patients. Our analysis would begin with the question: What was the context? Could the patients have refused the job offer freely, or were they coerced into accepting it by a power-dependency relationship? Were they exploited or otherwise harmed? Regardless of these valuable heuristic inquiries, boards of registration make their own decisions. The psychiatrist was ostracized by his clinic, suspended, stripped of his department chairmanship, and made the subject of numerous rumors that hurt his practice and reputation; he eventually had to resign and relocate.

There are several cautionary dimensions to this sad tale. Even assuming a small error was made in employing the former patient, a highly reputable clinician may become a pariah, because the public may not distinguish between a minor boundary crossing with an ex-patient and someone who has sex with a current patient. Similarly, hospitals may act conservatively and reject one's application for privileges. Note that an unidentified expert witness testified that boundary *violations* had occurred. That claim, of course, would have to rest on the evidence of harm or exploitation of the patient, but no such evidence was presented.

Another important aspect is the role of third parties in complaints. This therapist was not conscious of any wrongdoing, nor did the patient feel a reason to complain; instead, the complaint was brought by a third party outside the therapeutic relationship. Consultative experience reveals that this third party may be a vindictive ex-spouse or ex-partner of the therapist, as here; the patient's subsequent treater, who, by whatever standard, interprets the previous therapist's behavior as a boundary problem; people in the community (including current or past patients of the therapist) who literal-mindedly take boundary standards from the Internet; the patient's best friend; or other parties entirely.

The Lure of Simplicity

Like the lure of reductionism noted above, the "list of forbidden acts" offers an illusory promise of simplicity. This appeals to decision makers and to patients offended by or dissatisfied with some aspect of their therapy.

Minor violations can be claimed to be harmful. It is as if the "slippery slope" had been replaced by a "slippery cliff"—one step and you are over the edge. Less metaphorically, some decision makers appear to have the attitude that any minor deviation is *tantamount to* a major one; thus, calling a patient by his or her first name is seen as equivalent to having sexual intercourse with that patient. To those unfamiliar with the workings of boards of registration in the more punitive states, this idea may seem a hyperbolic exaggeration, but unfortunately it is proven by experience.

"BOUNDARIES ARE TOO TIGHT": THE "BACKLASH" RESPONSE

A "backlash" against the preoccupation with boundary maintenance surfaced in the literature during the mid- and late 1990s. A series of articles, book chapters, and books (e.g., Combs & Freedman, 2002; Greenspan, 1996; Heyward, 1993; Kroll, 2001; A. A. Lazarus, 1994; Martinez, 2000; Ragsdale, 1996; Williams, 1997) share the common theme that orthodox regulation of therapeutic boundaries is "too tight." In other words, by purportedly imposing a rigid code of permitted behaviors, boundary theory is said to be too restrictive and to have suppressed innovative approaches, humane gestures, novel developments, and evolution of the field of psychotherapy.

Why did this revisionist viewpoint surface just when it did? One answer (admittedly speculative but based on extensive consultative experience and a large forensic caseload) is that—thanks to increased attention to the problem—actual incidents of intercourse by therapists with patients appear to have declined. Meanwhile, there has been an increase in civil cases, ethics complaints, and board complaints about boundary transgressions short of sexual relations. That is, therapists are now quite aware of the prohibition against sex with patients but may not be as clear about boundary issues short of that. At the same time, a public exposed to disillusioning accounts of sexual misconduct by therapists appears to have become suspicious about therapists' actions, even in the case of milder crossings. In this atmosphere, patients ready to blame therapists for all sorts of reasons have been able to employ alleged boundary violations as the vehicle for doing so. This resultant trend toward what must be viewed as more subtle cases has focused critical attention on the theory behind boundary maintenance and its regulation.

Another factor in prompting a backlash has been the complaints to various decision makers about minor boundary crossings and questionable boundary violations. Ostensibly trivial complaints to professional ethics committees (such as those listed by J. Lazarus, 1993; see also Chapter 1) have prompted concerns that boundary theory is too rigid to accommodate the vagaries of clinical practice. Jeremy Lazarus's list, which was merely descriptive, prompted three letters to *Psychiatric News*, all chiding the article's author for appearing to promote rigidity. We quote from each of these letters here to show the intensity of debate over this issue. The first letter, by L. James Grold (1994), described observed examples of benign boundary crossings, including physical contact, by Karl Menninger, MD. The author noted: "Being warm, friendly and personable does not constitute boundary violations" (p. 22). The author went on to caution against dehumanization in the name of avoiding litigation, concluding, "As part of a culture currently dedicated to self-scrutiny and censorship, we psychiatrists must maintain a professional objectivity to assist those individuals who are caught up in this reactionary frenzy" (p. 22).

The second letter was by Judd Marmor (1994), the author of influential articles two decades earlier that had made clear the unethical, exploitative nature of therapist–patient sex (Marmor, 1972, 1976). Regarding the Lazarus list, Marmor commented: "Thus, to take an ethical prohibition [against extratherapeutic and posttherapeutic contact with patients] that is meaningful and appropriate in long-term dyadic treatment and extend it to all patient–psychiatrist contacts for life is stretching the precept to the point of absurdity" (Marmor, 1994, p. 23).

The third letter stated: "The clear implication is that psychiatrists who do not accept psychoanalysis as their role model run the risk of being considered unethical. I find that implication reprehensible" (Klein, 1994, p. 23).

Understandable as are the concerns they addressed—concerns that continue to be aired in professional forums and in legal proceedings—these correspondents may have missed three points. First, as a consultant to the ethics committee of the American Psychiatric Association (APA), Dr. Lazarus was simply keeping his colleagues informed by reporting on the kinds of incidents that had come across his desk. Second, Dr. Lazarus may have used the term "boundary violation" loosely to describe a number of incidents, some of which might better be termed "crossings." Third, to complain to the APA ethics committee is not a matter of a simple phone call; instead, some effort must be expended over time to obtain and fill out the written complaint forms. Whether or not their claims are meritorious, the patients in those examples, for whatever reasons (including a climate of hysteria), felt strongly enough to make those efforts.

The response to Jeremy Lazarus's article reflected a larger movement questioning the wisdom of excessively rigid regulation of therapeutic boundaries. In a paper provocatively titled "How Certain Boundaries and Ethics Diminish Therapeutic Effectiveness," Arnold Lazarus (1994) boldly attempted to turn the ethical discussion on its head: "If I am to summarize my position in one sentence, I would say that one of the worst professional or ethical violations is that of permitting current risk management principles to take precedence over human interventions" (p. 260). Lazarus conflated the rigidity with which some boards of registration view boundary issues with the flexibility and context dependence that we and other writers in the field recommend. His argument also failed to grasp that ethical and effective risk management, rather than being opposed to clinical effectiveness, works precisely because it rests on a solid clinical foundation. The best risk management is high-quality clinical care, that is, treatment that is good for the patient.

Most significantly, such an argument can encourage the common tendency to accept the benign *intent* with which a boundary is crossed or even violated ("I didn't mean any harm") without sufficiently considering the *impact* on a patient with a particular psychological organization (Gutheil, 1994a). Pope et al.'s (2006) cautionary example of the therapist who played tennis with a patient while avoiding confronting the patient's problems—a common motivation (however unconscious) for therapeutic boundary violations—underscores the insufficiency of good intentions alone. Clearly the foreseeable effect of a boundary incursion is the critical variable in assessing whether or not the event was problematic for the patient or whether the therapist's conduct met professional standards. The latter criteria would be relevant to the evaluation of particular applications of Lazarus's "multimodal" approaches (A. A. Lazarus, 1989, 2006) even if, in a particular case, no bad outcome resulted from the actions in question.

Another article laid down a direct challenge to orthodoxy in its title: "Boundary Violations: Do Some Contended Standards of Care Fail to Encompass Commonplace Procedures of Humanistic, Behavioral and Eclectic Psychotherapies?" In it Williams (1997) pointed to what he saw as a contradiction in the accepted understanding of boundaries:

> On the one hand, authors argue that ethics concerns dictate a need for careful maintenance of boundaries as well as a need to sanction practitioners who violate. On the other hand, the traditions and practices of some forms of psychotherapy dictate that certain boundaries be routinely crossed. (p. 238)

Examples of crossings that Williams cites include hugging, dining with, and self-disclosing to patients (the risks of which are exemplified by the case, in Chapter 9, of the woman being treated with CBT for social anxiety disorder). For example, humanistic therapy, Williams points out, "has been devoted *not to maintaining but to tearing down the boundaries between therapist and patient*" (pp. 241–242; emphasis in original) in order to achieve an authentic encounter between therapist and patient. (See Farber, 2006, on the historical role of humanistic and client-centered therapy in promoting greater self-disclosure by therapists.) Similarly, reality therapy (Glasser, 1965) routinely involves specific self-disclosures by the therapist. Gestalt therapy (Perls, 1969) invoked the use of therapists' first names, hugging, and some socializing with patients, especially in therapeutic retreats.

Regarding behavior therapy, Williams cites what appears to be an outdated source. According to Marquis (1972), as summarized by Williams:

> Nothing in the theory of behavior therapy would or should preclude socializing with patients, taking meals with them, giving them gifts, or treating them in their homes, schools, or offices. Hugging patients might reinforce the therapist's potency as a reinforcer for the patient and, thus, might be supported theoretically. (p. 244)

Not many cognitive-behavioral therapists today would subscribe to this position. Although the actions described might make the therapist temporarily a more potent reinforcer, they have considerable potential for producing aversive consequences. Thus, they often can be characterized as "therapy-interfering behaviors" (Linehan, 1993).

In a different vein, some practitioners of feminist therapy (e.g., Jordan, 1995; Miller & Stiver, 1997) and "narrative therapy" (Freedman & Combs, 1996; Monk, Winslade, Crocket, & Epston, 1997) conceive of therapy in terms of "relationships" of collaboration and interdependence rather than "boundaries," a term that connotes separation and alienation. This reframing, of course, accommodates an ethical concern with the way the therapeutic relationship is conducted (Combs & Freedman, 2002).

All these paradigms, and others, are themselves contexts in which the actions of therapists may be considered. To repeat an earlier example, it is a clear deviation for a classical psychoanalyst to visit a public bathroom together with a patient, but not for a CBT practitioner effecting the final step of the treatment of paruresis. There are, on the other hand, boundary questions and liability risks specific to behavior therapy (Goisman & Gutheil,

1992). Thus, concern that the standards of psychoanalysis are being imposed on practitioners of other kinds of therapy can be addressed by emphasizing the distinctive contexts of particular practices, as reflected in their therapeutic contracts. All, however, are subject to the ethical standard that the therapist must always act in the interest of the patient. Every legitimate form of therapy accepts this fiduciary responsibility.

Kroll (2001) uses the term "backlash" to describe the original intense concern with boundary maintenance rather than resistance to it, as we are using it here. He traces the emergence of boundary guidelines to a backlash against therapy movements of the 1960s and 1970s that were perceived as permissive. As a result, he contends, conservative limits on therapists' conduct have been imposed even though they may not reflect the consensus of practitioners in the field. He suggests that boundary definitions, which he characterizes as culturally shaped or culture-bound, have proliferated beyond the point of helpfulness. According to Kroll, excessive restrictions have been placed on ordinary therapy in an overreaction to sexual misconduct episodes. He asserts that even the term "boundary crossings" is pejorative, although the latter are considered benign. Clearly, the context of the restrictions Kroll describes would be central to determining whether those restrictions are excessive.

Kroll also appears to misread, as others have done, the notion of the "slippery slope." This term, adapted from legal theory, is a description of an observed progression of boundary transgressions in actual cases as well as a caution to practitioners (Gutheil & Simon, 2002). Kroll criticizes the term as signifying an *inevitable* progression from mild to serious boundary incursions, as if a commonly observed pattern could be applied deterministically to any individual case. This is a misconception; indeed, later in this chapter we will address the issue of recovery from boundary problems. In addition to self-disclosure, a subject of considerable recent discussion among mainstream as well as revisionist thinkers (see Chapter 5), Kroll focuses on three boundary issues: therapist neutrality, relative anonymity, and a stable fee policy (see Chapters 2 and 4). He sees these guidelines as excessively rigid, as they may be in some context-dependent cases. For example, neutrality may be translated by some practitioners as coldness, which neither boundary theory nor accepted practice requires.

Not surprisingly, two leading boundary theorists who responded to Kroll's critique wrote that they in fact practice and advocate the very flexibility that Kroll finds to be lacking in psychotherapeutic orthodoxy (Gabbard, 2001; Simon, 2001). Blatt (2001) explains: "Neutrality is not an alternative to empathy; rather, neutrality is maintained through an empathic nonjudgmental focus on articulating patients' thoughts and feelings—

their experiential field." Likewise, "The issue is not whether to maintain anonymity, but to maintain the focus on the phenomenal field of the patient as the central therapeutic task. Thus, it is important to put into words the patient's curiosity about aspects of the therapist and to ask the patient, as well as oneself, to consider what the patient really wants to know and why" (p. 292). Some approaches to CBT openly depart from neutrality in their recommendation of "cheerleading" by the therapist for successful completion of therapy tasks (Linehan, 1993). Notwithstanding this outward divergence, analytically oriented therapists often give patients reinforcement for therapeutic progress, and CBT practitioners have taken an interest in the interpersonal dynamics of therapy, including (under whatever rubrics) transference and countertransference (see Kohlenberg & Tsai, 2007; Wachtel, 2007).

Whether the "boundary" question is self-disclosure by the therapist or an adjustment of the fee structure, the clinical and ethical significance of the boundary excursion (whether contemplated, requested, or enacted) lies primarily in its meaning for the patient (cf. Schultz-Ross et al., 1992; Waldinger, 1994). For this and other reasons, informed consent is essential when establishing, changing, or deviating from the treatment contract. As Samuel and Gorton (2001) emphasize, "Cautious exploration of the potential risks, benefits, and multiple meanings of any significant change in the framework or conduct of the treatment should take place, both with consultant colleagues . . . and with the patient. " (p. 68).

Kroll cites a fascinating case from Waldinger and Gunderson's text (1987) in which a patient with borderline personality disorder, marooned by a blizzard at the therapist's home office, was invited to dinner by the therapist's children (Freud, of course, did the same, but that was long ago). The therapist's dismay and fears for the therapy were allayed because the patient found the home and family mundane and ordinary, and this observation allegedly calmed the patient, decreasing the amount of time the patient spent badgering the therapist for personal information. But despite this benign outcome, clinically experienced readers are quite familiar with how even minor exposures to a therapist's reality can inflame borderline patients into rage, envy, and a burning desire to learn ever more personal data, and may feed the fantasy of belonging to the therapist's family. Indeed, our caseload includes a naive male neurologist who attempted to disabuse an idealizing, personality-disordered patient about his "specialness" by showing her the ordinariness of his house; tragically, this attempt to "demythologize" himself produced a false charge of rape. The examples do, however, capture the individualized nature of responses to boundary crossings.

Martinez (2000) critiques the "rule-based approach to ethical decision making" (p. 43) allegedly inherent in boundary theory. His proposed graded-risk model actually involves a highly sophisticated and appropriately contextualized approach to decision making about boundaries; thus, his critique resolves the very questions it raises. Like the authors quoted previously in this section, Martinez asserts:

> The current "slippery slope" model and rule-based decision-making approach emphasize negative consequences of boundary crossings while inadvertently minimizing potential benefits. However, many boundary crossings are motivated by and result in constructive developments in the professional–patient relationship. (p. 50)

Like Lazarus and to some degree Kroll, Martinez here focuses on both benevolent intent and positive results from boundary crossings. This captures an important point: that the lesson of boundary theory is not to avoid any crossings at all costs, especially humane ones. If a patient falls to the floor by tripping on your office rug, help him or her up and do not fear that any physical touch is always forbidden.

Martinez provides a model of four levels of boundary crossings, from severe to mild. Each is graded on the following factors: risk of harm to the patient and to the therapeutic relationship; coercive and exploitative elements; potential benefits; the professional's intentions and motives; the professional ideals involved; and the recommended professional response or action (i.e., encouraged or discouraged). Complex and highly context-dependent, this model exemplifies a calculus in decision making that rests on valid clinical principles, including avoidance of exploitation or harm. One can imagine that a decision-making agency might find this calculus useful.

CLINICAL MISUNDERSTANDING AND CAVEATS

Consultative practice reveals a recurring problem in boundary management by clinicians. To certain types of patients even mild boundary crossings seem like a promise of further intimacies that the clinician cannot appropriately keep. Clinicians themselves sometimes seem trapped by this same view. Consider this composite example:

> A patient who has had a very positive experience or achieved a significant insight during a session impulsively hugs the therapist in the office doorway upon departing. The therapist accepts or does not re-

ject the hug. Some therapists—although they acknowledge that this was not an appropriate response—think that they are now committed to hugging that patient ever after, because not to do so would feel like a rejection and be harmful to the patient or to the alliance. The therapist feels trapped into behavior that he or she does not approve of, but can imagine no way to step back from and to resume the status quo. The therapist may ask the consultant: "If I hugged the patient once, do I have to do it thereafter? Will the patient be mad at me if I later refuse? Will I be expected to go further in boundary transgressions?"

On such occasions either the patient or the therapist may say or feel that "I have come so far, I cannot retreat—I cannot go back." Indeed, some serious boundary violations begin in this way. Some categories of patients will argue persuasively in favor of such an escalation, but that neither necessitates nor justifies a therapist's abdication of responsibility. To the contrary, one can always retreat; one can always stop doing something that is not helpful and may be harmful. Here, the therapist appears to assume that the alliance must remain stuck on whatever course it has taken, even if that course is an error. In these cases, the "slippery slope" is a self-imposed rationalization rather than a legal calculus. In reality, then, the "slippery slope" is not an inevitable escalation of uncontrolled behavior but an observation of the tendency of human behavior to expand under permissive circumstances.

A therapist's concern about having "signed on" for an ongoing deviation is a problem for the treatment. At least some of this concern may well derive from fear of being faulted by a patient complaint or fear of the patient's quitting therapy out of pique at the therapist's "retraction." As Epstein and Simon (1990) make clear, "The therapist's ability to deal with exploitive enticement, whether emanating from within or from without, is a fundamental component of the treatment process and a vital aspect of maintaining its integrity" (p. 463). Moreover, "Even in instances where exploitation originates from the therapist alone, recognition and empathic acknowledgment of its occurrence to the patient may be appropriate and can facilitate substantial therapeutic benefit" (p. 464).

For those who fear they have "crossed the Rubicon" by committing or participating in even a minor boundary violation, Epstein (1994) recommends reparative responses for most categories of boundary violations. We encourage responses such as the following (usually preceded by consultation with a supervisor or colleague) to the range of reconsidered boundary crossings:

- "I did hug you [or whatever the boundary crossing was], but now that I think about it, it was probably not helpful to your treatment."
- "I was wrong to do so, and I apologize."
- "You are right. I did it once, but having reflected further (and/or gotten consultation), I think it was not helpful, and we should not do it again."

All these responses should be followed both by clinical debriefing (e.g., exploration of the patient's experience, meaning, fantasies, and subsequent views of the event) and by careful documentation. Failure to do either creates a significant problem from the standpoint of both treatment and ethics.

In addition to the foregoing measures, technical psychotherapeutic skills may also be useful. These include analysis of the dynamics of the therapeutic dyad, now sadly in danger of being lost (Schultz-Ross et al., 1992). Epstein and Simon (1990) remind us that "If detected and properly understood, minor errors are usually helpful in understanding the patient's problem, especially when the therapist is responding to transferentially derived cues" (pp. 463–464). Person (2003) describes how the patient can experience such benefits:

> Compared with other transferences the erotic transference has always been tainted by unsavory associations and continues to be thought of as slightly disreputable. However, we should not lose sight of the fact that it may confer on the patient a new appreciation of the possibilities inherent in relationships (sometimes through an identification with a therapist's empathy and kindness). (p. 31)

Safran and Muran (2003) have developed a comprehensive framework for negotiating and repairing alliance ruptures and strains for therapeutic benefit. Their approach, which draws on the contemporary psychoanalytic theories known as "relational" as well as humanistic and cognitive therapies, gives clinicians a theoretical and practical foundation for effectively addressing boundary crossings and violations (cf. Leahy, 2001, 2003b).

An excellent summary—both sensible and sobering—of the dilemmas posed for mental health professionals by both the public's hypersensitivity to therapeutic boundaries and the reaction against this concern is provided by Waldinger (1994):

> For a great many of our patients, standard models of the professional relationship are all that is required. Yet some patients—including many

more-disturbed people—at times need forms of engagement with us that go beyond the usual, just as some patients require experimental uses of medications. Our ability to respond creatively to our patients' needs is vital to our work. . . . Equally vital is our adherence to professional standards and maintenance of clearly defined roles as doctor and patient. This tension between creativity and structure, between flexibility and boundaries, is neither new nor particular to psychiatry as a medical specialty. But the exploration of this tension, and our need to define the limits of acceptable clinical behavior, have taken on a particular urgency as our public image deteriorates. (p. 225)

Samuel and Gorton (2001) add:

In a nutshell, in order not to deceive either ourselves or our patients, we must, for the perpetuity of our practice, be open to other interpretations, perspectives, and judgments regarding our professional work such that nothing we do will ever be so sacred, so perfectly known and understood, so inviolate, that it cannot be thrown into question on both our patients', our own, and our profession's behalf. (p. 70)

In the reality of clinical and forensic work, the oscillation of the pendulum between "Boundaries are too loose" and "Boundaries are too tight" has not ceased or reached a useful midpoint even to this day. Variations on this battle are continually being fought before licensing boards, ethics committees, and courts of law. In this book we have tried to locate the pendulum at a moderate point that supports clinical effectiveness while avoiding harm to patients.

KEY REMINDERS

- Nuanced critical discussion of boundary issues has been made difficult by the influence of simplistic reductionism, gender bias, and political correctness.

- The pendulum of professional opinion has swung between the punitive position that "boundaries are too loose" and the inevitable reaction that "boundaries are too tight."

- Clinicians can best avoid the oversimplifications at both extremes, in the interest of providing effective clinical care, by maintaining an open-minded critical awareness of the importance of context in the assessment of boundary issues.

- The "slippery slope" of boundary violations is best understood not as an inevitable escalation of uncontrolled behavior but as an observation of the tendency of human behavior to expand under permissive circumstances.

- Reparative measures have been developed to overcome many types of boundary violations and to repair the therapeutic alliance for the patient's benefit.

CHAPTER 12

Liabilities

For both individual and organizational risk management purposes, every clinician should have some knowledge of the legal liabilities and administrative sanctions applicable to cases of treatment boundary violations. Moreover, even though most clinicians are not directly involved in evaluating claims of boundary violations, it is useful to have a general understanding of how such claims are evaluated, in the event that an allegation is made against you or a colleague (cf. Pope & Vasquez, 2007, pp. 102–109). Finally, if you have a patient who has brought suit or filed a complaint—or is considering doing so—against a previous therapist for sexual misconduct or other boundary violations, it can be helpful to understand the process as it affects the patient/complainant. Needless to say, the impact on clinicians as to their future career and functioning is also extremely significant. As shown by case examples throughout this book, many kinds of boundary violations besides sexual misconduct can result in severe legal and professional sanctions.

Regrettably, the manner in which such claims are evaluated by licensing boards, courts, and professional ethics committees often diverges from the more complex and realistic methods and criteria of trained forensic evaluators. Therefore, this chapter has a dual focus: first, forensic evaluation as it should be properly carried out; second, the kinds of dispositions actually made by less informed decision makers, who are often far less sensitive to context.

This chapter covers the most common avenues of patient action—namely, complaints to ethics committees of professional associations, complaints to state professional licensing boards, and civil litigation.

Criminal prosecution for therapist sexual misconduct is also an available remedy in sixteen states. Needless to say, complaints to a clinician's employing agency or institution (e.g., a university department) and informal complaints to a clinician's supervisors or colleagues also occur and are dealt with as provided for by the organization in question.

PROFESSIONAL ASSOCIATIONS
AND LICENSING BOARDS

The first resort for an aggrieved patient is to file an ethics complaint with the clinician's state and/or national professional organization (e.g., American Psychiatric Association, American Psychological Association, National Association of Social Workers, American Medical Association, American Psychoanalytic Association) or with the state licensing board that regulates practitioners (Friedman & Boumil, 1995, pp. 65–71; Gabbard, 1994b; Appelbaum & Gutheil, 2007, p. 144; Strasburger, 1999). For the patient, taking this route requires much less of a personal investment than filing a lawsuit. For one thing, it is not necessary to hire an attorney. Although typically the complainant must sign a complaint and may be questioned (and in some cases cross-examined) in a committee or board hearing, the process usually does not entail the same degree of public exposure for an already traumatized patient as does a lawsuit. For the clinician, however, the consequences may be very serious. However costly and stressful—even traumatic—it may be to go through a malpractice lawsuit, an adverse decision by a state board may result in loss of license and livelihood.

   In an ethics committee hearing, the question at issue is whether the clinician's alleged conduct, if corroborated, violated the professional organization's code of ethics. Ethics committees, especially at the state level, often proceed slowly, because they lack sufficient legal and staff resources. A clinician who is found to have committed a serious violation of the code of ethics, such as sexual misconduct involving a patient, may be suspended or expelled from membership in the organization. Although such sanction does not prevent the offender from practicing, it can seriously damage a practitioner's standing in the community. Suspension or expulsion usually is reported to boards of registration and to the National Practitioner Data Bank, thus affecting all future employment of the offender. In lieu of suspension or expulsion, the ethics committee may request or mandate that the therapist be supervised, accept limitations on his or her practice, or enter psychotherapy or a substance abuse program. In addition, depending on the profession and the jurisdiction, complaints (resolved or pending) to professional societies may, as a matter of law, be reported to the state licensing board at the time of reapplication for license.

In a licensing board complaint, the issue is whether the clinician is competent and fit to practice or is a danger to the public at large. As in the case of disciplinary proceedings by professional societies, sanctions may include reprimand, censure, mandated supervision or psychotherapy, or limitations on practice. If these measures are deemed insufficient or are not agreed to by the clinician, the board can (and, in the present climate, often does) suspend or revoke the clinician's license to practice. Nonetheless, in most jurisdictions one who is no longer permitted to call oneself a "physician" or "psychologist" or to avail oneself of third-party reimbursements and other perquisites of those professions can still practice as an unlicensed "psychotherapist." Moreover, in some states, clinicians with other licenses (e.g., as a counselor or social worker) may continue to practice under those licenses, in part because boards tend not to communicate with one another.

Licensing board procedures vary considerably in different jurisdictions and professions. In a typical generic case (presented hypothetically here for illustrative purposes), a complaint is made online. Complainants may be directed to a link on the state's website for psychology, social work, medicine, or whatever profession is involved. They are then instructed to download a complaint form, on which the complainant and the defendant are to be identified and the complaint described. The complainant may also be asked, "How would you like this complaint to be resolved?" (e.g., the defendant should lose his or her license, be reprimanded, be evaluated for fitness to practice, or face other sanctions). The complaint is signed, notarized, and sent to the licensing board, which reviews it to determine whether more information is needed. If so, an investigator may be sent by the board to speak with the complainant and the defendant. If the board determines that there is a potential violation, the case may be sent to a prosecutorial division of an agency with a name such as the Bureau of Professional and Occupational Affairs, which oversees all licensed professionals within the state or jurisdiction. At this point an attorney is assigned to the case, additional information is gathered, and a decision is made as to whether formal action will be taken. The prosecutorial division often relies on expert consultants in crafting a formal motion. At the board hearing that typically follows, the defendant can appear with or without legal representation. Although the complaint form may allow the complainant to remain anonymous, he or she typically will need to be identified if the complaint is to be heard formally.

Some complainants elect to drop the complaint at that stage rather than face the defendant.

A number of case examples in this book have involved dispositions (for better or worse) by licensing boards. There are no uniform standards governing board proceedings in different states and professions. Licensing boards are not bound by statutes of limitations. Nor are accused practitioners protected by due process—for example, with respect to the types of testimony allowed. Granting the power to impose punitive sanctions without judicial restraints is a formula for inconsistency and arbitrariness. Outcomes can depend on who sits on the board at a given time and which way the winds of politics and media publicity are blowing.

Historically, the mental health professions have been quite limited in their ability to deal appropriately with deviant or impaired members. As a result, they tend to overreact in particular cases. Boards have been observed to oscillate between periods of relative inactivity or "benign neglect" and overzealous crackdowns. The latter can happen after a sensational case generates unfavorable publicity. Although board proceedings ostensibly constitute review by professional peers, psychiatrists face a special problem—namely, that members of medical licensing boards may have insufficient familiarity with psychiatric practice and may show varying degrees of conscientiousness in accessing psychiatric (let alone forensic psychiatric) expertise.

Clinicians should be aware that the same alleged offense can prompt an ethics complaint to a professional organization, a licensing board complaint, a malpractice claim in civil court, and (where applicable) criminal charges. These separate actions involve different (though often related) questions to resolve, different standards to apply, and different procedures for resolution. Indeed, plaintiffs' attorneys usually advise their clients to file a complaint with the ethics committee and the licensing board in addition to a civil suit, so that the patient will not appear to be motivated exclusively by financial gain. The attorney can then use the cost-free public investigation at taxpayers' expense to obtain discovery data for the lawsuit. Moreover, the committee or board determination typically carries weight during a subsequent legal proceeding, since a breach of the governing professional code of ethics or standards of conduct may be grounds for civil liability.

MALPRACTICE LITIGATION

In a civil court action, establishing malpractice liability entails proving the occurrence of a *dereliction* of *duty directly* causing *damages*—referred to as the "four Ds" (Gutheil, 1999b). That is, it is necessary to prove not only that the clinician deviated from the standard of care (dereliction) but also that a clinician–patient relationship existed to which the standard of care applied (duty). Moreover, the plaintiff must have suffered harm (damages), and the negligent conduct must be shown to have caused those damages (directly). The defense can seek to disprove any of these four requisite components of the plaintiff's case.

Conduct found to have violated the code of ethics of the clinician's profession constitutes a departure from the standard of care. Therefore, having sex with a patient is a dereliction of the clinician's duty in any mental health profession. Indeed, some states have enacted civil statutes establishing that sexual contact with a patient is, per se, a breach of the therapist's duty (Haspel et al., 1997). Beyond that point, the legal determinations become less clear. Other boundary violations besides sex also violate professional codes of ethics and standards of care. However, as demonstrated throughout this book, whether a particular act constitutes a boundary violation, as opposed to a boundary crossing, is a contextual determination contingent on circumstances, the patient's needs, and the type, purpose, and process of therapy as specified in the therapeutic contract (questions that many jurors and judges are ill equipped to resolve). Moreover, the factual question of whether an alleged act occurred may be disputed—a case of "he said, she said." Finally, the defense can claim that the therapist did not have a duty to care for the patient, because no therapeutic relationship existed at the time of the violation. In most cases, however, such a defense is correctly perceived as opportunistic hair-splitting and therefore fails.

Once a deviation from the standard of care has been shown, the case enters the often murky waters of damages and causation. As discussed in Chapter 9, sexual and other boundary violations can cause serious harms, including depression, suicidal ideation, anxiety, distrust of future treaters, loss of consortium resulting from broken marriages and relationships, and the loss of a window of opportunity for beneficial treatment. However, patients who come to therapy with significant symptoms and impairments must prove that the alleged damages were caused by the therapist's misconduct or negligent treatment rather than by the natural course of a preexisting condition or, for that matter, by the termination of the therapy. For example, against a defense claim that the plaintiff already was chronically depressed and suicidal, the plaintiff needs to show that these symptoms were exacerbated by the therapist's boundary violations, or else that reasonable treatment would likely have resulted in an improvement in his or her condition. Nonetheless, the public's sympathy for victims of boundary violations, especially sexual boundary violations, makes it less difficult than it might seem for plaintiffs to meet this burden of proof. As a result, many cases are settled before they ever get to a jury.

The Insurance Wrinkle and the Basis of Liability

Suing a clinician for malpractice on the basis of sexual misconduct would seem to be a straightforward matter. However, malpractice insurance policies generally cover only liability that arises from the provision of, or failure to provide, professional services. Having sex with a patient is not a recognized, approved clinical service. Therefore, malpractice insurance companies have excluded or severely limited coverage for sexual misconduct claims on the basis that sexual misconduct is not a form of negligent treatment; rather, it is an intentional wrongful act (intentional tort or civil wrong), analogous to assault and battery (Jorgenson, Bisbing, & Sutherland, 1992; Stone & MacCourt, 1999). Malpractice insurance usually covers sins of omission, not sins of commission. In addition, there are strong social policy arguments for not insuring intentional torts (or, for that matter, what are criminal offenses in those states that criminalize sexual misconduct).

Plaintiffs' attorneys, thereby denied access to the "deep pockets" of malpractice insurers, have had to reframe sexual misconduct claims as negligent rather than intentional torts so as to make large damage awards available to their clients. A common way of doing so is to fall back on the theory of "concurrent proximate causation," as applied to therapist sexual misconduct litigation in *Cranford Insurance Co. v. Allwest Insurance Co.* (1986). This legal doctrine holds that when an insured risk and an excluded risk are simultaneously among the causes of an injury the insurer is liable for the insured risk (Jorgenson et al., 1992; Jorgenson & Sutherland, 1993). Since sexual misconduct virtually always is preceded or accompanied by other forms of professional negligence, those concurrent deviations from the standard of care can be claimed as the basis of liability. Such deviations can include nonsexual boundary violations and related acts (e.g., deception, role reversals, failure to set behavioral limits, negligent use of drugs or alcohol) as well as misdiagnosis, failure to provide appropriate treatment, failure to obtain consultation or referral, improper termination, and abandonment.

By asserting a claim based only on other forms of alleged therapeutic negligence, one risks losing the clarity and concreteness (not to mention emotional salience for the jury) of a sexual misconduct claim. Under the theory of concurrent proximate causation, one can at least attempt to gain the sympathy of the jury by including the alleged sexual misconduct in the factual narrative even though it is not the claimed basis of liability.

That approach, however, has not satisfied many plaintiffs' attorneys, who have sought to implicate the sexual misconduct directly as a form of professional negligence by redefining it as mishandling of the transference and countertransference (Hardegree, 1989). This formulation was used successfully in prominent, precedent-setting cases (*Simmons v. U.S.*, 1986; *St. Paul Fire & Marine Insurance Co. v. Love*, 1989; *Zipkin v. Freeman*, 1968).

Although clearly expedient for plaintiffs' attorneys and beneficial to some deserving victims, this tactic is conceptually flawed and problematic in its implications (Gutheil, 1992b, 1999b). For one thing, it is unfairly applied to the growing number of therapists who seek to understand the clinician–patient relationship in nonpsychodynamic terms and thus are unable to utilize the psychoanalytically derived concepts of transference and countertransference. Frequently, defendants in cases of alleged sexual or other boundary violations are so unaccustomed to thinking in terms of these concepts that, when questioned, they are genuinely unable to discuss them.

It may well be—as this book assumes and as is recognized in standard texts on cognitive-behavioral therapy (Dimeff & Koerner, 2007; Kohlenberg & Tsai, 2007; Leahy, 2003a, 2004; Linehan, 1993; Safran & Segal, 1996)—that therapists of any theoretical orientation are better equipped to help their patients while avoiding boundary violations if they have some understanding of relational dynamics in therapy. Nonetheless, to charge nonpsychodynamic therapists and counselors with mismanaging transference is to hold those practitioners to a standard of care they do not acknowledge or to compromise the impact of their intentions. In one example among many, the Supreme Court of Alaska held that misuse of transference constituted negligent treatment on the part of a pastoral counselor who kissed and fondled a counselee during sessions and later had intercourse with her, even though the pastoral counseling was not shown to have anything to do with psychoanalytic principles (*Doe v. Samaritan Counseling Center*, 1990). The point here is not, of course, to excuse sexual misconduct and other self-serving, exploitative actions, which are unethical in any school or philosophy of practice. In psychodynamic therapy itself, such conduct is wrong even if the transference is negative, hostile, or disparaging.

Rarely if ever do patients bring suit because they consciously believe that a therapist has mismanaged the transference and countertransference. Rather, they typically do so because they feel violated, degraded, and betrayed by the sexual contact and/or by its traumatic cessation. Thus, turning psychoanalytic concepts into a legal formula is almost always an artificial exercise from both the clinician's and the patient's point of view. Furthermore, it carries the implication, sometimes made explicit in legal arguments, that the patient is the equivalent of a child who lacks autonomous will and therefore is incompetent to consent to the sexual or other boundary-violating relationship. On the contrary, a competent adult patient may, for whatever reasons, choose to participate in such a relationship, but such consent and participation are not a defense for the clinician against the charge of unethical conduct. Thus, the adoption of the transference model for legal purposes not only is misleading but also may subtly contribute to the stigmatization of people seeking mental health treatment (and, in many cases, of women). It also represents the law taking sides in a scientific dispute, i.e., whether or not the model of unconscious functioning inherent in the terms "transference" and "counter-transference" is a universally valid one that should be imposed on clinicians using other frameworks (Malmquist & Notman, 2001).

A sounder and more useful model for ethical and legal determinations (referred to in connection with the axioms presented in Chapter 1) is to view boundary violations as breaches of fiduciary responsibility by the exercise of undue influence (Gutheil, 1992b; Jorgenson, 1995d; Jorgenson et al., 1997; Jorgenson & Randles, 1991). One court has defined a fiduciary relationship as follows:

> The essence of a fiduciary relationship is that one party places trust and confidence in another who is in a dominant or superior position. A fiduciary relationship arises between two persons when one person is under a duty to act for or give advice for the benefit of another on matters within the scope of their relationship. (F.G. v. MacDonell et al., 1997)

We all depend on the ethical exercise of fiduciary responsibility by stockbrokers, attorneys, bankers, contractors, executors, physicians, psychotherapists, and counselors, in whom we entrust some aspect of our welfare because they know more than we do in their area of expertise. A clinician who exploits a patient is taking unfair advantage of this position of power and trust. This model does not imply that the patient is impaired or incapable of autonomous choice. Many people, under internal or external pressure, make unwise, ill-considered decisions without being incompetent or psychotic—or, for that matter, having any psychiatric diagnosis.

Statute of Limitations

If the statute of limitations were applied strictly to cases of alleged misconduct by mental health clinicians, those claiming such misconduct typically would be required to file suit within 2 or 3 years or lose the opportunity to pursue a civil remedy. Increasingly, however, the statute of limitations has been seen as placing an unfair burden on abused patients, who, given their vulnerability to undue influence, may remain unaware for years of the wrong done them and its consequences. This vulnerability is especially great in psychotherapy because of the special nature of the trust extended in the patient–therapist relationship. Moreover, the complex, subtle nature of psychological damages and the difficulty (in some cases) of separating the effects of malpractice from preexisting impairments can prevent abused patients from identifying clearly the harms they have suffered. For example, patients previously abused in their family of origin may have been conditioned to accept abuse as a normal (or at least familiar) way of relating and may fail to identify resultant harms. Indeed, those very harms can include a traumatic paralysis (i.e., ongoing undue influence or psychological intimidation) that disables the patient from recognizing the maltreatment that occurred.

Fortunately, fiduciary theory provides a foundation for allowing victims to seek redress even after the time period allowed by the statute of limitations (Jorgenson & Appelbaum, 1991; Jorgenson & Randles, 1991). It utilizes the "discovery rule," which holds that the time period specified by the statute of limitations does not begin to run until a reasonably prudent person in the patient's position would have discovered the harm he or she has suffered as a result of the therapist's misconduct. This suspension of the statute of limitations is referred to as "tolling." The discovery rule has been applied to mental health malpractice involving boundary violations since the landmark cases of *Greenberg v. McCabe* (1978) and *Simmons v. U.S.* (1986).

In a widely cited example of the expanding use of the discovery rule in such cases, a male psychiatrist allegedly introduced alcohol, marijuana, and Valium into therapy sessions with a male patient. On more than one occasion the psychiatrist used a pseudotherapeutic rationale to persuade the patient to have sexual relations with him. The patient reportedly became very dependent on the psychiatrist, whom he referred to as "God." After he was abruptly abandoned by the psychiatrist (a typical case of "cessation trauma"), the patient developed severe emotional problems and began to drink heavily and abuse drugs. Nonetheless, in subsequent litigation he claimed that he had not recognized the causal link between the psychiatrist's unethical conduct and his symptoms until 4 years after termination, when he saw a different therapist and was put in touch with another former patient who had been similarly abused by the same psychiatrist. The Supreme Judicial Court of Massachusetts, reversing a lower court's ruling that the statute of limitations had run out, held that it was up to a jury to determine when the ex-patient became aware of his injury. The court explained that "if the defendant's conduct would, in an ordinary reasonable person, cause an injury which by its very nature prevents the discovery of its cause, the action cannot be said to have accrued" (*Riley v. Presnell*, 1991). In other words, the plaintiff's impaired understanding and judgment are to be taken into account in tolling the statute of limitations.

If the discovery rule is inapplicable in a particular jurisdiction or set of circumstances, the doctrine of "fraudulent concealment" provides another basis for extending the time period in which a lawsuit can be filed. This doctrine applies when the therapist withholds material facts or makes false representations about the treatment provided. In *Riley v. Presnell*, the court found that the psychiatrist's deceptive statements about the therapy might constitute independent grounds for allowing the plaintiff to bring suit after the statutory time limit. In this particular case, the psychiatrist said that a special kind of therapy—having sex with him—would help the patient work through his feelings about his father. In some contexts this is known as the "therapeutic deception" and may accrue additional sanctions. Any claim by a therapist that sex between therapist and patient is not unethical or harmful, let alone that it is therapeutic, may be found to constitute fraudulent concealment.

CRIMINAL PROSECUTION

From the 1980s to the present, 16 states have enacted laws making sexual misconduct by mental health professionals a criminal act. Some of these statutes included relationships with former as well as current patients. Such legislation was intended to protect public safety by deterring potential perpetrators, removing the defense of consent that applies in prosecutions for rape, and disabling offenders from practicing, even as unlicensed psychotherapists (Haspel et al., 1997; Strasburger, Jorgenson, & Randles, 1991).

Notwithstanding the desire of the public's representatives to make a clear statement condemning morally repugnant behavior, serious questions have been raised about the wisdom of criminalizing this particular behavior (Barker, 1990; Deaton, Illingworth, & Bursztajn, 1992; Illingworth, 1995; Samuel & Gorton, 2001; Strasburger, 1999). Criminalization has been characterized as a selectively punitive response to public furor, singling out the mental health professions for special retribution while most other breaches of fiduciary duty are left to civil law and professional regulation. Enacting criminal sanctions may simply draw attention away from strengthening existing remedies at the same time as it risks driving the abuses underground. Colleagues and even some patients may be less likely to report offenders when criminal prosecution may ensue. Patients/plaintiffs have described wanting abusing therapists to lose their licenses but not wanting them to go to prison.

Patients may be deprived of civil damage awards when malpractice insurance policies exclude coverage for the commission of a felony. Moreover (because criminal cases usually are tried before civil cases), once a defendant is found not guilty "beyond a reasonable doubt," it may be more difficult for the plaintiff to win a civil lawsuit against the same clinician even by the less strict standard of "preponderance of the evidence." Fear of prosecution may deter admissions of guilt that can lead to restitution and rehabilitation, and criminal conviction may deny those offenders who are capable of rehabilitation the opportunity to return to practice for the benefit of the public. Finally, making therapist sexual misconduct a crime raises subtle questions about power, consent, freedom of choice, and the extent of undue influence in the therapeutic relationship. Thus, criminalization may reinforce paternalistic, disempowering conceptions of psychotherapy by stigmatizing patients as incapable of self-determination and autonomous choice.

These questions are potentially resolvable by monitoring the effects of the statutes in practice (e.g., Kane, 1995; Roberts-Henry, 1995), but they may by now be academic. Criminal prosecutions for therapist sexual misconduct have been sufficiently few in number that these statutes may be seen to have served more of a public education function than a legal one. Although the consequences of a criminal conviction can be severe, civil actions for malpractice and complaints to professional licensing boards and ethics committees are still the primary sanctions that practitioners realistically can expect to face.

EMPLOYER AND SUPERVISORY LIABILITY

As in other areas of malpractice litigation, plaintiffs' attorneys typically cast a wide net for defendants in a civil claim alleging sexual misconduct or other boundary violations. Those who employ or supervise other mental health clinicians, whether of the same or other disciplines, are potentially liable under two legal theories. The first is *respondeat superior* ("let the master reply [for the servant's deeds]"), or vicarious liability, by which the employer is automatically liable for the employee's negligent or wrongful conduct irrespective of the presence or absence of specific negligence on the employer's part. The second theory is actual negligence in hiring, training, supervision, or retention of the offending employee (Jorgenson, 1995b). One may also be held liable for the acts of one's partners in a private group practice.

A detailed discussion of supervisory and organizational liability is beyond the scope of this book. Nonetheless, those who are or may be responsible for the actions of others in a clinical practice setting need to be aware of statutory requirements, legal standards, regulations, and standard practices in their jurisdiction. These may vary widely, since there are no uniform standards of employer liability in common law. Some states, however, have enacted civil statutes setting specific standards in this area. For example, the Minnesota statute shields an employer of psychotherapists from liability in civil actions resulting from alleged sexual misconduct if the employer has (1) checked the background of prospective employees by contacting the applicant's employers for the preceding 5 years, (2) responded to such background checks from other employers, and (3) taken appropriate and timely remedial action in response to patient complaints or other indications of misconduct (Haspel et al., 1997). These are useful ethical and risk management guidelines in any region or locality.

Risk management is an institutional as well as individual responsibility. Administrators and staff members involved in setting, implementing, and monitoring organizational policies and procedures can consult texts that outline organizational liabilities and administrative safeguards (Carroll, 2006; Caudill, 1997a; Jorgenson, 1995b; Reamer, 2001; Schoener, 1995b). The impact (professional and personal) of actual or alleged sexual exploitation of patients on colleagues of an accused clinician is treated by Regehr and Glancy (1995).

ASSESSMENT OF FALSE ALLEGATIONS

False accusations of sexual misconduct and other serious boundary violations by therapists, although constituting only a small proportion of such complaints, represent a troubling phenomenon (Gutheil, 1991, 1992a; Hall & Hall, 2001; Sederer & Libby, 1995; Smith & Gutheil, 1993; Williams, 2000). False claims not only cause great harm to innocent clinicians but also greatly complicate the tasks of identifying abusing practitioners, obtaining justice for exploited patients, and preventing others from being victimized. A small number of claims are found to be specious by virtue of convincing alibi evidence, deliberate or inadvertent recantation (e.g., through diaries or unguarded remarks), discorroborating witnesses, or definitive factual discrepancies. Others are deemed suspect on the basis of forensic evaluation. In a national survey of psychologists involving nearly 1,000 cases in which patients reported sexual intimacy with previous therapists, respondents judged about 4% of those reports to have been false (Pope & Vetter, 1991). The incidence may be greater in some high-risk caseloads. Whatever the percentage, however, a commitment to objectivity as well as to justice demands careful evaluation.

This determination of the truth or falsity of an allegation of misconduct ultimately is made by the court, licensing board, or ethics committee that receives the complaint. As a practical matter, such determinations are made provisionally by staff members who first receive the complaint. Subsequently, forensic experts commonly are asked to review the totality of a claim for its merit, which results in opinions presented to the court. Of course, there are forensic evaluators on both sides of the case who may reach opposing conclusions to be resolved by the formal proceedings.

A patient who makes an allegation of misconduct loses the right to keep the therapist's records out of the proceedings, a right conferring privacy protection, which is referred to as privilege. As distinct from confidentiality, which is a general obligation on fiduciaries such as mental health clinicians or attorneys to keep in confidence what a patient "confides" to them in their professional role, the term "privilege" stands for a patient's right to bar information from a legal or quasi-legal forum. People's communications with their therapists, health care providers, and attorneys are protected in this way. However, when a patient brings suit against a clinician this triggers the so-called patient–litigant exception to testimonial privilege. By this exception, the patient, having sued the therapist, cannot prevent the therapist's medical records—a foundation of the therapist's defense—from being produced in court. Moreover, the patient usually cannot bar other relevant medical and mental health records from being entered into evidence if they are held by the court to bear upon either the facts alleged by the patient or the patient's claims of medical or emotional damage.

As in any other forensic evaluation to which the possibility of malingering is relevant, that possibility must be considered. A systematic assessment includes numerous considerations (Gutheil, 1992a) that we will outline here.

Motivation for False Claims

Establishing a motivational basis for a false claim is the single most important component of the assessment, without which it is difficult to determine with confidence that a claim is false. Several alternative scenarios commonly emerge.

Revenge or Retaliation

Revenge or retaliation is the most common scenario. Its usual precipitant is termination or limit setting (which may involve the threat of termination). In a typical example, a therapist explains to a patient that therapy cannot continue if the patient spends every session trying to talk the therapist into a sexual relationship. The patient, angrily accusing the therapist of "breaking your promise" to continue the therapy for a specified time, stalks out and files a claim alleging that the desired sexual relationship with the therapist actually happened. False claims have also served as a form of retaliation in billing disputes.

Object Retention

In the case of object retention, the patient tries to hold on to a therapist who is terminating, even for such an innocuous reason as retirement or moving to another state. Through a lawsuit, the patient keeps the therapist involved in a relationship, albeit a hostile-dependent one. It is as if the patient were saying, "Don't think you can get rid of me *that* easily. I'll make sure you *never* forget me!"

Competition with Others

A patient may falsely claim sexual misconduct as a means of feeling closer to the therapist than other patients (or, in some cases, the therapist's spouse or family). Competition among patients can play itself out in either true or false scenarios. On the one hand, multiple misconduct claims made independently can provide corroborative evidence of predatory behavior by a therapist (Jorgenson, Sutherland, & Bisbing, 1995). Even when there is no actual misconduct, a therapist may unwittingly encourage dynamics by which dependent patients vie for his or her attention. As the line between fantasy and reality becomes blurred, this competition may escalate to false claims of sexual boundary violations. Simultaneous claims by members of the same therapy group, as occurred in one case, suggest the possibility of a competition as to which of several borderline patients is most "special."

Fantasy or Distortion

Even without the incitement of group competition, a patient with a powerful longing for intimacy with a therapist may spin an elaborate fantasy (sometimes recorded in a private journal) that comes to be treated as reality. This wish fulfillment is to be distinguished from a psychotic delusion. More plausible false claims have been made in therapeutic relationships that become so boundaryless and erotized that the allegation of sexual relations, while literally inaccurate, takes on an underlying truth (Gutheil, 1999b).

Delusion

Contrary to the claims of some abusing therapists, false accusations arising from psychotic delusions are quite rare. Occasionally such a case results from the projection of the patient's erotomania. A patient may assume that his or her own sexual arousal means that sex has occurred. In one notorious case, a schizophrenic patient who read the erotic novel *The Story of O* concluded that the narrative was a factual record of her relationship with her psychiatrist. Her malpractice case was fairly well advanced before her attorneys recognized the plot line and dropped the suit. Other cases stem from previous abuses in the patients' lives, causing them to develop what is known as an "encapsulated" delusional system, which at times may appear so real to them that they actually pass a polygraph test (Langleben, Dattilio, & Gutheil, 2006). In yet another potential obstacle to truth detection, the authors have formed the impression that some patients with dissociative identity disorders may experience a present benign situation as a past abusive one in an altered state of consciousness. That is, the altered scenario occurs in the altered mental state and therefore describes an event as happening in the office that actually happened in a completely different context in the past.

Extortion

Regrettably, there have been cases in which a patient overtly threatened to file a sexual misconduct complaint unless the clinician complied with a demand made by the patient, such as giving a favorable disability evaluation.

Financial Gain or Avoidance of Responsibility

More often than not, greed occurs in combination with other motivations such as dependency or revenge. Nonetheless, financial gain cannot be overlooked as a potential motivator of the accusing patient (or significant others). Three manifestations of economic opportunism are *coat-tailing*, whereby a patient adds his or her false allegation to a high-profile claim against the same clinician; *contamination*, in which plaintiffs who are thrown together (e.g., in a law office) suggest incidents and symptoms to one another in a form of contagion; and *conspiracy*, in which two or more patients plot to discredit a clinician with seemingly corroborative claims (Gutheil, 1999b). In another expression of economic entitlement, a patient who owes a therapist a substantial amount of money may file a lawsuit based on a trivial allegation, hoping that the settlement will cancel out the debt.

Escape from Treatment

Patients have been found to make false allegations against clinicians when therapy becomes too difficult or threatening. This gambit should be suspected in cases in which the patient was compelled to undertake the treatment by a court, employer, or family members. In one such instance, a teenage girl in treatment for amphetamine abuse accused her therapist of sexual misconduct in order to be able to discontinue treatment and see other therapists who were unaware of her continued drug use (Williams, 2000).

The Role of Borderline Personality Disorder in False Accusations

The subgroup of false complainants is dominated by patients with borderline personality disorder—a diagnosis in most cases made long before the alleged abuse (Gutheil, 1991). The dynamics (of rage, neediness, dependency, boundary confusion, manipulativeness, and entitlement) by which these patients become involved in both actual and fabricated cases of therapist sexual misconduct were outlined in Chapter 10 (see Gutheil, 1989, 2005b, 2005c). The following cases (taken from Gutheil & Alexander, 1992) illustrate how some of the motivations for false accusations discussed above can grow out of borderline dynamics.

> Enraged at her therapist for treating her "like a welfare case," a patient with borderline personality disorder claimed that the therapist had sexually molested her during a therapy session. She later con-

fided to her attorney that she had fabricated the claim as a way of getting back at her therapist for treating her disrespectfully. Her attorney dropped the lawsuit.

Responding to a patient's helpless demeanor and acute loneliness, a therapist became excessively, although not sexually, involved with her in ways that fed her magical wishes to be part of his family. For example, over a period of several weeks while she was without a car, he drove her home after each therapy session. On one occasion, she asked to see him over a holiday weekend. He refused, explaining that he had plans with his family. Her fantasy rudely shattered, the enraged patient sued the therapist for sexual abuse. Later she told a friend that she had lied, and the friend revealed her deceit to her attorney.

Neither of these therapists was guilty of sexual misconduct. However, the second therapist apparently did contribute to the breakdown of boundaries. In the first case, the patient's feeling of being mistreated was not traceable to any actions on the therapist's part that might reasonably be interpreted as mistreatment. By contrast, in the second case the therapist's errors in clinical judgment reinforced the patient's fantasy that the therapist had "special feelings" for her that led him to favor her over other patients as well as his family. In a nonsexual instance of "cessation trauma" (described in Chapter 9), the patient was set up for a perceived personal rejection, for which she retaliated with a false accusation. By allowing therapeutic boundaries to become too loose, her therapist apparently fed her intense disappointment and rage.

Factual Evidence and Other Considerations for Evaluation

The factual context of the allegations may seem more the province of the attorney and hired investigators than of a forensic mental health evaluator. Even so, factual evidence constitutes valuable corroborative or discorroborative data that can either support or call into question the evaluator's hypotheses. In an objective, comprehensive forensic analysis, considerations such as the following are not to be overlooked.

Internal Inconsistency

A person (accuser or accused) who is not telling the truth can readily be caught in contradictions (in spoken and/or written statements) with respect to details such as dates, times, places, and the nature of the physical contact that allegedly occurred.

Implausibility

When a hospital examining room in which a clinician allegedly took extended sexual liberties with a patient turned out to be a curtained-off bed in an open area behind the nurses' station, the allegation lost credibility. Likewise, an often intoxicated patient's claim of repeated instances of sexual abuse by an outpatient psychologist in private practice foundered on the discovery that the psychologist always asked his secretary to stay until the patient had left. Since the partition that separated the psychologist's office from the secretary's filing area was thin, providing less than fully adequate sound-proofing, the secretary could hardly have failed to pick up the sounds of the energetic trysts described by the patient.

Exploiting therapists (leaving aside the "lovesick" variety) are known to select victims likely to comply and keep secrets (Rutter, 1989a). Therefore, a patient known for indiscriminate self-disclosure when drinking is an unlikely choice of prey. Whereas a patient who is mildly demented or developmentally disabled may be vulnerable to exploitation by a certain kind of predator (e.g., a technician in a psychiatric hospital), a patient who is physically unattractive and not very bright is unlikely to become an object of passion for a considerably younger therapist with a desirable spouse. Although some of these considerations are admittedly subjective, they can be cited validly to fill out a picture replete with implausible claims, such as that the therapist was wildly smitten with the patient and even consulted the patient on professional matters. Another kind of implausible claim is an alleged sexual scenario that corresponds to the patient's "ideal fantasy" (e.g., prolonged, fully clothed hugging and holding without intercourse) but appears to offer the therapist little exploitive gratification to compensate for the risks to his or her career.

Uncharacteristic Object Choice

A particular implausibility that is often disregarded occurs when the allegation involves a deviation from the clinician's (and sometimes the patient's) usual sexual orientation. Habitual gender choice tends to be a high barrier for an offending clinician to hurdle, unless deeper evaluation of the therapist reveals a possible tendency to use the therapeutic situation to experiment sexually or to act out ambivalence about gender choice or bisexuality. The few bisexual abusers tend to be bisexual to begin with.

In the case in Chapter 8 in which a female therapist trained in counseling psychology was accused of sexual boundary violations by a female patient diagnosed with borderline personality disorder and possible dissociative identity disorder, both the therapist and patient were stably married. To commit the alleged acts, this therapist would have had to violate her gender preference, her marriage, and her professional and ethical commitments—all of which (as shown by history and examination) she took seriously. In this case, the unlikelihood of the alleged lesbian affair was corroborated by other ego-dystonic aspects of the behavior pattern alleged. Yet, the licensing board seemed not to consider that for the alleged acts to have occurred between two stably married heterosexual women was rather implausible. But the board members did not engage in this kind of analysis. Instead, they simply compiled a list of potential boundary problems.

Ability to Describe Therapist's Body

If the alleged scenario involved the patient's seeing the therapist unclothed in adequate light, corroboration can hinge in part on the patient's ability to identify distinguishing bodily markings or features, such as tattoos or scars, as well as the type of underwear or concealed jewelry worn by the therapist.

History of Deception, Lying, or Fraud

Pathological lying, which is commonly part of the psychopathology of borderline personality disorder, can fuel false accusations (Snyder, 1986). For this and more general reasons, the patient's records should be examined for a pattern of dishonesty and fraud. At the same time, as in any "he said, she said" disputes, it is necessary to look into the accused clinician's background (including his or her conduct in the case at issue) for potential deception, fraud, or perjury.

Indoctrination by Subsequent Therapists

Tragically, a patient can become a battlefield for competing philosophies or schools of psychotherapy (psychodynamic, cognitive-behavioral, humanistic, relational, feminist, etc.). Such rivalries can erupt in the form of disagreements between current and previous therapists about what constituted appropriate "boundaries." This dynamic is especially common in "recovered memory" cases (Williams, 2000). To take a minor example, a therapist who insisted that a patient use his last name explained that the patient's previous therapist's use of his first name was seductive and inappropriate.

Empirical Comparison with Other Cases

As these cited examples illustrate, orienting facts and perspectives are honed into directions for analysis as a forensic evaluator's caseload grows. Given a sufficient database (culled from personal experience as well as the literature in the field), a given case's congruence or incongruence with previously observed patterns can provide useful starting points, although by no means a definitive judgment.

Truth is elusive, no matter how skilled and experienced the evaluator. A plaintiff's case may appear credible until the plaintiff's deposition—or, worse yet, courtroom testimony—exposes its falsity. Conversely, a case may give every indication of being a false accusation until the defendant clinician breaks down and remorsefully admits the misconduct. A mark of forensic expertise is to be ready always to be surprised.

What an Attorney Looks for

Linda Jorgenson, a very experienced attorney specializing in cases of alleged boundary violations, provides this list of relevant evidence (Jorgenson, personal communication, 2007).

1. *Admissions by therapist or patient.* Has the therapist made incriminating admissions to the attorney, to a colleague or supervisor, or in some written form? Has the patient made damaging disclosures to the attorney, a friend, or a subsequent therapist (as in above cases involving false allegations)?

2. *Credible witnesses.* Are there witnesses, not compromised by an interest in the outcome of the case (as a spouse might be), who can attest to damaging admissions made by the patient or therapist, or to statements made by either party against his or her interest? Are there direct eyewitnesses to negligent or inappropriate behavior, office irregularities, other boundary violations plausibly leading up to the alleged acts, or even the alleged acts themselves?

3. *Role reversals.* Is the patient in possession of personal information about the therapist, such as information about therapist's life history, home, bedroom, possessions, or body? Could the patient have obtained this information by any means other than through the alleged extrathera-

peutic contact? Has the therapist made confidentiality-breaching disclosures about other patients to this patient?

4. *Documentary evidence.* Are the alleged boundary violations corroborated or discorroborated by cards and letters, tapes from answering machines or answering services, gifts, photographs, checks written by the therapist to the patient, or receipts or other records from hotels, restaurants, or ATMs? Written records to be examined include the patient's or therapist's notes, journals, or diaries or a supervisor's notes.

5. *Repeat offenders.* Absence of evidence of past offenses is not necessarily "evidence of absence," inasmuch as a "lovesick" therapist may have strayed from the reservation on a single occasion or a repeat offender may have expertly covered his or her tracks. However, evidence of past offenses on the part of the therapist does make the present allegations more credible by indicating either a predatory pattern, serious psychiatric disorder, or personal maladjustment. On the other hand, a history of similar unsubstantiated allegations on the patient's part calls into question the credibility of the present allegations.

Defenses against False Accusations

Any clinician is potentially vulnerable to false accusations. There is no absolute defense against someone who is willing to lie under oath in the absence of other witnesses. However, careful documentation of boundary challenges, including what actions were taken and why, can lay the foundation for a defense. Moreover, in any case in which the relationship becomes sexually charged or beset by persistent boundary challenges of any kind, the clinician should start presenting the case regularly to a supervisor. Such documentation and consultation are, first, good clinical practice and, second, good risk management.

In addition, three "context defenses" can help insulate a clinician against false charges. These are thoroughgoing professionalism in all areas of one's practice, avoidance of any form of boundary violations, and the absence of any allegations of sexual harassment. Although the last consideration is not in itself a treatment boundary issue, a history of sexual harassment can be used by the plaintiff's attorneys to discredit a clinician with respect to professional and interpersonal boundaries generally (Gutheil, 1992a).

Finally, there is no substitute for prevention. You may never know about the false accusations that patients did not make because you followed the recommendations for prevention in the next chapter (including—at least in private practice—prescreening patients for serious pathologies) as well as the guidelines presented throughout this book for maintaining the therapeutic frame and appropriate limit setting in such areas as time, physical setting, and dress.

Common Misjudgments

As has been made clear in this and previous chapters, board members in licensing hearings or jurors in the courtroom cannot be relied on to weigh all the factors that seasoned forensic evaluators and legal specialists consider. Elementary errors made in administrative and legal dispositions include disregarding data that make an allegation implausible, mistaking boundary crossings for violations (i.e., failing to consider the innocuousness or legitimate therapeutic purpose of an action that falls outside of customary practice), and assuming incorrectly that "where there's smoke, there's fire" (i.e., that evidence of precursor boundary violations proves that sexual misconduct occurred). Licensing boards (not to mention plaintiffs' attorneys) are also notorious for applying the standards of one kind of practice, such as classical psychodynamic therapy, to a different kind of practice, such as a behavioral desensitization program. In one example, a complaint against a Christian therapist for supplementing individual therapy with group prayer meetings at his house—which was included in the therapy contract—was evaluated by board members who knew nothing about Christian therapy. A related error is to fail to take the perspective of a clinician who is not trained to anticipate the dynamic fallout from naive good intentions, like the neurologist in the preceding chapter who showed a patient his home and was falsely charged with rape.

Remember that there are "four Ds" to prove in malpractice litigation: *dereliction* of *duty directly* causing *damages*. As explained in Chapter 9, uncritical invocation of the "therapist–patient sex syndrome" can amount to an unwarranted inference that the alleged misconduct actually occurred or that it caused the observed damages (Gutheil, 1992c). Conversely, a jury outraged by a therapist's misconduct (or simply clinical misjudgment) may overlook the critical question of whether the acts in question caused the alleged harms (Williams, 2000).

Justice for both accuser and accused, as well as high standards of clinical and ethical care, will better be served if all participants in the legislative, judicial, and regulatory process respect the complex and variable contexts in which boundary issues play themselves out. Mechanistic litanies of forbidden acts are not as useful as careful case-by-case evaluation and reasonable, flexible application of guidelines aimed at preventing situations of potential harm (Gutheil & Gabbard, 1992, 1998).

RESPONSIBILITIES OF SUBSEQUENT THERAPISTS

Guidance with respect to the clinical treatment of victims of abuse by previous therapists can be found in other sources (e.g., Apfel & Simon, 1985b; Atkins & Stein, 1993; Gabbard, 1994b; Jorgenson, 1995a; Kluft, 1989; Luepker, 1995; Nestingen, 1995; Notman & Nadelson, 1994; Pope, 1994; Wohlberg & Reid, 1996). Providers of such treatment can benefit from the victims' own perspectives (Wohlberg, 1997; Wohlberg, McCraith, & Thomas, 1999). Our concern here is with certain specific responsibilities as well as hazards that can arise for subsequent treating clinicians at the intersection of the clinical and legal arenas (see Edelwich & Brodsky, 1991, pp. 225–229).

Mandatory Reporting

A number of states have enacted statutes requiring clinicians to report sexual exploitation of a patient by a mental health professional, just as child abuse must be reported. While addressing important public safety concerns, mandatory reporting statutes raise troubling questions about patient confidentiality and informed choice. Some states have recognized this dilemma by requiring the patient's permission for the therapist to report the abuse. Where the patient's permission is not required, the therapist needs to work through the implications of the reporting requirement as part of the informed-consent process. Since the patient may experience mandatory reporting as compromising the confidentiality of any disclosures made in therapy, it is sometimes best to refer the patient to another clinician, either to make the report as a consultant or to continue the therapy (Haspel et al., 1997; Notman & Nadelson, 1994; Stone, 1983; Strasburger, 1999).

"Informed Consent" to Litigation

Therapists who regularly advise patients to bring suit or file licensing board complaints against therapists who violate treatment boundaries risk crossing a boundary themselves from a clinical into an advocacy role (Apfel & Simon, 1985b). Taking action against the abuser by "going public" can be empowering for the victim, but it is also likely to be—for a prolonged period of time—a stressful, sometimes threatening, and even traumatic or retraumatizing experience (one described in vivid detail, from the patient's viewpoint, in Bates and Brodsky, 1989). Clinicians with little court experience often markedly underestimate the extent, degree, and stress of exposure that accompany most litigation, especially on a sexual subject. Attorneys experienced with such cases often understand the need to prepare patients for the emotional and personal hazards of litigation, a process analogous to informed consent in the clinical realm. However, not all attorneys can be relied on to assume this responsibility. In any case, it remains the role and function of a therapist not to promote a particular course of action for ideological reasons, but to explore the patient's experiences and feelings (including fears, anxieties, and concerns for personal privacy) so that the patient can make an informed choice in his or her best interest (see Apfel & Simon, 1985b; Atkins & Stein, 1993).

Avoiding the Treater–Expert Role Conflict

Another way in which a treating psychotherapist may be tempted to step outside the clinical role is to testify as an expert witness as to the damage the therapist's patient has suffered as a result of a previous therapist's boundary violations. According to Strasburger et al. (1997), "The psychotherapist's wish to help the patient too often carries over into more direct, active forms of 'helping' that (however well-motivated) are contrary to the therapeutic mission," such that "in particular, a therapist's venturing into forensic terrain may be understood as a boundary violation that can compromise therapy as surely and as fatally as other, more patently unethical transgressions" (p. 455).

The role conflicts inherent in serving as treating clinician and forensic evaluator with respect to the same person have been outlined by various commentators (Bursztajn, Scherr, & Brodsky, 1994; Bush, Connell, & Denney, 2006; Drogin, in press; Goldstein, 2003; Greenberg & Shuman, 1997; Gutheil, 1998; Hornsby, Drogin, & Barrett, 1997; Iverson, 2000; Knapp & VandeCreek, 2003; Shuman, Greenberg, Heilbrun, & Foote, 1998; Strasburger et al., 1997; Wettstein, 2001). These two roles entail very different and usually incompatible ways of understanding a person—namely, a therapist's empathy and a forensic expert's objectivity. Thus, serving in one role is likely to compromise any attempt to perform the other, especially when the lack of confidentiality in forensic evaluation is taken into account.

> Simply put, there is a danger that when you provide treatment after a forensic evaluation, you have already committed yourself to an opinion which may color the goals and progress of treatment, and a judge or jury may find your motivations suspect. When you provide a forensic evaluation after treatment or standard clinical assessment, you may undermine the validity and persuasiveness of your opinion, because a judge or jury

may feel you have an interest in remaining consistent with conclusions
you have already reached in a psychological report or progress notes.
(Hornsby et al., 1997, p. 8)

For these reasons, it is advisable to refer the patient (or the patient's
attorney) to a qualified forensic mental health expert for evaluation. The
treating therapist does need to be aware of any legal or administrative
process in which the patient is or may be involved and to communicate
and coordinate appropriately (while safeguarding patient confidentiality)
with other professionals involved in that process (Atkins & Stein, 1993).
Nonetheless, maintaining clear role boundaries, communicated to and
agreed upon with the patient, provides a model of role clarity from which
the patient can derive future benefits.

KEY REMINDERS

- The actions most commonly taken by patients alleging boundary
  violations are complaints to ethics committees of professional associations, complaints to state professional licensing boards, and
  civil litigation.

- The manner in which such claims are evaluated by licensing
  boards, courts, and professional ethics committees often diverges
  from the more complex and realistic methods and criteria of
  trained, context-sensitive forensic evaluators.

- Complaints to state regulatory boards have the most serious potential consequences for the clinician, in that an adverse decision
  by a state board may result in loss of license and livelihood.

- In a civil court action, establishing malpractice liability entails
  proving the occurrence of a *dereliction* of *duty directly* causing
  damages—referred to as the "four Ds."

- False accusations of sexual misconduct and other boundary violations by therapists, although constituting only a small proportion of such complaints, have potentially devastating consequences and require careful evaluation for the sake of justice as
  well as objectivity.

- Therapists can best protect themselves against false accusations
  through thoroughgoing professionalism in their practice generally as well as in maintaining the therapeutic frame in any particular case.

CHAPTER 13

Prevention

Prevention of boundary violations through an understanding of underlying psychological and interpersonal processes has been the primary purpose of this book. There is no shortcut to prevention, no formula for avoiding difficulties and dilemmas. Rather, the discussions, analyses, and case examples in the preceding chapters have been developed to help equip the clinician to think clearly and productively about boundary questions that arise in practice. This approach reflects a conviction that the most effective form of prevention is an alert, anticipatory, and questioning attitude toward challenging clinical situations. This concluding chapter reviews central guidelines for boundary maintenance and summarizes practical preventive measures derived from them, including early warning signs of potential boundary compromises.

ETERNAL VIGILANCE: "FOR WHOSE BENEFIT?"

Boundary violations are best prevented by maintaining an awareness of clinical dynamics and practicing with sensitivity to the boundary challenges that inevitably arise. This means keeping an observing eye on one's own practice, the patient's behavior, and the interaction between the two. It also includes evaluating one's behavior according to the boundaries dictated by the type of therapy one is practicing; as we have discussed in previous chapters, proper therapist behavior in psychodynamic psychotherapy may or may not be the same as proper therapist behavior in cognitive-behavioral treatment in any given instance.

Yet, transcending all questions of theoretical orientation or ideology, a spot check for actual or potential boundary violations is the question posed in Chapter 1: *"Cui bono?"* (For whose benefit?) "Is this for my own gain or gratification, or is it *for the patient*? And is it for the patient's benefit as defined by the therapeutic contract, as opposed to simply satisfying the patient's immediate demands?" Whatever supports the development of the healthy side of the patient can be presumed to be appropriate and ethical. This is in contrast to indulging the side of the patient that seeks to avoid confronting issues by bribing, seducing, or overpowering the therapist or otherwise compromising therapy.

Often, however, the question of benefit is only the beginning, not the end, of exploration. How sure can we be about what is for the patient's benefit? As discussed in Chapter 10, a vulnerable therapist can all too readily rationalize that an intervention is for the patient's benefit when an objective observer would conclude otherwise (Bollas & Sundelson, 1995; Gabbard, 1996; Riker, 1997; Samuel & Gorton, 2001). After all, many therapists have rationalized that sex with a therapist is good for the patient. Far short of that extreme, a therapist's clinical and ethical judgment may be undermined by personal needs, life circumstances, or feelings about a particular patient.

In other words, boundary determinations can be as simple as *"Cui bono?"* and as complex as many of the discussions that have led up to this chapter. Therefore, one needs to develop an educated sense of "the patient's benefit" through clinical experience mediated by interaction with consultants, supervisors, and peers. Such interaction can help guard not only against unexamined boundary slippage but also against the opposite extreme, that of overdoing the vigilance at the expense of common sense and humanity. While exercising caution and prudence, it is essential not to lose clinical effectiveness and an ethical, compassionate focus on patients' well-being.

DOCUMENTATION AND CONSULTATION

Experienced clinicians practice and teach the maxim "Never worry alone." Patient and therapist alike benefit from bringing difficult questions into a less private, more open, space of interpersonal exchange and consideration. Because we are fallible and because we cannot fully know ourselves, everything we do—and why we do it—needs to be open to examination from perspectives other than our own (Samuel & Gorton, 2001). This is especially true inasmuch as the privacy and intimacy of the patient–therapist dyad (exacerbated, for some, by the isolation of private practice) are major risk factors for boundary violations. To correct for this isolation, clinicians have resources available for sorting out and managing boundary dilemmas.

Documentation and consultation (supplemented by peer support and, where needed, ongoing supervision) are not only major pillars of liability prevention; they are also pillars of responsible clinical and ethical care.

Documentation

Appropriate documentation leaves a record that a therapist has practiced according to professional standards and exercised reasonable clinical judgment. Even when an error has been made or a bad outcome occurs, the documentary record can establish that the clinician acted in the patient's best interest by assessing risks and benefits in light of the patient's condition and circumstances and intervening appropriately.

The value of documentation is not just after the fact, as a form of risk management. A therapist who fails to document a significant interaction with a patient because of an emotional conflict is at risk for losing focus. By contrast, ongoing documentation helps keep the treatment process on track by leaving it open to examination and review. That is, the very act of putting one's actions and rationales in writing redirects the patient–therapist relationship to the proper clinical realm rather than allowing it to go off into the "magic bubble" of fantasy (Gutheil, 1989). Thus, writing it down, like consulting a colleague or supervisor, is a test of—and a corrective for—the risk of stepping out of role and losing the appropriate clinical and ethical stance.

Documentation of clinical reasoning belongs in the patient's chart, not in informal personal journals. Entries that pertain directly to the care of the patient should go in the progress notes. Background thoughts for the purpose of better understanding the patient and considering possible consequences of different treatment strategies can be recorded in separate process notes (Appelbaum & Gutheil, 2007). Personal journals, on the other hand, are of ambiguous evidentiary value and should be considered a personal activity with little clinical or forensic relevance.

Consultation, Supervision, and Peer Support

Nearly all psychotherapists find the burdens of their "perilous calling" (Sussman, 1995a) too heavy to bear alone. It is essential to be able to call on the support of colleagues or supervisors to help deal with the pressures of this work, including challenges to the boundaries of the therapeutic frame. Ongoing supervision is recommended for managing a difficult course of treatment (Walker & Clark, 1999). Consultation with a supervisor or a knowledgeable, respected colleague is called for when sexual feelings enter into the relationship, when the patient demands or seeks to elicit boundary-breaking behavior from the therapist, or when the therapist is tempted to deviate from normal practice.

At any serious indication of patient dissatisfaction (or confusion about whether to be dissatisfied), it is advisable to call your insurer and seek the advice of an underwriter. Then, if legal action follows, you will have given the insurer timely notice. Another precaution is to get an anonymous advisory from the professional ethics committee or licensing board. You can ask, for example, "A patient of mine asked me to endorse a book he just wrote. Is this a potential problem? Is this the kind of thing you look into if it's brought to your attention?"This does not mean that one should wait to seek consultation until a crisis is brewing. From a risk management viewpoint, the most frustrating cases are those in which a therapist seeks consultation too late for the consultant to say anything except "Call your insurer and start planning your defense." On the contrary, consultation should be a regular practice, an outgrowth of normal clinical vigilance. Discussing routine as well as complicated interactions with patients lowers the threshold for seeking consultation and makes it easier to anticipate and prevent complications.

Consultation is beneficial on several levels. First, an informed but disinterested perspective can correct any distortions, misperceptions, or emotional overinvolvement on the therapist's part. (The consultant needs to be someone in a position to give an objective opinion rather than be predisposed to agree with the therapist.) Second, obtaining consultation is itself consistent with the standard of care and can help establish a record of acceptable professional practice. Third, a therapist who is willing to subject his or her judgment to peer scrutiny is less vulnerable to attributions of recklessness, narcissistic grandiosity, concealment, or clandestine activity. As emphasized in the preceding chapter, the best protection against false accusations, misattributions of motive, or misinterpretations of therapeutic efforts is an attitude of unwavering professionalism, maintained both inwardly and outwardly. When an accusation of improper conduct is made, one wants to have the kind of reputation that leads colleagues immediately to say "He [or she] didn't do it."

A low threshold for consultation is recommended whether it is the patient or therapist who takes the initiative. If a patient requests a consultation, the therapist should welcome the opportunity to broaden the exploration of issues that have arisen. In other circumstances the therapist may find a confidential or anonymous consultation useful. (Patients' names are not revealed to outside consultants without permission.) Among the clearest signs of a need for consultation are a conviction that consultation is not needed in a particular case and resentment at the suggestion that consultation might be advisable. In other words, the very reluctance to share information and seek advice signals a need to do so (Gabbard, 2001, 2005; Norris et al., 2003).

A therapist who has access to regular supervision through a training program or organizational hierarchy will normally use that supervisory relationship for needed consultations. To intervene effectively, however, a supervisor needs to understand the dynamics of boundary maintenance and boundary crossings and violations (Bursztajn, 1990; Norris et al., 2003; Waldinger, 1994; Walker & Clark, 1999). Such understanding cannot be presumed, as the following case illustrates:

> [A] senior forensic psychiatrist was asked to consult about the dangerousness of a [therapist's] former patient who was a possible stalker. Unraveled, the case proved to be one of a patient who began to experience erotic feelings for his female therapist—feelings that she did not know how to handle. Two successive layers of supervisors could not deal with this issue either, and the therapist terminated the psychotherapy on their recommendation. In reality, the baffled patient had taken to hanging about the clinic trying to get a straight answer about what had happened—hence, he was a "stalker." (Norris et al., 2003, p. 521)

As in this instance, you may need to go up the hierarchy—or reach out beyond it—to find a consultant experienced in the management of the therapeutic frame. When in doubt, you can call on a recognized clinical or forensic expert.

For therapists in private practice who do not have an established structure for supervision, a "buddy system" can be the first line of defense. If you have a colleague whose judgment you respect, each of you can serve as consultant of first resort for the other. In recent years such mutual support has expanded into peer supervision groups for solo practitioners and others seeking ongoing consultation. Groups of practitioners meet weekly, biweekly, or monthly to present cases for discussion (although cases involving sufficient discomfort or embarrassment may need to be presented to an outside consultant). In addition to the usual benefits of consultation, group members can become sufficiently familiar with one another to detect and question deviations from normal practice (Gabbard, 2005).

Such questioning need not be limited to formal supervision groups. Whether within an agency staff or among independent practitioners, the professional community should actively monitor reported or observed deviations from the standard of care. If there is reason for concern about an individual's practice, two colleagues can meet with that therapist and ask, "Are you aware that this is what has been reported about you?" The therapist will then know that others are aware of the rumors and will have the opportunity to explore the situation in a consultative way—or, if the allegations are false, to defend himself or herself (Gabbard, 2005).

Tips for the Novice

Novice clinicians should exercise extra care with respect to boundaries and maintain a much lower threshold for consultation and supervision. Notwithstanding the personal vulnerabilities that clinicians may manifest in midlife and beyond, a therapist who has faced down a thousand boundary challenges is not very likely to be thrown into confusion and panic by the thousand-and-first. Novice therapists are also advised to be cautious about attempting unusual interventions that experienced therapists are better prepared to keep from turning into boundary violations. Inexperienced and experienced therapists alike should keep in mind the criteria for evaluating prospective treatment interventions presented in the context of home visits in Chapter 3: (1) the therapist's intentions (clinical rationale); (2) foreseeable impact on the patient; (3) consistency with therapy contract or informed-consent process; and (4) appearance to third parties.

SCREENING AND REFERRAL

One form of preventive maintenance is careful screening to rule out serious psychopathologies to which a clinician's training and expertise are not well suited. Psychological testing and review of previous records can be helpful in finding an appropriate match between patient and clinician. A referral to a clinician with greater expertise or experience in dealing with a particular type of high-risk patient (e.g., someone skilled in alliance formation with patients with personality disorders) can benefit the patient as well as the referring therapist. Considerations of safety and comfort enter into screening decisions as well. For example, it can be reasonable for a female therapist to refer a serial rapist to a male therapist.

Clinicians employed in agencies typically cannot choose their patients. However, there may be pathways and protocols for referrals within the agency. In addition, one can take advantage of the safety features built into the agency setting and structure (such as established procedures for patient–clinician interaction, the presence of observers, and readily available consultation) to protect against boundary challenges.

EDUCATION AND TRAINING

As Apfel and Simon (1985a) note, "The privileged intimacy in the psychotherapist–patient relationship, the ineluctable issues of power, the human frailty of the players, and the extraordinary capacities of therapist and patient to rationalize and deny are all factors that make the elimination of patient–therapist sex unlikely" (p. 57). The same is true, by extension, of boundary violations generally. Although elimination of boundary violations is not a realistic goal, we can strive to reduce the incidence of such violations by preparing clinicians for the challenges they will face in practice. No amount of education will stop antisocial predators, but those individuals sometimes can be identified and screened out in training. At the same time, ethical practitioners can be armed with a conceptual framework and guidelines for practice (Gabbard, 1999a, 2005).

The design and specific content of training programs are beyond the scope of this book. (For more detailed discussion of actual or proposed training programs and curricula, see Ad Hoc Committee on Physician Impairment, 1994; Averill et al., 1989; Blackshaw & Patterson, 1992; Bridges, 1995a; Duckworth, Kahn, & Gutheil, 1994; Garfinkel, Dorian, Sadavoy, & Bagby, 1997; Gorton, Samuel, & Zembrowski, 1996; Hamilton & Spruill, 1999; Housman & Stake, 1999; Kay & Roman, 1999; Milgrom, 1992; Morrison & Morrison, 2001; Plaut, 1997; Robinson & Stewart, 1996a, 1996b; Rodolfa, Kitzrow, Vohra, & Wilson, 1990; Roman & Kay, 1997; Schoener, 1999). Here we will simply summarize themes and principles (consistent with the preceding chapters) that should inform the training of clinicians.

1. Clinicians in training should receive explicit guidance in the ethical, clinical, and legal issues surrounding boundary violations and sexual misconduct. A majority of psychiatry residency training directors and psychology internship directors surveyed in the 1990s indicated that such training should be mandatory (Gorton & Samuel, 1996; Samuel & Gorton, 1998, 2001). The importance of boundaries should be taught in terms of the protection of patients and the therapeutic frame rather than mecha-

nistic lists of prohibited acts (Gutheil & Gabbard, 1998). Students should be educated as to what facilitates therapy and what blocks or compromises it.

2. Ethics should be taught in the context of clinical understanding, allowing for different treatment philosophies and practices (Gabbard, 1996; Gutheil & Gabbard, 1998; Gutheil & Simon, 2002). Whether the relevant interpersonal and intrapsychic processes are understood in terms of psychoanalytic theory (Gabbard & Lester, 2002) or cognitive-behavioral therapy (Kohlenberg & Tsai, 2007; Linehan, 1993; Safran & Segal, 1996), clinical training should incorporate a basic understanding of the relational dynamics of therapy, including the power imbalance and the patient's vulnerability to exploitation (Duckworth et al., 1994; Gutheil, 1992b; Norris et al., 2003).

3. The concepts of fiduciary duty and undue influence (still greatly underutilized in professional training programs) have the depth, relevance, and broad applicability to serve as the best foundation for training in boundary maintenance and monitoring, whatever the discipline or approach to treatment (Samuel & Gorton, 2001).

4. The "slippery slope" from small to large boundary violations should be taught not in a simplistic, deterministic manner but as an empirical observation of an avoidable pitfall (Gutheil & Simon, 2002; Strasburger, Jorgenson, & Sutherland, 1992). The aim should be both to sensitize trainees to the potential harms resulting from even minor boundary transgressions and to show how the slide down the slippery slope can be halted by reflection and intervention.

5. Trainees need to be guided and supported in accepting, understanding, and working with—rather than acting out—their feelings (sexual and otherwise) toward patients (Bridges, 1994, 1995a, 1998; Duckworth et al., 1994; Edelwich & Brodsky, 1991; Hamilton & Spruill, 1999; Pope et al., 1993).

6. Trainees should receive practical instruction in the management of treatment impasses and maintenance of interpersonal boundaries through alliance-based interaction and intervention, allowing for the different conceptions and manifestations of the treatment alliance in different schools of therapy (Leahy, 2003b; Meissner, 1996; Safran & Muran, 1998, 2003). This is especially important in the treatment of patients who have a tendency toward blurring of boundaries, excessive dependency, and emotional instability (Gutheil, 1989).

7. Trainees need to be sensitized to the impact of cultural differences on boundary dynamics. The patient's and clinician's cultural backgrounds can affect body image, the meaning of touch, male–female relations, con-

ceptions of territoriality and violation, attitudes toward gender and sex-ual orientation, and the perceived role of the clinician. Immigrants and economically disadvantaged patients regularly require active interven-tions that might be viewed as boundary violations in a more affluent private-practice clientele, such as walking a patient through the welfare office, visiting an indigent patient at home to assess the living environ-ment, or regularly making phone calls to monitor and facilitate the pa-tient's attendance at sessions (Gabbard & Nadelson, 1995; Twemlow, 1997).

DECISION-MAKING GUIDELINES

An extensive literature has explored the troubling reality of multiple rela-tionships between mental health professionals and patients (Adleman & Barrett, 1990; Bader, 1994; Baer & Murdock, 1995; Barnett & Yutrzenka, 1994; Borys, 1994; Borys & Pope, 1989; Brown & Cogan, 2006; Burian & O'Connor-Slimp, 2000; Campbell & Gordon, 2003; Clarkson, 1994; Ebert, 1997; Faulkner & Faulkner, 1997; Haas, Malouf, & Mayerson, 1988; Helbok, Marinelli, & Walls, 2006; Horst, 1989; Kagle & Giebelhausen, 1994; Kitchener, 1988, 2000; Lamb, Catanzaro, & Moorman, 2004; Lazarus & Zur, 2002; Meara, Schmidt, & Day, 1996; Moleski & Kiselica, 2005; O'Connor-Slimp & Burian, 1994; Pope & Vetter, 1991; Pope & Wedding, 2008; Rinella & Gerstein, 1994; Roll & Millen, 1981; Ryder & Hepworth, 1990; Simon & Williams, 1999; Sonne, Borys, Haviland, & Ermshar, 1998; Welfel, 2002; Williams, 1997). Systematic decision-making guides are now available for clinicians who face the possibility of such multiple (nonsex-ual) relationships. Sonne (2005), drawing on theoretical models, research findings, and clinical guidelines, outlines four categories of factors to be considered in determining how to handle such a situation: therapist fac-tors, client factors, therapy relationship factors, and other relationship fac-tors. Gottlieb (1993) presents a model to help translate ethical principles into practical guidelines, acknowledging (as does the American Psycho-logical Association's code of ethics) that psychotherapists inevitably face dilemmas involving multiple relationships. Gottlieb's model helps the cli-nician structure the decision while allowing latitude for professional judgment. It involves assessment of both the current and the contem-plated relationship along three dimensions: power, duration of relation-ship, and clarity (i.e., finality) of termination. Consultation with a knowl-edgeable colleague and discussion of the decision with the patient are called for. Pope and Keith-Spiegel (in press) have developed a nine-step process for making decisions about boundary crossings. They also list common errors of thinking and judgment with respect to boundary decisions and recommend reparative measures when a boundary crossing creates difficulties. Younggren (2002) advises therapists to ask the following questions when the prospect of a dual relationship arises:

- Is the dual relationship necessary?
- Is the dual relationship exploitative?
- Whom does the dual relationship benefit?
- Is there a risk that the dual relationship could damage the patient?
- Is there a risk that the dual relationship could disrupt the therapeutic relationship?
- Am I being objective in my evaluation of this matter? (Answering this question requires consultation.)
- Have I adequately documented the decision-making process?
- Did the client give informed consent regarding the risks of the dual relationship?

These questions are consistent with the precautions recommended throughout this book (see Younggren & Gottlieb, 2004). Other widely used decision-making guides apply specifically to multiple relationships in rural communities (Campbell & Gordon, 2003; Faulkner & Faulkner, 1997; Simon & Williams, 1999). Lamb and Catanzaro's (1998) model extends to multiple relationships with supervisees and students as well as patients.

WARNING SIGNS

An important preventive measure for clinicians, as well as for supervisors, colleagues, and consultants, is timely recognition of potential boundary compromises (Simon, 1995). Early warning signs of boundary problems can be found throughout the case vignettes and discussions in the preceding chapters. A general preventive strategy that encompasses many of those specific red flags is to give careful attention to any slippage in one's usual way of practicing. When you catch yourself thinking "Why don't I change the time frame for our sessions?" or "I noticed I wanted to hug the patient after that last session" or "Why did I feel like telephoning the patient after the session?", your next thought should be "I wonder why that occurred to me at just this moment. I think I'll talk to my supervisor or consultant about it."

A widely used compilation of early warning indicators is Epstein and Simon's "Exploitation Index" (Epstein, 1994, pp. 275–280; Epstein & Simon, 1990; Epstein et al., 1992). The Exploitation Index consists of 32 self-assessment questions grouped into the following categories:

- *Generalized boundary violations* (role conflicts that blur the line between a therapeutic relationship and a personal, social, or business relationship)
- *Eroticism* (indulging in self-gratifying romantic feelings about a patient)
- *Exhibitionism* (boasting or otherwise obtaining personal gratification from a patient's accomplishments or notoriety)
- *Dependency* (feeling a need for a patient to continue in therapy or to give the therapist personal emotional support)
- *Power seeking* (a need for mastery and control over the patient, in or out of therapy)
- *Greediness* (seeking financial benefits from a patient beyond the contracted fee for therapy)
- *Enabling* (allowing "rescue fantasies" and a need to "cure" to lead one to make exceptions for a patient who is felt to be "special")

In addition to the warning signs listed in the Exploitation Index, the following common indicators of boundary confusion or compromise are taken from other sources (Friedman & Boumil, 1995, pp. 45–60; Gutheil & Simon, 1995; Menninger & Holzman, 1973; Norris et al., 2003) and from clinical and forensic experience:

- Engaging in idle, nontherapeutically focused conversation with a patient
- Arguing or attempting dogmatically to impose one's views (about politics, philosophy, religion, etc.) on a patient
- Becoming inappropriately directive about a patient's personal choices, especially with respect to intimate relationships
- Attempting to impress a patient
- Allowing or engaging in inappropriate personal familiarity and disclosures with a patient at the beginning or end of sessions, when the patient is entering or leaving the office
- Feeling that one is solely responsible for a patient's life
- Feeling that one has allowed a patient to take over the management of his or her case
- Selective or omitted documentation of significant interactions, occurrences, or dynamics in treatment

- Reluctance to discuss a case with a consultant or supervisor for fear of revealing one's errors or disrupting a "special" relationship with a patient
- Discouraging a patient from obtaining a consultation or seeking a second opinion
- Insisting on secrecy about what goes on in therapy

Although not all of these warning signs indicate that a boundary violation has occurred or will occur, all are triggers for consultation or for colleagues to look into the situation.

PREVENTION AT THE INSTITUTIONAL LEVEL

As discussed in Chapter 12, an organization is ethically and legally responsible to its clients for the acts of its employees. An agency's or institution's fiduciary duty extends to everything its staff members do on the job. There is much that clinics, hospitals, university departments, and other organizations can and must do—not only in training but also in hiring, supervision, and retention—to uphold accepted standards of care, support clinicians in practicing ethically, and prevent unethical or impaired individuals from practicing. Representative guidelines for organizational policy and procedure are those outlined by Edelwich and Brodsky (1991, pp. 229–231).

1. The agency needs a written policy that is clear, specific, enforceable, and consistent with governing law and professional codes of ethics. The policy should be signed by every new employee upon hiring and placed in the employee's permanent file.

2. The agency should have documented in-service training sessions at least twice a year on clinical, ethical, and policy issues, including principles and practice of clinical ethics, fiduciary responsibility, undue influence, the dynamics of clinician–patient interaction as understood within the relevant schools of therapy, and the importance of documentation and consultation. Ongoing supervision offers clinicians continuity of support between training programs (see Bursztajn, 1990).

3. The administration must be able to intervene in a timely manner before or as transgressions or questionable acts occur. This is accomplished through appropriate supervision, monitoring, and prompt investigation when there are reasonable grounds for suspicion.

For additional treatment of these and other administrative safeguards (including hiring, record keeping, complaint resolution, and peer review), the reader is referred to other sources (Carroll, 2006; Gabbard, 1994b; Gabbard & Lester, 2002, ch. 10; Gabbard & Peltz, 2001; Reamer, 2001; Schoener, 1989a, 1995b; Strasburger et al., 1992).

REHABILITATION OF OFFENDERS

Although the assessment and rehabilitation of clinicians who have committed sexual misconduct or other serious boundary violations is beyond the scope of this book, a starting point for assessment can be found in the typologies of vulnerable therapists in Chapter 10. Each category of perpetrator (e.g., naive or "lovesick" vs. sociopathic or narcissistic) is assessed as having a greater or lesser potential for rehabilitation. However, a thorough mental health evaluation is necessary to develop an individualized rehabilitation plan (Gabbard, 1994a, 1994b). Models for such in-depth assessment are described by Celenza & Gabbard (2003), Gonsiorek (1995a), Irons (1995), and Schoener (1995a).

Glen Gabbard, who has written extensively on this subject, outlines the following components of an effective rehabilitation plan: personal psychotherapy and (as needed) pharmacotherapy, assignment of a rehabilitation coordinator (a mental health professional other than the psychotherapist), practice limitations, supervision, and continuing education. In some cases mediation between the offending therapist and the patient/victim proves useful to both parties. This rehabilitation process may go on for 3–5 years, with yearly evaluations of progress (Gabbard, 1994a, 1994b, 1999a, 2005; Gabbard & Lester, 2002, pp. 182–191).

Treatment and rehabilitation of boundary-violating therapists can be undertaken using either a psychodynamic (Celenza, 1991; Gabbard, 1995b; Gabbard & Lester, 2002, pp. 182–191) or cognitive-behavioral (Abel, Barrett, & Gardos, 1992; Abel & Osborn, 1999; Abel, Osborn, & Warberg, 1995) approach. Frick, McCartney, and Lazarus (1995) provide guidelines for supervision as part of a rehabilitation plan. Jorgenson (1995c) discusses rehabilitation from a risk management perspective, outlining the potential liability of rehabilitation providers and subsequent employers. Jorgenson (1995c), Pope (1990a, 1994), and Samuel and Gorton (2001) raise questions about whether and how the effectiveness of rehabilitation can be measured. (For additional information on rehabilitation and remedial training, see Irons, 1991; Schoener, 1999.)

PUBLIC EDUCATION

While educating and training clinicians, we should not overlook opportunities to educate and inform patients. For example, brochures that provide straightforward explanations about therapy and its boundaries, making clear that some things are "never OK," can be made available in office waiting rooms. An informed consumer is more likely to walk out of the office and report a therapist who acts unethically. There has, of course, been progress since the 1980s in making the public aware that sex between therapist and patient is impermissible and that therapeutic boundaries are to be respected. The voices of victims of misconduct by therapists are an invaluable resource in educating the public as well as professionals (Wohlberg, 1997; Wohlberg et al., 1999). A challenge that remains is to disabuse the public of rigid caricatures of therapeutic boundaries that trigger misguided complaints.

Websites now provide information for patients about professional misconduct and what to do if one believes one has been a victim of exploitation. One such resource is known as the "Advocate Web: Helping Overcome Professional Exploitation." This site can be visited at *www. advocateweb.org./hope/default.asp*. Other support networks include the following: Boston Associates to Stop Treatment Abuse (BASTA!) *www.advocateweb. org/basta/*; Therapy Exploitation Link Line (TELL) *www.therapyabuse.org/*; Treatment Exploitation Recovery Network (TERN) *www.advocateweb./ tern/*.

Websites come and go, of course, and there is no guarantee that a particular site will remain available. However, the number of such resources is likely to increase in the coming years, and any one of them can serve as a gateway to others.

An extraordinary resource for the professions and the public has been the website (*http://kspope.com*) maintained by psychologist Kenneth Pope, a leading researcher on boundary issues in the mental health fields. This site links to a growing library of publications on boundary violations, multiple relationships, professional ethics and standards, and many related subjects.

PERSONAL INTERVENTIONS

A vital component of prevention is self-care (Gabbard, 1994b, 2005; R. Hilton, 1997a). When psychotherapists attend to their physical and mental health and maintain a balanced, satisfying life, they have less need to seek personal emotional gratification from patients. Strean (1993) reported that none of the boundary-transgressing therapists he treated had intimate relationships that were warm, close, and spontaneous. These therapists were as useful to their patients as a drowning lifeguard is to a swimmer in trouble.

Those who have studied "burnout" among mental health professionals emphasize the importance of meeting one's own needs for fun, rest and relaxation, intimacy, and social connection (Edelwich & Brodsky, 1980; Grosch & Olsen, 1994, 1995). These are protective factors against vulnerability to clinical boundary violation. In addition, personal psychotherapy can be a valuable tool for coming to terms with the pain, disappointment, and longing hidden beneath the therapist's professional role, as well as for understanding one's reactions to difficult patients (Gabbard, 1994b; R. Hilton, 1997a). Norcross and Guy (2007) have developed a comprehensive program of self-care (physical, emotional, spiritual, and environmental) that can reduce stress and increase clinical effectiveness for psychotherapists. At times of increased stress (e.g., divorce, serious illness, bereavement) when one's abilities are compromised and one's effectiveness foreseeably reduced, a leave of absence may be advisable.

COMMUNAL AND SOCIETAL INTERVENTIONS

Ultimately, this prescription for self-nurturance within a supportive community of family and friends needs to be extended to a collective nurturance in the professional community and the larger society. Samuel and Gorton (2001) speak of an emerging "culture of awareness" in which the mental health professions' painful self-examination has compelled them to acknowledge the humanity of their members. Samuel and Gorton refer to this cultural movement as "a watershed period in the revolution in human species self-awareness" (p. 76). Only in community, notes Genova (2001), do human beings have any chance to cope with the pressures that have produced widespread therapeutic boundary violations. Yet, the therapeutic dyad is too often isolated from community, even as both members need the resources that community offers. This book is offered as a contribution to the creation of the highly developed humane moral atmosphere envisioned by those in our field who see farthest and deepest.

KEY REMINDERS

- Boundary violations are best prevented by maintaining an awareness of clinical dynamics and practicing with sensitivity to the boundary challenges that inevitably arise.

- A spot check for actual or potential boundary violations is the question *"Cui bono?"* (For whose benefit?). "Is this for my own gain or gratification, or is it *for the patient*? And is it for the patient's benefit as defined by the therapeutic contract, as opposed to simply satisfying the patient's immediate demands?"

- Documentation and consultation (supplemented by peer support and, where needed, ongoing supervision) are not only major pillars of liability prevention but also pillars of responsible clinical and ethical care.

- Consultation is called for when sexual feelings enter into the relationship, when the patient demands or seeks to elicit boundary-breaking behavior from the therapist, or when the therapist is tempted to deviate from customary practice.

- The best protection against false accusations, misattributions of motive, or misinterpretations of therapeutic efforts is an attitude of unwavering professionalism, maintained both inwardly and outwardly.

- Novice clinicians should exercise extra care with respect to boundaries and maintain a much lower threshold for consultation and supervision.

- Clinicians in training should receive explicit guidance in the ethical, clinical, and legal issues surrounding boundary violations and sexual misconduct as well as practical instruction in the management of treatment impasses and maintenance of interpersonal boundaries through alliance-based interaction and intervention.

- Timely recognition of potential boundary compromises is an important preventive measure for clinicians as well as for supervisors, colleagues, and consultants.

- Good health, a balanced, satisfying life, and personal psychotherapy are protective factors against vulnerability to violating clinical boundaries.

Afterword

We have conceived of this book as a "supervisor on a bookshelf." A book cannot, however, take the place of a flesh-and-blood supervisor or consultant. It is impossible to identify and prescribe solutions for every type of boundary challenge that may arise in clinical practice. Moreover, given the virtually unlimited variety of clinical contexts in which readers find themselves, we do not think it helpful to offer lists of "musts" and "must-nots." Instead, we have sought to model a way of thinking about boundaries that takes into account contexts of practice, vulnerabilities of patients and therapists, the importance of informed consent, and the serious consequences that both patients and therapists may suffer when boundaries are not properly maintained. Although this book cannot be everything for everybody, we hope it will strengthen the knowledge, skills, and clinical judgment that make therapy beneficial, not harmful, and thereby will foster useful collaborations between therapists and patients.

Some key principles have emerged from this exploration:

1. Boundaries play a meaningful part in almost every form of therapy, but the particular boundaries to be observed differ in different clinical contexts.
2. Contexts of practice that affect the determination of boundaries include the type of therapy, the setting of the practice, the patient's presenting problems and diagnosis, and characteristics of the patient and therapist (e.g., age, gender, cultural background).

3. In any form of therapy, the underlying principle of ethical boundary maintenance is that any therapeutic intervention be for the benefit of the patient.
4. The responsibility for setting and maintaining boundaries always belongs to the therapist, not the patient.
5. Assessment of whether an intervention constitutes a boundary violation depends not only on the therapist's intent, but also on the impact (actual or foreseeable) on the patient.
6. Good therapy is the best form of risk management.
7. Never worry alone. If in doubt, consult a supervisor or experienced colleague.
8. Always be professional, and always be human.

References

A. B. v. C. D., Va., Albemarle County Cir. Ct., No. 5871-L, April 24, 1996.

Abel, G. G., Barrett, D. H., & Gardos, P. S. (1992). Sexual misconduct by physicians. *Journal of the Medical Association of Georgia, 81,* 237–246.

Abel, G. G., & Osborn, C. A. (1999). Cognitive-behavioral treatment of sexual misconduct. In J. D. Bloom, C. C. Nadelson, & M. T. Notman (Eds.), *Physician sexual misconduct* (pp. 225–246). Washington, DC: American Psychiatric Press.

Abel, G. G., Osborn, C. A., & Warberg, B. (1995). Cognitive-behavioral treatment for professional sexual misconduct. *Psychiatric Annals, 25,* 106–112.

Ad Hoc Committee on Physician Impairment. (1994). Report of the Federation's Ad Hoc Committee on Physician Impairment. *Federal Bulletin, 81,* 229–242.

Adleman, J., & Barrett, S. E. (1990). Overlapping relationships: Importance of the feminist ethical perspective. In H. Lerman & N. Porter (Eds.), *Feminist ethics in psychotherapy* (pp. 87–91). New York: Springer.

Akamatsu, T. J. (1988). Intimate relationships with former clients: National survey of attitudes and behavior among practitioners. *Professional Psychology: Research and Practice, 19,* 454–458.

Alyn, J. H. (1988). The politics of touch in therapy: A response to Willison and Masson. *Journal of Counseling and Development, 66,* 432–433.

American Association for Marriage and Family Therapy. (2001). *AAMFT code of ethics.* Alexandria, VA: Author.

American Psychiatric Association. (2006). *The principles of medical ethics with annotations especially applicable to psychiatry.* Arlington, VA: Author.

American Psychological Association. (2002). *Ethical principles of psychologists and code of conduct.* Washington, DC: Author.

Anderson, S. K., & Kitchener, K. S. (1996). Nonromantic, nonsexual posttherapy relationships between psychologists and former clients: An exploratory study of critical incidents. *Professional Psychology: Research and Practice, 27,* 59–66.

Anderson, S. K., & Kitchener, K. S. (1998). Nonsexual posttherapy relationships: A conceptual framework. *Professional Psychology: Research and Practice, 29,* 91–99.

Apfel, R. J., & Simon, B. (1985a). Patient–therapist sexual contact: I. Psychodynamic perspectives on the causes and results. *Psychotherapy and Psychosomatics, 43,* 57–62.

303

Apfel, R. J., & Simon, B. (1985b). Patient–therapist sexual contact: II. Problems of subsequent psychotherapy. *Psychotherapy and Psychosomatics, 43,* 63–68.

Appelbaum, P. S., & Gutheil, T. G. (2007). *Clinical handbook of psychiatry and the law* (4th ed.). Philadelphia, PA: Lippincott Williams & Wilkins.

Appelbaum, P. S., & Jorgenson, L. (1991). Psychotherapist–patient sexual contact after termination of treatment: An analysis and a proposal. *American Journal of Psychiatry, 148,* 1466–1473.

Appelbaum, P. S., Jorgenson, L., & Sutherland, P. K. (1994). Sexual relationships between physicians and patients. *Archives of Internal Medicine, 154,* 2561–2565.

Arlow, J. (1969). Fantasy, memory and reality testing. *Psychoanalytic Quarterly, 38,* 28–51.

Aron, L. (1996). *A meeting of minds: Mutuality in psychoanalysis.* Hillsdale, NJ: Analytic Press.

Atkins, E. L., & Stein, R. (1993). When the boundary is crossed: A protocol for attorneys and mental health professionals. *American Journal of Forensic Psychiatry, 14*(3), 51–69.

Averill, S. C., Beale, D., Benfer, B., Collins, D. T., Kennedy, L., Myers, J., Pope, D., Rosen, I., & Zoble, E. (1989). Preventing staff–patient sexual relationships. *Bulletin of the Menninger Clinic, 53,* 384–393.

Bader, E. (1994). Dual relationships: Legal and ethical trends. *Transactional Analysis Journal, 24*(1), 64–66.

Baer, B. E., & Murdock, N. L. (1995). Nonerotic dual relationships between therapists and clients: The effects of sex, theoretical orientation, and interpersonal boundaries. *Ethics and Behavior, 5,* 131–145.

Barish, K. (2004). The child therapist's generative use of self. *Journal of Infant, Child, and Adolescent Psychotherapy, 3,* 270–282.

Barker, J. A. (1990). Professional–client sex: Is criminal liability an appropriate means of enforcing professional responsibility? *UCLA Law Review, 40,* 1275–1339.

Barnett, J. E., & Yutrzenka, B. A. (1994). Nonsexual dual relationships in professional practice, with special applications to rural and military communities. *The Independent Practitioner, 14,* 243–248.

Barrett, M. S., & Berman, J. S. (2001). Is psychotherapy more effective when therapists disclose information about themselves? *Journal of Consulting and Clinical Psychology, 69,* 597–603.

Bartell, P. A., & Rubin, L. J. (1990). Dangerous liaisons: Sexual intimacies in supervision. *Professional Psychology: Research and Practice, 21,* 442–450.

Bates, C. M., & Brodsky, A. M. (1989). *Sex in the therapy hour: A case of professional incest.* New York: Guilford Press.

Beal, S. W. (1989). Patient–therapist sex [letter]. *American Journal of Psychiatry, 146,* 1518–1519.

Beck, A. T. (1991). *Cognitive therapy and the emotional disorders.* New York: Penguin.

Belote, J. (1974). Sexual intimacy between female clients and male psychotherapists: Masochistic sabotage. Doctoral dissertation, California School of Professional Psychology, San Francisco, CA. *Dissertation Abstracts International.* 1977. *38,* 887B.

Benowitz, M. (1995). Comparing the experiences of women clients sexually exploited by female versus male psychotherapists. In J. C. Gonsiorek (Ed.), *Breach of trust: Sexual exploitation by health care professionals and clergy* (pp. 213–224). Thousand Oaks, CA: Sage.

Berg, J. W. (2002). Ethics and e-medicine. *St. Louis University Law Journal, 46,* 61–83.

Berg, J. W., Appelbaum, P. S., Lidz, C. W., & Parker, L. S. (2001). *Informed consent: Legal theory and clinical practice* (2nd ed.). New York: Oxford University Press.

Berne, E. (1972). *What do you say after you say hello? The psychology of human destiny.* New York: Grove Press.

Bernsen, A., Tabachnick, B. G., & Pope, K. S. (1994). National survey of social workers' sexual attraction to their clients: Results, implications, and comparison to psychologists. *Ethics and Behavior, 4,* 369–388.

Bienen, M. (1990). The pregnant therapist: Countertransference dilemmas and willingness to explore transference material. *Psychotherapy, 27,* 607–612.

Blackshaw, S. L., & Patterson, P. G. R. (1992). The prevention of sexual exploitation of patients: Educational issues. *Canadian Journal of Psychiatry, 37,* 350–353.

Blanton, S. (1971). *Diary of my analysis with Sigmund Freud.* New York: Hawthorn Books.

Blatt, S. J. (2001). Commentary: The therapeutic process and professional boundary guidelines. *Journal of the American Academy of Psychiatry and the Law, 29,* 290–293.

Bleger, J. (1966). Psychoanalysis of the psychoanalytic frame. *International Journal of Psychoanalysis, 48,* 511–519.

Bollas, C., & Sundelson, D. (1995). *The new informants: The betrayal of confidentiality in psychoanalysis and psychotherapy.* Northvale, NJ: Aronson.

Borenstein, D. B., & Fintzy, R. T. (1980–1981). Postanalytic encounters. *International Journal of Psychoanalytic Psychotherapy, 8,* 151–164.

Borys, D. S. (1994). Maintaining therapeutic boundaries: The motive is therapeutic effectiveness, not defensive practice. *Ethics and Behavior, 4,* 267–273.

Borys, D. S., & Pope, K. S. (1989). Dual relationships between therapist and client: A national study of psychologists, psychiatrists, and social workers. *Professional Psychology: Research and Practice, 20,* 283–293.

Bouhoutsos, J., Holroyd, J., Lerman, H., Forer, B. R., & Greenberg, M. (1983). Sexual intimacy between psychotherapists and patients. *Professional Psychology: Research and Practice, 14,* 185–196.

Boynton, R. S. (2002, December 15). The interpretation of Khan. *Boston Globe,* pp. C1–C3.

Bridges, N. A. (1994). Meaning and management of attraction: Neglected areas of psychotherapy training and practice. *Psychotherapy, 31,* 424–433.

Bridges, N. A. (1995a). Managing erotic and loving feelings in therapeutic relationships: A model course. *Journal of Psychotherapy Practice and Research, 4,* 329–339.

Bridges, N. A. (1995b). Psychotherapy with therapists: Countertransference dilemmas. In M. B. Sussman (Ed.), *A perilous calling: The hazards of psychotherapy practice* (pp. 175–187). New York: Wiley.

Bridges, N. A. (1998). Teaching psychiatric trainees to respond to sexual and loving feelings: The supervisory challenge. *Journal of Psychotherapy Practice and Research, 7,* 217–226.

Bridges, N. A. (2001). Therapist self-disclosure: Expanding the comfort zone. *Psychotherapy, 38,* 21–30.

Bridges, N. A., & Smith, J. M. (1988). The pregnant therapist and the seriously disturbed patient: Managing long-term psychotherapeutic treatment. *Psychiatry, 51,* 104–109.

Brown, J. L., & Cogan, K. D. (2006). Ethical clinical practice and sport psychology: When two worlds collide. *Ethics and Behavior, 16,* 15–23.

Brown, L. S. (1985). Power, responsibility, boundaries: Ethical concerns for the lesbian feminist therapist. *Lesbian Ethics, 1,* 30–45.

Brown, L. S. (1988). Harmful effects of posttermination sexual and romantic relationships between therapists and their former clients. *Psychotherapy, 25,* 249–255.

Brownlee, K. (1996). The ethics of nonsexual dual relationships: A dilemma for the rural mental health professional. *Community Mental Health Journal, 32,* 497–503.

Burgess, A. W., & Hartman, C. R. (Eds.). (1986). *Sexual exploitation of patients by health professionals.* New York: Praeger.

Burian, B. K., & O'Connor-Slimp, A. (2000). Social dual-role relationships during internship: A decision-making model. *Professional Psychology: Research and Practice, 31,* 332–338.

Burke, W. F. (1992). Countertransference disclosure and the asymmetry/mutuality dilemma. *Psychoanalytic Dialogues, 2,* 241–271.

Bursztajn, H. J. (1985). More law and less protection: "Critogenesis," "legal iatrogenesis," and medical decision-making. *Journal of Geriatric Psychiatry, 18,* 143–153.

Bursztajn, H. J. (1990, June). Supervisory responsibility for prevention of supervisee sexual misconduct. Presentation at International Congress of Psychiatry and the Law, Toronto, Ontario.

Bursztajn, H. J., Feinbloom, R. I., Hamm, R. M., & Brodsky, A. (1990). *Medical choices, medical chances: How patients, families, and physicians can cope with uncertainty.* New York: Routledge.

Bursztajn, H. J., Gutheil, T. G., Brodsky, A., & Swagerty, E. L. (1988). "Magical thinking," suicide, and malpractice litigation. *Bulletin of the American Academy of Psychiatry and the Law, 16,* 369–377.

Bursztajn, H. J., Scherr, A. E., & Brodsky, A. (1994). The rebirth of forensic psychiatry in light of recent historical trends in criminal responsibility. *Psychiatric Clinics of North America, 17,* 611–635.

Bush, S. S., Connell, M. A., & Denney, R. L. (2006). *Ethical practice in forensic psychology: A systematic model for decision making.* Washington, DC: American Psychological Association.

Butler, S., & Zelen, S. L. (1977). Sexual intimacies between therapists and patients. *Psychotherapy: Theory, Research, and Practice, 14,* 139–145.

Campbell, C., & Gordon, M. (2003). Acknowledging the inevitable: Understanding multiple relationships in rural practice. *Professional Psychology: Research and Practice, 34,* 430–434.

Canning, S., Hauser, M. J., Gutheil, T. G., & Bursztajn, H. J. (1991). Communications in psychiatric practice: Decision making and the use of the telephone. In T. G. Gutheil, H. J. Bursztajn, A. Brodsky, & V. G. Alexander (Eds.). *Decision making in psychiatry and the law* (pp. 227–235). Baltimore, MD: Williams & Wilkins.

Carroll, R. (Ed.). (2006). *Risk management handbook for health care organizations* (5th ed., 3 vols.). San Francisco: Jossey-Bass.

Casement, P. J. (1985). *On learning from the patient.* London: Tavistock.

Casement, P. J. (1990). The meeting of needs in psychoanalysis. *Psychoanalytic Inquiry, 10,* 325–346.

Caudill, O. B., Jr. (1997a). Can therapists be vicariously liable for sexual misconduct? In L. E. Hedges, R. Hilton, V. W. Hilton, & O. B. Caudill, Jr. (Eds.), *Therapists at risk: Perils of the intimacy of the therapeutic relationship* (pp. 269–273). Northvale, NJ: Aronson.

Caudill, O. B., Jr. (1997b). The mind business. In L. E. Hedges, R. Hilton, V. W. Hilton, & O. B. Caudill, Jr. (Eds.), *Therapists at risk: Perils of the intimacy of the therapeutic relationship* (pp. 275–284). Northvale, NJ: Aronson.

Caudill, O. B., Jr. (1997c). The seduction of the innocent therapist. In L. E. Hedges, R. Hilton, V. W. Hilton, & O. B. Caudill, Jr. (Eds.), *Therapists at risk: Perils of the intimacy of the therapeutic relationship* (pp. 87–98). Northvale, NJ: Aronson.

Celenza, A. (1991). The misuse of countertransference love in cases of sexual intimacies between therapists and patients. *Psychoanalytic Psychology, 8,* 501–509.

Celenza, A. (1998). Precursors to sexual misconduct: Preliminary findings. *Psychoanalytic Psychology, 15,* 378–395.

Celenza, A. (2007). *Sexual boundary violations: Therapeutic, supervisory, and academic contexts.* Lanham, MD: Aronson.

Celenza, A., & Gabbard, G. O. (2003). Analysts who commit sexual boundary violations: A lost cause? *Journal of the American Psychoanalytic Association, 51,* 617–636.

Celenza, A., & Hilsenroth, M. (1997). Personality characteristics of mental health professionals who have engaged in sexualized dual relationships: A Rorschach investigation. *Bulletin of the Menninger Clinic, 61,* 90–107.

Claman, J. M. (1987). Mirror hunger in the psychodynamics of sexually abusing therapists. *American Journal of Psychoanalysis, 47,* 35–40.

Clarkson, P. (1994). In recognition of dual relationships. *Transactional Analysis Journal, 24* (1), 32–38.

Clayton, A. H., Weeks, R. B., & Vieweg, W. V. R. (1991). Medical students' attitudes toward sexual contact with patients and supervisors. *Academic Psychiatry, 15* (2), 80–86.

Coale, H. W. (1998). *The vulnerable therapist: Practicing psychotherapy in an age of anxiety.* New York: Haworth Press.

Coleman, P. (1988). Sex in power dependency relationships: Taking unfair advantage of the "fair" sex. *Albany Law Review, 53,* 95–141.

Collins, D. T., Mebed, A. A. K., & Mortimer, R. L. (1978). Patient–therapist sex: Consequences for subsequent treatment. *McLean Hospital Journal, 3,* 24–36.

Combs, G., & Freedman, J. (2002). Relationships, not boundaries. *Theoretical Medicine and Bioethics, 23,* 203–217.

Conte, H. R., Plutchik, R., Picard, S., & Karasu, T. B. (1989). Ethics in the practice of psychotherapy: A survey. *American Journal of Psychotherapy, 43,* 32–42.

Cranford Insurance Co. v. Allwest Insurance Co., 645 F. Supp. 1440 (N.D. Cal. 1986).

Croarkin, P., Berg, J., & Spira, J. (2003). Informed consent for psychotherapy: A look at therapists' understanding, opinions, and practices. *American Journal of Psychotherapy, 57,* 384–400.

D'Addario, L. J. (1977). Sexual relations between female clients and male therapists. Doctoral dissertation, California School of Professional Psychology, San Diego, CA. *Dissertation Abstracts International.* 1978. *38,* 5007B.

Dahlberg, C. C. (1970). Sexual contact between patient and therapist. *Contemporary Psychoanalysis, 6,* 107–124.

Davidson, V. M. T. (1991). Touching patients: Implications of the handshake, the hug, and the embrace. *Psychodynamic Letter, 1*(3), 5–7.

Davies, D., & Gabriel, L. (2000). The management of ethical dilemmas. In D. Davies & C. Neal (Eds.), *Issues in therapy with lesbian, gay, bisexual and transgender clients* (pp. 35–54). Buckingham, UK: Open University Press.

Deaton, R. J. S., Illingworth, P. M. L., & Bursztajn, H. J. (1992). Unanswered questions about the criminalization of therapist–patient sex. *American Journal of Psychotherapy, 46,* 526–531.

Derlega, V. J., Hendrick, S. S., Winstead, B. A., & Berg, J. H. (1991). *Psychotherapy as a personal relationship.* New York: Guilford Press.

Derlega, V. J., Metts, S., Petronio, S., & Margulis, S. T. (1993). *Self-disclosure.* Newbury Park, CA: Sage.

Derrig-Palumbo, K., & Zeine, F. (2005). *Online therapy: A therapist's guide to expanding your practice.* New York: Norton.

Dewald, P. A., & Clark, R. W. (2001). *Ethics case book of the American Psychoanalytic Association*. New York: American Psychoanalytic Association.

DeYoung, M. (1981). Case reports: The sexual exploitation of incest victims by helping professionals. *Victimology: An International Journal, 6*, 92–101.

Dimeff, L. A., & Koerner, K. (Eds.). (2007). *Dialectical behavior therapy in clinical practice: Applications across disorders and settings*. New York: Guilford Press.

Doe v. Samaritan Counseling Center, 791 P.2d 344 (Alaska 1990).

Doyle, K. (1997). Substance abuse counselors in recovery: Implications for the ethical issue of dual relationships. *Journal of Counseling and Development, 75*, 428–432.

Drogin, E. Y. (in press). Determining the need for, identifying, and selecting experts. In D. Faust (Ed.), *Ziskin's coping with psychiatric and psychological testimony*. New York: Oxford University Press.

Drude, K., & Lichstein, M. (2005, August). Psychologists' use of e-mail with clients: Some ethical considerations. *Ohio Psychologist*, pp. 13–17.

Dryden, W. (1990). Self-disclosure in rational-emotive therapy. In G. Stricker & M. Fisher (Eds.), *Self-disclosure in the therapeutic relationship* (pp. 61–74). New York: Plenum.

Duckworth, K. S., Kahn, M. W., & Gutheil, T. G. (1994). Roles, quandaries, and remedies: Teaching professional boundaries to medical students. *Harvard Review of Psychiatry, 1*, 266–270.

Eber, M., & Kunz, L. B. (1984). The desire to help others. *Bulletin of the Menninger Clinic, 48*, 125–140.

Ebert, B. W. (1997). Dual-relationship prohibitions: A concept whose time never should have come. *Applied and Preventive Psychology, 6*, 137–156.

Edelwich, J., & Brodsky, A. (1980). *Burnout: Stages of disillusionment in the helping professions*. New York: Human Sciences Press.

Edelwich, J., & Brodsky, A. (1982). *Sexual dilemmas for the helping professional*. New York: Brunner/Mazel.

Edelwich, J., & Brodsky, A. (1991). *Sexual dilemmas for the helping professional* (2nd ed.). New York: Brunner/Mazel.

Elise, D. (1991). When sexual and romantic feelings permeate the therapeutic relationship. In C. Silverstein (Ed.), *Gays, lesbians, and their therapists* (pp. 52–67). New York: Norton.

Ellis, A. (2001). *Overcoming destructive beliefs, feelings, and behaviors: New directions for Rational Emotive Behavior Therapy*. Amherst, NY: Prometheus Books.

Epstein, R. S. (1994). *Keeping boundaries: Maintaining safety and integrity in the psychotherapeutic process*. Washington, DC: American Psychiatric Press.

Epstein, R. S., & Simon, R. I. (1990). The Exploitation Index: An early warning indicator of boundary violations in psychotherapy. *Bulletin of the Menninger Clinic, 54*, 450–465.

Epstein, R. S., Simon, R. I., & Kay, G. G. (1992). Assessing boundary violations in psychotherapy: Survey results with the Exploitation Index. *Bulletin of the Menninger Clinic, 56*, 150–166.

Eth, S. (1990). Ethical problems regarding sex between therapist and patient. In R. Rosner & R. Weinstock (Eds.), *Ethical practice in psychiatry and the law* (pp. 175–182). New York: Springer.

Evanier, D. (2002, March 3). Shrinking. *New York Times Magazine*. Retrieved November 20, 2007, from query.nytimes.com/gst/fullpage.html?res=9E0DE0D81F3EF930 A35750C0A9649C8B63.

Eyman, J. R., & Gabbard, G. O. (1991). Will therapist–patient sex prevent suicide? *Psychiatric Annals, 21*, 669–674.

Farber, B. A. (2006). *Self-disclosure in psychotherapy: Patient, therapist, and supervisory perspectives*. New York: Guilford Press.

Faulkner, K. K., & Faulkner, T. A. (1997). Managing multiple relationships in rural communities: Neutrality and boundary violations. *Clinical Psychology: Science and Practice, 4,* 225–234.

Federation of State Medical Boards. (2002). FSMB model guidelines for the appropriate use of the Internet in medical practice. Available at *www.fsmb.org.*

Feldman-Summers, S., & Jones. G. (1984). Psychological impacts of sexual contact between therapists or other health care practitioners and their clients. *Journal of Consulting and Clinical Psychology, 52,* 1054–1061.

Fenster, S., Phillips, S. B., & Rapoport, E. R. G. (1986). *The therapist's pregnancy: Intrusion in the analytic space.* Hillsdale, NJ: Analytic Press.

F.G. v. MacDonell et al., 150 N.J. 550; 696 A.2d 697; 1997 N.J. LEXIS 222.

Folman, R. Z. (1991). Therapist–patient sex: Attraction and boundary problems. *Psychotherapy, 28,* 168–173.

Frayn, D. H., & Silberfeld, M. (1986). Erotic transferences. *Canadian Journal of Psychiatry, 31,* 323–327.

Freedman, J., & Combs, G. (1996). *Narrative therapy: The social construction of preferred realities.* New York: Norton.

Freeman, L., & Roy, J. (1976). *Betrayal.* New York: Stein and Day.

Freud, S. (1958a). Recommendations to physicians practicing psychoanalysis. In J. Strachey (Trans. & Ed.), *The standard edition of the complete psychological works of Sigmund Freud* (Vol. 12, pp. 111–120). London: Hogarth Press. (Original work published 1912)

Freud, S. (1958b). On beginning the treatment: Further recommendations on the technique of psychoanalysis. In J. Strachey (Trans. & Ed.), *The standard edition of the complete psychological works of Sigmund Freud* (Vol. 12, pp. 123–144). London: Hogarth Press. (Original work published 1913)

Freud, S. (1958c). Observations on transference-love: Further recommendations on the technique of psychoanalysis III. In J. Strachey (Trans. & Ed.), *The standard edition of the complete psychological works of Sigmund Freud* (Vol. 12, pp. 159–171). London: Hogarth Press. (Original work published 1915)

Frick, D. E., McCartney, C. F., & Lazarus, J. A. (1995). Supervision of sexually exploitative psychiatrists: APA district branch experience. *Psychiatric Annals, 25,* 113–117.

Friedman, J., & Boumil, M. M. (1995). *Betrayal of trust: Sex and power in professional relationships.* Westport, CT: Praeger.

Gabbard, G. O. (1982). The exit line: Heightened transference–countertransference manifestations at the end of the hour. *Journal of the American Psychoanalytic Association, 30,* 579–598.

Gabbard, G. O. (Ed.). (1989). *Sexual exploitation in professional relationships.* Washington, DC: American Psychiatric Press.

Gabbard, G. O. (1990). Therapeutic approaches to erotic transference. *Directions in Psychiatry* (Vol. 10, lesson 4). New York: Hatherleigh.

Gabbard, G. O. (1991). Technical approaches to transference hate in the analysis of borderline patients. *International Journal of Psycho-Analysis, 72,* 625–637.

Gabbard, G. O. (1993). An overview of countertransference with borderline patients. *Journal of Psychotherapy Practice and Research, 2,* 7–18.

Gabbard, G. O. (1994a). Psychotherapists who transgress sexual boundaries with patients. *Bulletin of the Menninger Clinic, 58,* 124–135.

Gabbard, G. O. (1994b). Sexual misconduct. In J. M. Oldham & M. B. Riba (Eds.), *American Psychiatric Press review of psychiatry* (Vol. 13, pp. 433–456). Washington, DC: American Psychiatric Press.

Gabbard, G. O. (1995a). The early history of boundary violations in psychoanalysis. *Journal of the American Psychoanalytic Association, 43,* 1115–1136.

Gabbard, G. O. (1995b). Transference and countertransference in the psychotherapy of therapists charged with sexual misconduct. *Journal of Psychotherapy Practice and Research, 4,* 10–17.

Gabbard, G. O. (1996). Lessons to be learned from the study of boundary violations. *American Journal of Psychotherapy, 50,* 311–321.

Gabbard, G. O. (1999a). Boundary violations. In S. Bloch, P. Chodoff, & S. A. Green (Eds.), *Psychiatric ethics* (3rd ed., pp. 141–160). Oxford, UK: Oxford University Press.

Gabbard, G. O. (Ed.). (1999b). *Countertransference issues in psychiatric treatment.* Washington, DC: American Psychiatric Press.

Gabbard, G. O. (2001). Commentary: Boundaries, culture, and psychotherapy. *Journal of the American Academy of Psychiatry and the Law, 29,* 284–286.

Gabbard, G. O. (2003, July). Boundary violations in psychotherapy. *Psychiatric Times,* pp. 71, 74.

Gabbard, G. O. (2005, October). Patient–therapist boundary issues. *Psychiatric Times* (special edition), pp. 28–33.

Gabbard, G. O., & Lester, E. P. (2002). *Boundaries and boundary violations in psychoanalysis.* Washington, DC: American Psychiatric Publishing.

Gabbard, G. O., & Nadelson, C. (1995). Professional boundaries in the physician–patient relationship. *Journal of the American Medical Association, 273,* 1445–1449.

Gabbard, G. O., & Peltz, M. L. (2001). Speaking the unspeakable: Institutional reactions to boundary violations by training analysts. *Journal of the American Psychoanalytic Association, 49,* 659–673.

Gabbard, G. O., & Pope, K. S. (1989). Sexual intimacies after termination: Clinical, ethical, and legal aspects. In G. O. Gabbard (Ed.), *Sexual exploitation in professional relationships* (pp. 115–127). Washington, DC: American Psychiatric Press.

Gabbard, G. O., & Wilkinson, S. M. (1994). *Management of countertransference with borderline patients.* Washington, DC: American Psychiatric Press.

Gabel, S., Oster, G., & Pfeffer, C. R. (Eds.). (1988). *Difficult moments in child psychotherapy.* New York: Plenum.

Gaines, R. (2003). Therapist self-disclosure with children, adolescents, and their parents. *Journal of Clinical Psychology: In Session, 59,* 589–598.

Gardner, R. A. (1993). *Psychotherapy with children.* Northvale, NJ: Aronson.

Garfinkel, P. E., Dorian, B., Sadavoy, J., & Bagby, R. M. (1997). Boundary violations and departments of psychiatry. *Canadian Journal of Psychiatry, 42,* 764–770.

Gartner, R. B. (1996). Incestuous boundary violations in families of borderline patients. *Contemporary Psychoanalysis, 32,* 73–80.

Gartrell, N. K. (1992). Boundaries in lesbian therapy relationships. *Women and Therapy, 12* (3), 29–50.

Gartrell, N., Herman, J., Olarte, S., Feldstein, M., & Localio, R. (1986). Psychiatrist–patient sexual contact: Results of a national survey, I: Prevalence. *American Journal of Psychiatry, 143,* 1126–1131.

Gartrell, N., Herman, J., Olarte, S., Feldstein, M., & Localio, R. (1987). Reporting practices of psychiatrists who knew of sexual misconduct by colleagues. *American Journal of Orthopsychiatry, 57,* 287–295.

Gartrell, N., Herman, J., Olarte, S., Localio, R., & Feldstein, M. (1988). Psychiatric residents' sexual contact with educators and patients: Results of a national survey. *American Journal of Psychiatry, 145,* 690–694.

Gartrell, N. K., Milliken, N., Goodson, W. H. III, Thiemann, S., & Lo, B. (1992). Physician–patient sexual contact: Prevalence and problems. *Western Journal of Medicine, 157,* 139–143.

Gates, K., & Speare, K. (1990). Overlapping relationships in the rural community. In H. Lerman & N. Porter (Eds.), *Feminist ethics in psychotherapy* (pp. 97–101). New York: Springer.

Gay, P. (1988). *Freud: A life for our time.* New York: Norton.

Gechtman, L. (1989). Sexual contact between social workers and their clients. In G. O. Gabbard (Ed.), *Sexual exploitation in professional relationships* (pp. 27–38). Washington, DC: American Psychiatric Press.

Geller, J. D. (2003). Self-disclosure in psychoanalytic-existential therapy. *Journal of Clinical Psychology: In Session, 59,* 541–554.

Geller, J. D. (2005). Style and its contribution to a patient-specific model of therapeutic technique. *Psychotherapy: Theory/Research/Practice/Training, 42,* 469–482.

Genova, P. (2001). Boundary violations and the fall from Eden. *Psychiatric Times, 18,* 64, 66.

Gentile, S. R., Asamen, J. K., Harmell, P. H., & Weathers, R. (2002). The stalking of psychologists by their clients. *Professional Psychology: Research and Practice, 33,* 490–494.

Gill, M. (1982). *Analysis of transference* (Vol. 1). New York: International Universities Press.

Gitelson, M. (1952). The emotional position of the analyst in the psychoanalytic situation. *International Journal of Psychoanalysis, 33,* 1–10.

Glaser, R. D., & Thorpe, J. S. (1986). Unethical intimacy: A survey of sexual contact and advances between psychology educators and female graduate students. *American Psychologist, 41,* 43–51.

Glass, L. L. (2003). The gray areas of boundary crossings and violations. *American Journal of Psychotherapy, 57,* 429–444.

Glasser, W. (1965). *Reality therapy.* New York: Harper & Row.

Goisman, R. M., & Gutheil, T. G. (1992). Risk management in the practice of behavior therapy: Boundaries and behavior. *American Journal of Psychotherapy, 46,* 532–543.

Golden, G. A., & Brennan, M. (1995). Managing erotic feelings in the physician–patient relationship. *Canadian Medical Association Journal, 153,* 1241–1245.

Goldstein, A. (2003). Overview of forensic psychology. In I. B. Weiner (Series Ed.) & A. M. Goldstein (Vol. Ed.), *Comprehensive handbook of psychology: Vol. 11. Forensic psychology* (pp. 3–20). Hoboken, NJ: Wiley.

Gonsiorek, J. C. (1989). Sexual exploitation by psychotherapists: Some observations on male victims and sexual orientation issues. In G. R. Schoener, J. H. Milgrom, J. C. Gonsiorek, E. T. Luepker, & R. M. Conroe (Eds.), *Psychotherapists' sexual involvement with clients: Intervention and prevention* (pp. 113–119). Minneapolis, MN: Walk-In Counseling Center.

Gonsiorek, J. C. (1995a). Assessment for rehabilitation of exploitative health care professionals and clergy. In J. C. Gonsiorek (Ed.), *Breach of trust: Sexual exploitation by health care professionals and clergy* (pp. 145–162). Thousand Oaks, CA: Sage.

Gonsiorek, J. C. (1995b). Boundary challenges when both therapist and client are gay males. In J. C. Gonsiorek (Ed.), *Breach of trust: Sexual exploitation by health care professionals and clergy* (pp. 225–233). Thousand Oaks, CA: Sage.

Gonsiorek, J. C., & Brown, L. S. (1989). Post therapy sexual relationships with clients. In

G. R. Schoener, J. H. Milgrom, J. C. Gonsiorek, E. T. Luepker, & R. M. Conroe (Eds.), *Psychotherapists' sexual involvement with clients: Intervention and prevention* (pp. 289–301). Minneapolis, MN: Walk-In Counseling Center.

Goodman, M., & Teicher, A. (1988). To touch or not to touch. *Psychotherapy, 25,* 492–500.

Gorkin, M. (1985). Varieties of sexualized countertransference. *Psychoanalytic Review, 72,* 424–440.

Gorkin, M. (1987). *The uses of countertransferences.* Northvale, NJ: Aronson.

Gorton, G. E., & Samuel, S. E. (1996). National survey of psychiatric residency training directors on education for prevention of psychiatrist–patient sexual exploitation. *Academic Psychiatry, 20,* 92–98.

Gorton, G. E., Samuel, S. E., & Zembrowski, S. M. (1996). A pilot course for residents on sexual feelings and boundary maintenance in treatment. *Academic Psychiatry, 20,* 43–55.

Goss, S., & Anthony, K. (Eds.). (2003). *Technology in counseling and psychotherapy: A practitioner's guide.* New York: Palgrave Macmillan.

Gottlieb, M. C. (1993). Avoiding exploitive dual relationships: A decision-making model. *Psychotherapy: Theory, Research, Practice, Training, 30,* 41–48.

Greenberg, J. R. (1995). Psychoanalytic technique and the interactive matrix. *Psychoanalytic Quarterly, 64,* 1–22.

Greenberg, S. A., & Shuman, D. W. (1997). Irreconcilable conflict between therapeutic and forensic roles. *Professional Psychology: Research and Practice, 28,* 50–57.

Greenberg v. McCabe, 453 F.Supp. 765, (E.D. Pa. 1978), *aff'd without op.,* 594 F.2d 854 (3d Cir.), *cert. denied,* 444 U.S. 840 (1979).

Greenson, R. R. (1967). *The technique and practice of psychoanalysis* (Vol. 1). New York: International Universities Press.

Greenspan, M. (1996). Out of bounds. In K. H. Ragsdale (Ed.), *Boundary wars: Intimacy and distance in healing relationships* (pp. 129–136). Cleveland: Pilgrim Press.

Gregory. (2001, May 14). [Cartoon]. *The New Yorker,* 98.

Groesbeck, C. J., & Taylor, B. (1977). The psychiatrist as wounded physician. *American Journal of Psychoanalysis, 37,* 131–139.

Grold, L. J. (1994). Boundary violations [letter]. *Psychiatric News, 29*(6), 22.

Grosch, W. N., & Olsen, D. C. (1994). *When helping starts to hurt.* New York: Norton.

Grosch, W. N., & Olsen, D. C. (1995). Prevention: Avoiding burnout. In M. B. Sussman (Ed.), *A perilous calling: The hazards of psychotherapy practice* (pp. 275–287). New York: Wiley.

Gutheil, T. G. (1982a). On the therapy in clinical administration: Part II. The administrative contract, alliance, ultimatum and goal. *Psychiatric Quarterly, 54,* 11–17.

Gutheil, T. G. (1982b). The psychology of psychopharmacology. *Bulletin of the Menninger Clinic, 46,* 321–330.

Gutheil, T. G. (1985). Medicolegal pitfalls in the treatment of borderline patients. *American Journal of Psychiatry, 142,* 9–14.

Gutheil, T. G. (1986). Fees in beginning private practice. In D. W. Krueger (Ed.), *The last taboo: Money as symbol and reality in psychotherapy and psychoanalysis* (pp. 175–188). New York: Brunner/Mazel.

Gutheil, T. G. (1989). Borderline personality disorder, boundary violations, and patient–therapist sex: Medicolegal pitfalls. *American Journal of Psychiatry, 146,* 597–602.

Gutheil, T. G. (1991). Patients involved in sexual misconduct with therapists: Is a victim profile possible? *Psychiatric Annals, 21,* 661–667.

Gutheil, T. G. (1992a). Approaches to forensic assessment of false claims of sexual misconduct by therapists. *Bulletin of the American Academy of Psychiatry and the Law, 20,* 289–296.

Gutheil, T. G. (1992b). Some ironies in psychiatric sexual misconduct litigation: Editorial and critique. *AAPL Newsletter, 17,* 56–59.

Gutheil, T. G. (1992c). "Therapist-patient sex syndrome": The perils of nomenclature for the forensic psychiatrist. *Bulletin of the American Academy of Psychiatry and the Law, 20,* 185–190.

Gutheil, T. G. (1994a). Discussion of Lazarus's "How certain boundaries and ethics diminish therapeutic effectiveness." *Ethics and Behavior, 4,* 295–298.

Gutheil, T. G. (1994b). Risk management at the margins: Less familiar topics in psychiatric malpractice. *Harvard Review of Psychiatry, 2,* 214–221.

Gutheil, T. G. (1998). *The psychiatrist as expert witness.* Washington, DC: American Psychiatric Publishing.

Gutheil, T. G. (1999a, August). Clinical concerns in boundary issues. *Psychiatric Times,* 57–59.

Gutheil, T. G. (1999b). Issues in civil sexual misconduct litigation. In J. D. Bloom, C. C. Nadelson, & M. T. Notman (Eds.), *Physician sexual misconduct* (pp. 3–17). Washington, DC: American Psychiatric Press.

Gutheil, T. G. (2005a). Boundaries, blackmail, and double binds: A pattern observed in malpractice consultation. *Journal of the American Academy of Psychiatry and the Law, 33,* 476–481.

Gutheil, T. G. (2005b). Boundary issues. In J. M. Oldham, A. E. Skodol, & D. S. Bender (Eds.), *The American Psychiatric Publishing textbook of personality disorders* (pp. 421–429). Arlington, VA: American Psychiatric Publishing.

Gutheil, T. G. (2005c). Boundary issues and personality disorders. *Journal of Psychiatric Practice, 11,* 88–96.

Gutheil, T. G., & Alexander, V. (1992). Medicolegal issues between the borderline patient and the therapist. In D. Silver & M. Rosenbluth (Eds.), *The handbook of borderline disorders* (pp. 389–413). New York: International Universities Press.

Gutheil, T. G., Bursztajn, H. J., Brodsky, A., & Strasburger, L.H. (2000). Preventing "critogenic" harms: Minimizing emotional injury from civil litigation. *Journal of Psychiatry and Law, 28,* 5–18.

Gutheil, T. G., & Gabbard, G. O. (1992). Obstacles to the dynamic understanding of therapist–patient sexual relations. *American Journal of Psychotherapy, 46,* 515–525.

Gutheil, T. G., & Gabbard, G. O. (1993). The concept of boundaries in clinical practice: Theoretical and risk-management dimensions. *American Journal of Psychiatry, 150,* 188–196.

Gutheil, T. G., & Gabbard, G. O. (1998). Misuses and misunderstandings of boundary theory in clinical and regulatory settings. *American Journal of Psychiatry, 155,* 409–414.

Gutheil, T. G., & Hilliard, J. T. (2001). "Don't write me down": Legal, clinical, and risk-management aspects of patients' requests that therapists not keep notes or records. *American Journal of Psychotherapy, 55,* 157–165.

Gutheil, T. G., & Simon, R. I. (1995). Between the chair and the door: Boundary issues in the therapeutic "transition zone." *Harvard Review of Psychiatry, 2,* 336–340.

Gutheil, T. G., & Simon, R. I. (2002). Non-sexual boundary crossings and boundary violations: The ethical dimension. *Psychiatric Clinics of North America, 25,* 585–592.

Gutheil, T. G., & Simon, R. I. (2005). E-mails, extra-therapeutic contact, and early boundary problems: The internet as a "slippery slope." *Psychiatric Annals 35*, 952–960.

Haas, L. J., Malouf, J. L., & Mayerson, N. H. (1988). Personal and professional characteristics as factors in psychologists' ethical decision making. *Professional Psychology: Research and Practice, 19*, 35–42.

Hall, R. C. W., & Hall, R. C. W. (2001). False allegations: The role of the forensic psychiatrist. *Journal of Psychiatric Practice, 7*, 343–346.

Hamilton, J. C., & Spruill, J. (1999). Identifying and reducing risk factors related to trainee–client sexual misconduct. *Professional Psychology: Research and Practice, 30*, 318–327.

Hankins, G. C., Vera, M. I., Barnard, G. W., & Herkov, M. J. (1994). Patient–therapist sexual involvement: A review of clinical and research data. *Bulletin of the American Academy of Psychiatry and the Law, 22*, 109–126.

Hardegree, D. L. (1989). Why psychiatrist–patient sex is medical malpractice: The mishandling of the transference phenomenon. *American Journal of Trial Advocacy, 13*, 747–773.

Hartlaub, G. H., Martin, G. C., & Rhine, M. W. (1986). Recontact with the analyst following termination: A survey of 71 cases. *Journal of the American Psychoanalytic Association, 34*, 895–910.

Haspel, K. C., Jorgenson, L. M., Wincze, J. P., & Parsons, J. P. (1997). Legislative intervention regarding therapist sexual misconduct: An overview. *Professional Psychology: Research and Practice, 28*, 63–72.

Havens, L. (1989). *A safe place: Laying the groundwork of psychotherapy.* Cambridge, MA: Harvard University Press.

Havens, L. (1993). *Coming to life: Reflections on the art of psychotherapy.* Cambridge, MA: Harvard University Press.

Hedges, L. E., Hilton, R., Hilton, V. W., & Caudill, O. B., Jr. (Eds.). (1997). *Therapists at risk: Perils of the intimacy of the therapeutic relationship.* Northvale, NJ: Aronson.

Heinmiller v. Dept. of Health, 903 P.2d 433, Wash. 1995.

Helbok, C. M., Marinelli, R. P., & Walls, R. T. (2006). National survey of ethical practices across rural and urban communities. *Professional Psychology: Research and Practice, 37*, 36–44.

Herman, J. L., Gartrell, N., Olarte, S., Feldstein, M., & Localio, R. (1987). Psychiatrist–patient sexual contact: Results of a national survey: II. Psychiatrists' attitudes. *American Journal of Psychiatry, 144*, 164–169.

Herman, J. L., Perry, J. C., & Van der Kolk, B. A. (1989). Childhood trauma in borderline personality disorder. *American Journal of Psychiatry, 146*, 490–495.

Heru, A. M., Strong, D. R., Price, M., & Recupero, P. R. (2004). Boundaries in psychotherapy supervision. *American Journal of Psychotherapy, 58*, 76–89.

Heyward, C. (1993). *When boundaries betray us: Beyond illusions of what is ethical in therapy and life.* San Francisco: Harper.

Hill, C. E., & Knox, S. (2002). Self-disclosure. In J. C. Norcross (Ed.), *Psychotherapy relationships that work: Therapist contributions and responsiveness to patients* (pp. 255–265). New York: Oxford University Press.

Hilliard, J. T. (2001, November 30). Patients who violate boundaries. Presentation at conference on "Liability Prevention for Mental Health Clinicians: Strategies and Update." Massachusetts Mental Health Center and Harvard Medical School Department of Continuing Education, Boston.

Hilton, R. (1997a). The healing process for therapists: Some principles of healing and self recovery. In L. E. Hedges, R. Hilton, V. W. Hilton, & O. B. Caudill, Jr. (Eds.), *Therapists at risk: Perils of the intimacy of the therapeutic relationship* (pp. 147–157). Northvale, NJ: Aronson.

Hilton, R. (1997b). The perils of the intimacy of the therapeutic relationship. In L. E. Hedges, R. Hilton, V. W. Hilton, & O. B. Caudill, Jr. (Eds.), *Therapists at risk: Perils of the intimacy of the therapeutic relationship* (pp. 69–85). Northvale, NJ: Aronson.

Hilton, R. (1997c). Touching in psychotherapy. In L. E. Hedges, R. Hilton, V. W. Hilton, & O. B. Caudill, Jr. (Eds.), *Therapists at risk: Perils of the intimacy of the therapeutic relationship* (pp. 161–180). Northvale, NJ: Aronson.

Hilton, V. W. (1997). Sexuality in the therapeutic process. In L. E. Hedges, R. Hilton, V. W. Hilton, & O. B. Caudill, Jr. (Eds.), *Therapists at risk: Perils of the intimacy of the therapeutic relationship* (pp. 181–220). Northvale, NJ: Aronson.

Hoencamp, E. (1990). Sexual abuse and the abuse of hypnosis in the therapeutic relationship. *International Journal of Clinical and Experimental Hypnosis, 38,* 283–297.

Hoffer, A. (1985). Toward a definition of psychoanalytic neutrality. *Journal of the American Psychoanalytic Association, 33,* 771–795.

Hoffer, A. (1991). The Freud–Ferenczi controversy: A living legacy. *International Review of Psychoanalysis, 18,* 465–472.

Holladay v. Boyd, Ill., Cook Cty. Cir. Ct., No. 90 L 10098, April 24, 1995.

Holroyd, J. C., & Brodsky, A. M. (1977). Psychologists' attitudes and practices regarding erotic and nonerotic physical contact with patients. *American Psychologist, 32,* 843–849.

Holroyd, J. C., & Brodsky, A. M. (1980). Does touching patients lead to sexual intercourse? *Professional Psychology, 11,* 807–811.

Holub, E. A., & Lee, S. S. (1990). Therapists' use of nonerotic physical contact: Ethical concerns. *Professional Psychology: Research and Practice, 21,* 115–117.

Hornsby, M. M., Drogin, E. Y., & Barrett, C. L. (1997, Fall). The clinician–expert identity crisis: There's such a thing as being too helpful. *Kentucky Psychologist,* p. 8.

Horst, E. A. (1989). Dual relationships between psychologists and clients in rural and urban areas. *Journal of Rural Community Psychology, 10*(2), 15–24.

Horton, J. A., Clance, P. R., Sterk-Elitson, C., & Emshoff, J. (1995). Touch in psychotherapy: A survey of patients' experiences. *Psychotherapy, 32,* 443–457.

Housman, L. M., & Stake, J. E. (1999). The current state of sexual ethics training in clinical psychology: Issues of quantity, quality, and effectiveness. *Professional Psychology: Research and Practice, 30,* 302–311.

Hsiung, R. C. (2002). *E-therapy: Case studies, guiding principles, and the clinical potential of the Internet.* New York: Norton.

Hundert, E. M., & Appelbaum, P. S. (1995). Boundaries in psychotherapy: Model guidelines. *Psychiatry, 58,* 345–356.

Illingworth, P. M. L. (1995). Patient–therapist sex: Criminalization and its discontents. *Journal of Contemporary Health Law and Policy, 11,* 389–416.

Imber, R. R. (1990). The avoidance of countertransference awareness in a pregnant analyst. *Contemporary Psychoanalysis, 26,* 223–236.

Irons, R. R. (1995). Inpatient assessment of the sexually exploitative professional. In J. C. Gonsiorek (Ed.), *Breach of trust: Sexual exploitation by health care professionals and clergy* (pp. 163–175). Thousand Oaks, CA: Sage.

Irons, R. R., & Schneider, J. P. (1999). *The wounded healer: Addiction-sensitive approach to the sexually exploitative professional.* Northvale, NJ: Aronson.

Iverson, G. L. (2000). Dual relationships in psycholegal evaluations: Treating psychologists serving as expert witnesses. *American Journal of Forensic Psychology, 18,* 79–87.

Jackenthal v. Kirsch, N.Y., New York County Sup. Ct., No. 18423/90, Nov. 1, 1995.

Jaffe, D. (1986). Empathy, counteridentification, countertransference: A review, with some personal perspectives on the "analytic instrument." *Psychoanalytic Quarterly, 55,* 215–243.

Johnson, K. (2006, June 8). TV screen, not couch, is required for this session. *New York Times.* Retrieved November 16, 2007, from www.nytimes.com/2006/06/08/us/08teleshrink.html.

Johnston, S., & Farber, B. A. (1996). The maintenance of boundaries in psychotherapeutic practice. *Psychotherapy: Theory, Research, Practice, Training, 33,* 391–402.

Jordan, J. V. (1995). Female therapists and the search for a new paradigm. In M. B. Sussman (Ed.), *A perilous calling: The hazards of psychotherapy practice* (pp. 259–272). New York: Wiley.

Jordan, J. V., Kaplan, A., Miller, J. B., Stiver, I., & Surrey, J. (1990). More comments on patient-therapist sex (letter). *American Journal of Psychiatry, 147,* 129–130.

Jorgenson, L. M. (1995a). Countertransference and special concerns of subsequent treating therapists of patients sexually exploited by a previous therapist. *Psychiatric Annals, 25,* 525–534.

Jorgenson, L. M. (1995b). Employer/supervisor liability and risk management. In J. C. Gonsiorek (Ed.), *Breach of trust: Sexual exploitation by health care professionals and clergy* (pp. 284–299). Thousand Oaks, CA: Sage.

Jorgenson, L. M. (1995c). Rehabilitating sexually exploitative therapists: A risk management perspective. *Psychiatric Annals, 25,* 118–122.

Jorgenson, L. M. (1995d). Sexual contact in fiduciary relationships: Legal perspectives. In J. C. Gonsiorek (Ed.), *Breach of trust: Sexual exploitation by health care professionals and clergy* (pp. 237–283). Thousand Oaks, CA: Sage.

Jorgenson, L. M., & Appelbaum, P. S. (1991). For whom the statute tolls: Extending the time during which patients can sue. *Hospital and Community Psychiatry, 42,* 683–684.

Jorgenson, L. M., Bisbing, S. B., & Sutherland, P. K. (1992). Therapist–patient sexual exploitation and insurance liability. *Tort and Insurance Law Journal, 27,* 595–614.

Jorgenson, L. M., Hirsch, A. B., & Wahl, K. M. (1997). Fiduciary duty and boundaries: Acting in the client's best interest. *Behavioral Sciences and the Law, 15,* 49–62.

Jorgenson, L. M., & Randles, R. M. (1991). Time out: The statute of limitations and fiduciary theory in psychotherapist sexual misconduct cases. *Oklahoma Law Review, 44,* 181–225.

Jorgenson, L. M., & Sutherland, P. K. (1993, May). Psychotherapist liability: What's sex got to do with it? *Trial,* pp. 21–23.

Jorgenson, L. M., Sutherland, P. K., & Bisbing, S. B. (1995, May). Evidence of multiple victims in therapist sexual misconduct cases. *Trial,* pp. 30–37.

Jourard, S. M. (1971). *Self-disclosure: Experimental analysis of the transparent self.* New York: Wiley.

Kagle, J. D., & Giebelhausen, P. N. (1994). Dual relationships and professional boundaries. *Social Work, 39,* 213–220.

Kane, A. W. (1995). The effects of criminalization of sexual misconduct by therapists: Report of a survey in Wisconsin. In J. C. Gonsiorek (Ed.), *Breach of trust: Sexual exploitation by health care professionals and clergy* (pp. 317–337). Thousand Oaks, CA: Sage.

Kane, B., & Sands, D. Z. (1998). Guidelines for the clinical use of electronic mail with patients. *Journal of the American Medical Informatics Association, 5,* 104–111.

Kanter, S. S., & Kanter, J. A. (1977). Therapeutic setting and management of fees. *Psychiatric Annals, 7*(2), 23–34.

Kardener, S. H., Fuller, M., & Mensh, I. N. (1973). A survey of physicians' attitudes and practices regarding erotic and nonerotic contact with patients. *American Journal of Psychiatry, 130*, 1077–1081.

Kardener, S. H., Fuller, M., & Mensh, I. N. (1976). Characteristics of "erotic" practitioners. *American Journal of Psychiatry, 133*, 1324–1325.

Kay, J., & Roman, B. (1999). Prevention of sexual misconduct at the medical school, residency, and practitioner levels. In J. D. Bloom, C. C. Nadelson, & M. T. Notman (Eds.), *Physician sexual misconduct* (pp. 153–177). Washington, DC: American Psychiatric Press.

Kehoe, N., & Gutheil, T. G. (1984). Shared religious belief as resistance in psychotherapy. *American Journal of Psychotherapy, 38*, 579–585.

Kepner, J. I. (1987). *Body process: A gestalt approach to working with the body in psychotherapy.* New York: Gestalt Institute of Cleveland Press.

Kertay, L., & Reviere, S. L. (1993). The use of touch in psychotherapy: Theoretical and ethical considerations. *Psychotherapy, 30*, 32–40.

Kessler, L. E., & Waehler, C. A. (2005). Addressing multiple relationships between clients and therapists in lesbian, gay, bisexual, and transgender communities. *Professional Psychology: Research and Practice, 36*, 66–72.

Kitchener, K. S. (1988). Dual role relationships: What makes them so problematic? *Journal of Counseling and Development, 67*, 217–221.

Kitchener, K. S. (2000). *Foundations of ethical practice, research, and teaching in psychology.* Mahwah, NJ: Erlbaum.

Klein, D. F. (1994). Boundary violations [letter]. *Psychiatric News, 29* (6), 22, 23.

Kluft, R. P. (1989). Treating the patient who has been sexually exploited by a previous therapist. *Psychiatric Clinics of North America, 12*, 483–500.

Kluft, R. P. (Ed.). (1990). *Incest-related syndromes of adult psychopathology.* Washington, DC: American Psychiatric Press.

Knapp, S., & VandeCreek, L. (2003). *A guide to the 2002 revision of the American Psychological Association's ethics code.* Sarasota, FL: Professional Resource Press.

Knox, S., & Hill, C. E. (2003). Therapist self-disclosure: Research-based suggestions for practitioners. *Journal of Clinical Psychology: In Session, 59*, 529–540.

Kohlenberg, R. J., & Tsai, M. (2007). *Functional analytic psychotherapy: Creating intense and curative therapeutic relationships.* New York: Springer.

Kohut, H., & Wolf, E. S. (1977). The disorders of the self and their treatment. *International Journal of Psychoanalysis, 59*, 413–425.

Koocher, G. P. (2006). Foreword to the second edition: Things my teachers never mentioned. In K. S. Pope, J. L. Sonne, & B. Greene, *What therapists don't talk about and why: Understanding taboos that hurt us and our clients* (pp. xxi–xxii). Washington, DC: American Psychological Association.

Korn, M. (2003, July). A first-hand account of boundary violations in psychotherapy. *Psychiatric Times*, pp. 70–73.

Krassner, D. (2004). Gifts from physicians to patients: An ethical dilemma. *Psychiatric Services, 55*, 505–506.

Kraus, R., Zack, J., & Stricker, G. (2003). *Online counseling: A handbook for mental health professionals.* New York: Academic Press.

Kroll, J. (2001). Boundary violations: A culture-bound syndrome. *Journal of the American Academy of Psychiatry and the Law, 29*, 274–283.

Krueger, D. W. (Ed.). (1986). *The last taboo: Money as symbol and reality in psychotherapy and psychoanalysis.* New York: Brunner/Mazel.

Kumin, I. (1985–1986). Erotic horror: Desire and resistance in the psychoanalytic situation. *International Journal of Psychoanalytic Psychotherapy, 11,* 3–20.

Kupfermann, K., & Smaldino, C. (1987). The vitalizing and revitalizing experience of reliability: The place of touch in psychotherapy. *Clinical Social Work Journal, 15,* 223–235.

Lamb, D. H., & Catanzaro, S. J. (1998). Sexual and nonsexual boundary violations involving psychologists, clients, supervisors, and students: Implications for professional practice. *Professional Psychology: Research and Practice, 29,* 498–503.

Lamb, D. H., Catanzaro, S. J., & Moorman, A. S. (2004). A preliminary look at how psychologists identify, evaluate, and proceed when faced with possible multiple relationship dilemmas. *Professional Psychology: Research and Practice, 35,* 248–254.

Lamb, D. H., Strand, K. K., Woodburn, J. R., Buchko, K. J., Lewis, J. T., & Kang, J. R. (1994). Sexual and business relationships between therapists and former clients. *Psychotherapy, 31,* 270–278.

Lane, R., & Hull, J. (1990). Self-disclosure and classical psychoanalysis. In G. Stricker & M. Fisher (Eds.), *Self-disclosure in the therapeutic relationship* (pp. 31–46). New York: Plenum.

Langleben, D., Dattilio, F. M. D., & Gutheil, T. G. (2006). "True lies": Delusions and lie-detection technology. *Journal of Psychiatry and Law, 34,* 351–370.

Langs, R. J. (1973). *The technique of psychoanalytic psychotherapy* (Vol. 1). New York: Aronson.

Langs, R. J. (1976). *The bipersonal field.* New York: Aronson.

Langs, R. J. (1982). *Psychotherapy: A basic text.* New York: Aronson.

Langs, R. J. (1984–1985). Making interpretations and securing the frame: Sources of danger for psychotherapists. *International Journal of Psychoanalytic Psychotherapy, 10,* 3–23.

Lazarus, A. A. (1989). *The practice of multimodal therapy.* Baltimore: The Johns Hopkins University Press.

Lazarus, A. A. (1994). How certain boundaries and ethics diminish therapeutic effectiveness. *Ethics and Behavior, 4,* 255–261.

Lazarus, A. A. (2006). *Brief but comprehensive psychotherapy: The multimodal way.* New York: Springer.

Lazarus, A. A., & Zur, O. (Eds.). (2002). *Dual relationships and psychotherapy.* New York: Springer.

Lazarus, J. (1993, November 5). More on boundary violations. *Psychiatric News,* pp. 14, 27.

Leahy, R. L. (2001). *Overcoming resistance in cognitive therapy.* New York: Guilford Press.

Leahy, R. L. (2003a). *Cognitive therapy techniques: A practitioner's guide.* New York: Guilford Press.

Leahy, R. L. (Ed.). (2003b). *Roadblocks in cognitive-behavioral therapy: Transforming challenges into opportunities for change.* New York: Guilford Press.

Leahy, R. L. (Ed.). (2004). *Contemporary cognitive therapy: Theory, research, and practice.* New York: Guilford Press.

Lichtenberg, J. Ruderman, E., Shane, E., & Shane, M. (Issue Eds.). (2000). On touch in the psychoanalytic situation. *Psychoanalytic Inquiry, 20,* 1–186.

Linehan, M. M. (1993). *Cognitive-behavioral treatment of borderline personality disorder.* New York: Guilford Press.

Lipton, S. D. (1977). The advantages of Freud's technique as shown in his analysis of the Rat Man. *International Journal of Psychoanalysis, 58,* 255–273.

Little, M. (1951). Countertransference and the patient's response to it. *International Journal of Psychoanalysis, 32,* 32–40.

Little, M. I. (1990). *Psychotic anxieties and containment: A personal record of an analysis with Winnicott*. Northvale, NJ: Aronson.

Lomas, P. (1987). *The limits of interpretation: What's wrong with psychoanalysis?* New York: Penguin.

Luepker, E. T. (1989). Sexual exploitation of clients by therapists: Parallels with parent–child incest. In G. R. Schoener, J. H. Milgrom, J. C. Gonsiorek, E. T. Luepker, & R. M. Conroe (Eds.), *Psychotherapists' sexual involvement with clients: Intervention and prevention* (pp. 73–79). Minneapolis, MN: Walk-In Counseling Center.

Luepker, E. T. (1995). Helping direct and associate victims to restore connections after practitioner sexual misconduct. In J. C. Gonsiorek (Ed.), *Breach of trust: Sexual exploitation by health care professionals and clergy* (pp. 112–128). Thousand Oaks, CA: Sage.

Luepker, E. T. (1999). Effects of practitioners' sexual misconduct: A follow-up study. *Journal of the American Academy of Psychiatry and the Law, 27*, 51–63.

Lyn, L. (1995). Lesbian, gay, and bisexual therapists' social and sexual interactions with clients. In J. C. Gonsiorek (Ed.), *Breach of trust: Sexual exploitation by health care professionals and clergy* (pp. 193–212). Thousand Oaks, CA: Sage.

Maheu, M. M., & Gordon, B. (2000). Counseling and therapy on the Internet. *Professional Psychology: Research and Practice, 31*, 484–489.

Maheu, M. M., Pulier, M. L., Wilhelm, F. H., McMenamin, J. P., & Brown-Connolly, N. E. (2004). *The mental health professional and the new technologies: A handbook for practice today*. Mahwah, NJ: Erlbaum.

Malcolm, J. (1994). *Psychoanalysis: The impossible profession*. New York: Aronson.

Malcolm, J. G. (1992). Informed consent in the practice of psychiatry. In R. I. Simon (Ed.), *American Psychiatric Press review of clinical psychiatry and the law* (Vol. 3, pp. 223–281). Washington, DC: American Psychiatric Press.

Mallen, M. J., Day, S. X., & Green, M. A. (2003). Online versus face-to-face conversations: An examination of relational and discourse variables. *Psychotherapy: Theory, Research, Practice, Training, 40*, 155–163.

Mallow, A. J. (1998). Self-disclosure: Reconciling psychoanalytic psychotherapy and Alcoholics Anonymous philosophy. *Journal of Substance Abuse Treatment, 15*, 493–498.

Malmquist, C. P., & Notman, M. T. (2001). Psychiatrist–patient boundary issues following treatment termination. *American Journal of Psychiatry, 158*, 1010–1018.

Maltsberger, J. T. (1995). A career plundered. In M. B. Sussman (Ed.), *A perilous calling: The hazards of psychotherapy practice* (pp. 226–234). New York: Wiley.

Maltsberger, J. T., & Buie, D. (1974). Countertransference hate in the treatment of suicidal patients. *Archives of General Psychiatry, 30*, 625–633.

Marmor, J. (1972). Sexual acting-out in psychotherapy. *American Journal of Psychoanalysis, 32*, 3–8.

Marmor, J. (1976). Some psychodynamic aspects of the seduction of patients in psychotherapy. *American Journal of Psychoanalysis, 36*, 319–323.

Marmor, J. (1994). Boundary violations [letter]. *Psychiatric News, 29* (6), 22–23.

Maroda, K. J. (1994). *The power of countertransference: Innovations in analytic technique*. Northvale, NJ: Aronson.

Marquis, J. M. (1972). An expedient model for behavior therapy. In A. A. Lazarus (Ed.), *Clinical behavior therapy* (pp. 41–72). New York: Brunner/Mazel.

Martinez, R. (2000). A model for boundary dilemmas: Ethical decision-making in the patient–professional relationship. *Ethical Human Sciences and Services, 2* (1), 43–61.

Masters, W. H., & Johnson, V. E. (1970). *Human sexual inadequacy*. Boston: Little, Brown.

Masters, W. H., & Johnson, V. E. (1976). Principles of the new sex therapy. *American Journal of Psychiatry, 133,* 548–554.

May, R. (1986). Love in the counter-transference: The uses of the therapist's excitement. *Psychoanalytic Psychotherapy, 2,* 167–181.

McLaughlin, J. T. (1995). Touching limits in the analytic dyad. *Psychoanalytic Quarterly, 64,* 433–465.

Meara, N. M., Schmidt, L., & Day, J. D. (1996). Principles and virtues: A foundation for ethical decisions, policies, and character. *The Counseling Psychologist, 24,* 4–77.

Meek v. Holmes, Superior Court (Ariz.), Case No. 93–09341 (1995).

Meissner, W. W. (1996). *The therapeutic alliance.* New Haven, CT: Yale University Press.

Menninger, K., & Holzman, P. (1973). *Theory of psychoanalytic technique* (2nd ed.). New York: Basic Books.

Milgrom, J. H. (1989). Secondary victims of sexual exploitation by counselors and therapists: Some observations. In G. R. Schoener, J. H. Milgrom, J. C. Gonsiorek, E. T. Luepker, & R. M. Conroe (Eds.), *Psychotherapists' sexual involvement with clients: Intervention and prevention* (pp. 235–240). Minneapolis, MN: Walk-In Counseling Center.

Milgrom, J. H. (1992). *Boundaries in professional relationships: A training manual.* Minneapolis, MN: Walk-In Counseling Center.

Miller, A. (1981). *Prisoners of childhood: The drama of the gifted child and the search for the true self.* New York: Basic Books.

Miller, J. B., & Stiver, I. P. (1997). *The healing connection: How women form relationships in therapy and in life.* Boston: Beacon Press.

Miller, P. M., Commons, M. L., & Gutheil, T. G. (2006). Clinicians' perceptions of boundaries in Brazil and United States. *Journal of the American Academy of Psychiatry and the Law, 34,* 33–42.

Mogul, K. M. (1992). Ethics complaints against female psychiatrists. *American Journal of Psychiatry, 149,* 651–653.

Moleski, S. M., & Kiselica, M. S. (2005). Dual relationships: A continuum ranging from the destructive to the therapeutic. *Journal of Counseling and Development, 83,* 3–11.

Monk, G., Winslade, J., Crocket, K., & Epston, D. (Eds.). (1997). *Narrative therapy in practice: The archaeology of hope.* New York: Jossey-Bass.

Moon, L. (2005). Professional and ethical practice in the consulting room with lesbians and gay men. In R. Tribe & J. Morrissey (Eds.), *Handbook of professional and ethical practice for psychologists, counsellors and psychotherapists* (pp. 209–220). Hove, UK: Brunner-Routledge.

Morris v. State Board of Psychology, 697 A.2d 1034, Pa. 1997.

Morrison, J., & Morrison, T. (2001). Psychiatrists disciplined by a state medical board. *American Journal of Psychiatry, 158,* 474–478.

Munn, K. T. (1995). Making room for illness in the practice of psychotherapy. In M. B. Sussman (Ed.), *A perilous calling: The hazards of psychotherapy practice* (pp. 100–112). New York: Wiley.

Nadelson, C., Notman, M., Arons, E., & Feldman, J. (1974). The pregnant therapist. *American Journal of Psychiatry, 131,* 1107–1111.

National Association of Social Workers. (1999). *Code of ethics of the National Association of Social Workers.* Washington, DC: Author.

National Board for Certified Counselors. (2007). *The practice of Internet counseling.* Greensboro, NC: Author.

Nestingen, S. L. (1995). Transforming power: Women who have been exploited by a professional. In J. C. Gonsiorek (Ed.), *Breach of trust: Sexual exploitation by health care professionals and clergy* (pp. 81–90). Thousand Oaks, CA: Sage.

Norcross, J. C. (Ed.). (2002). *Psychotherapy relationships that work: Therapist contributions and responsiveness to patients.* New York: Oxford University Press.

Norcross, J. C., & Guy, J. D., Jr. (Eds.). (2007). *Leaving it at the office: A guide to psychotherapist self-care.* New York: Guilford Press.

Norcross, J. C., Hedges, M., & Prochaska, J. O. (2002). The face of 2010: A Delphi poll on the future of psychotherapy. *Professional Psychology: Research and Practice, 33,* 316–322.

Norris, D. M., Gutheil, T. G., & Strasburger, L. H. (2003). This couldn't happen to me: Boundary problems and sexual misconduct in the psychotherapy relationship. *Psychiatric Services, 54,* 517–522.

Notman, M. T., & Nadelson, C. C. (1994). Psychotherapy with patients who have had sexual relations with a previous therapist. *Journal of Psychotherapy Practice and Research, 3,* 185–193.

Novey, R. (1991). The abstinence of the psychoanalyst. *Bulletin of the Menninger Clinic, 55,* 344–362.

O'Connor-Slimp, A., & Burian, B. K. (1994). Multiple role relationships during internship: Consequences and recommendations. *Professional Psychology: Research and Practice, 25,* 39–45.

Ostrom, C. M. (2006, May 25). Woman ordered to pay physician $2.8 million. *Seattle Times.* Retrieved on November 20, 2007, from http://archives.seattletimes.nwsource.com/cgi-bin/texis.cgi/web/vortex/display?slug=momah25m&date=20060525&query=Woman+ordered+to+pay+physician.

Peele, S. (1998). *The meaning of addiction: An unconventional view.* San Francisco: Jossey-Bass.

Peele, S., & Brodsky, A. (1975). *Love and addiction.* New York: Taplinger.

Peele, S., Brodsky, A., & Arnold, M. (1991). *The truth about addiction and recovery: The life process program for outgrowing destructive habits.* New York: Simon & Schuster.

Peele, S., Bufe, C., & Brodsky A. (2000). *Resisting 12-step coercion: How to fight forced participation in AA, NA, or 12-step treatment.* Tucson, AZ: See Sharp Press.

Penn, L. S. (1986). The pregnant therapist: Transference and countertransference issues. In J. Alpert (Ed.), *Psychoanalysis and women: Contemporary reappraisals* (pp. 287–316). Hillsdale, NJ: Analytic Press.

Perlin, M. L. (1996). Power imbalances in therapeutic relationships. In *The Hatherleigh guide to psychotherapy* (pp. 215–229). New York: Hatherleigh.

Perls, F. (1969). *Gestalt therapy verbatim.* Lafayette, CA: Real People Press.

Perry, J. A. (1976). Physicians' erotic and nonerotic physical involvement with patients. *American Journal of Psychiatry, 133,* 838–840.

Person, E. S. (1985). The erotic transference in women and in men: Differences and consequences. *Journal of the American Academy of Psychoanalysis, 13,* 159–180.

Person, E. S. (2003, July). How to work through erotic transference. *Psychiatric Times,* pp. 29–31.

Peterson, M. R. (1992). *At personal risk: Boundary violations in professional–client relationships.* New York: Norton.

Pizer, B. (1995). When the analyst is ill: Dimensions of self-disclosure. *Psychoanalytic Quarterly, 64,* 466–495.

Plasil, E. (1985). *Therapist.* New York: St. Martin's Press.

Plaut, S. M. (1997). Boundary violations in professional-client relationships: Overview and guidelines for prevention. *Sexual and Marital Therapy, 12,* 77–94.

Pope, K. S. (1988). How clients are harmed by sexual contact with mental health professionals: The syndrome and its prevalence. *Journal of Counseling and Development, 67,* 222–226.

Pope, K. S. (1990a). Therapist–patient sex as sex abuse: Six scientific, professional, and practical dilemmas in addressing victimization and rehabilitation. *Professional Psychology: Research and Practice, 21,* 227–239.

Pope, K. S. (1990b). Therapist–patient sexual involvement: A review of the research. *Clinical Psychology Review, 10,* 477–490.

Pope, K. S. (1991). Dual relationships in psychotherapy. *Ethics and Behavior, 1,* 21–34.

Pope, K. S. (1994). *Sexual involvement with therapists: Patient assessment, subsequent therapy, forensics.* Washington, DC: American Psychological Association.

Pope, K. S. (2001). Sex between therapists and clients. In J. Worrell (Ed.), *Encyclopedia of women and gender: Sex* (pp. 955–962). New York: Academic Press.

Pope, K. S., & Bouhoutsos, J. C. (1986). *Sexual intimacy between therapists and patients.* New York: Praeger.

Pope, K. S., & Keith-Spiegel, P. (in press). A practical approach to boundaries in psychotherapy: Making decisions, bypassing blunders, and mending fences. *Journal of Clinical Psychology: In Session.*

Pope, K. S., Keith-Spiegel, P., & Tabachnick, B. G. (1986). Sexual attraction to clients: The human therapist and the (sometimes) inhuman training system. *American Psychologist, 41,* 147–158.

Pope, K. S., Levenson, H., & Schover, L. R. (1979). Sexual intimacy in psychology training: Results and implications of a national survey. *American Psychologist, 34,* 682–689.

Pope, K. S., Sonne, J. L., & Greene, B. (2006). *What therapists don't talk about and why: Understanding taboos that hurt us and our clients.* Washington, DC: American Psychological Association.

Pope, K. S., Sonne, J. L., & Holroyd. J. (1993). *Sexual feelings in psychotherapy: Explorations for therapists and therapists-in-training.* Washington, DC: American Psychological Association.

Pope, K. S., & Tabachnick, B. G. (1993). Therapists' anger, hate, fear, and sexual feelings: National survey of therapist responses, client characteristics, critical events, formal complaints, and training. *Professional Psychology: Research and Practice, 24,* 142–152.

Pope, K. S., Tabachnick, B. G., & Keith-Spiegel, P. (1987). Ethics of practice: The beliefs and behaviors of psychologists as therapists. *American Psychologist, 42,* 993–1006.

Pope, K. S., & Vasquez, M. J. T. (1998). *Ethics in psychotherapy and counseling: A practical guide* (2nd ed.). San Francisco: Jossey-Bass.

Pope, K. S., & Vasquez, M. J. T. (2007). *Ethics in psychotherapy and counseling: A practical guide* (3rd ed.). San Francisco: Jossey-Bass.

Pope, K. S., & Vetter, V. A. (1991). Prior therapist–patient sexual involvement among patients seen by psychologists. *Psychotherapy, 28,* 429–438.

Pope. K. S., & Wedding, D. (2008). Contemporary challenges and controversies. In R. J. Corsini & D. Wedding (Eds.), *Current psychotherapies* (8th ed., pp. 512–540). Belmont, CA: Thompson Brooks/Cole.

Psychiatrists' Program. (2002, May 17). Beware another kind of boundary violation. *Psychiatric News,* p. 33.

Psychopathology Committee of the Group for the Advancement of Psychiatry. (2001). Reexamination of therapist self-disclosure. *Psychiatric Services, 52,* 1489–1493.

Purcell, R., Powell, M. B., & Mullen, P. E. (2005). Clients who stalk psychologists: Prevalence, methods, and motives. *Professional Psychology: Research and Practice, 36,* 537–543.

Quadrio, C. (1996). Sexual abuse in therapy: Gender issues. *Australian and New Zealand Journal of Psychiatry, 30,* 124–133.

Racker, H. (1968). *Transference and countertransference.* New York: International Universities Press.

Ragsdale, K. H. (Ed.). (1996). *Boundary wars: Intimacy and distance in healing relationships.* Cleveland: Pilgrim Press.

Reamer, F. G. (2001). *Tangled relationships: Managing boundary issues in the human services.* New York: Columbia University Press.

Recupero, P. R. (2005). E-mail and the psychiatrist–patient relationship. *Journal of the American Academy of Psychiatry and the Law, 33,* 465–475.

Recupero, P. R. (2006). Legal concerns for psychiatrists who maintain web sites. *Psychiatric Services, 57,* 450–452.

Recupero, P. R., & Rainey, S. E. (2005a). Forensic aspects of e-therapy. *Journal of Psychiatric Practice, 11,* 405–410.

Recupero, P. R., & Rainey, S. E. (2005b). Informed consent to E-therapy. *American Journal of Psychotherapy, 59,* 319–331.

Regehr, C., & Glancy, G. (1995). Sexual exploitation of patients: Issues for colleagues. *American Journal of Orthopsychiatry, 65,* 194–202.

Renik, O. (1995). The ideal of the anonymous analyst and the problem of self-disclosure. *Psychoanalytic Quarterly, 64,* 466–495.

Rhode Island Senate Bill 96-S-2968 (1996).

Riker, J. H. (1997). *Ethics and the discovery of the unconscious.* Albany, NY: State University of New York.

Riley v. Presnell, 409 Mass. 239, 565 N.E.2d 780, 785–786 (1991).

Rinella, V. J., & Gerstein, A. I. (1994). The development of dual relationships: Power and professional responsibility. *International Journal of Law and Psychiatry, 17,* 225–237.

Roberts-Henry, M. (1995). Criminalization of therapist sexual misconduct in Colorado: An overview and opinion. In J. C. Gonsiorek (Ed.), *Breach of trust: Sexual exploitation by health care professionals and clergy* (pp. 338–347). Thousand Oaks, CA: Sage.

Robinson, G. E., & Stewart, D. E. (1996a). A curriculum on physician–patient sexual misconduct and teacher-learner mistreatment: Part 1. Content. *Canadian Medical Association Journal, 154,* 643–649.

Robinson, G. E., & Stewart, D. E. (1996b). A curriculum on physician–patient sexual misconduct and teacher–learner mistreatment: Part 2. Teaching method. *Canadian Medical Association Journal, 154,* 1021–1025.

Robinson, J. (1993). Sexual contact between gay male clients and male therapists. Unpublished doctoral dissertation, University of Southern California, Los Angeles, CA.

Rodolfa, E. R., Hall T., Holms, V., Davena, A., Komatz, D., Antunez, M., & Hall, A. (1994). The management of sexual feelings in therapy. *Professional Psychology: Research and Practice, 25,* 168–172.

Rodolfa, E. R., Kitzrow, M., Vohra, S., & Wilson, B. (1990). Training interns to respond to sexual dilemmas. *Professional Psychology: Research and Practice, 21,* 313–315.

Roll, S., & Millen, L. (1981). A guide to violating an injunction in psychotherapy: On seeing acquaintances as patients. *Psychotherapy: Theory, Research, and Practice, 18,* 179–187.

Roman, B., & Kay, J. (1997). Residency education on the prevention of physician–patient sexual misconduct. *Academic Psychiatry, 21,* 26–34.

Roth, P. (1974). *My life as a man.* New York: Holt, Rinehart & Winston.

Roy v. Hartogs, 366 N.Y.S. 2d 297, 81 Misc. 2d 350 (1975).

Rudy, D. R. (1986). *Becoming alcoholic: Alcoholics Anonymous and the reality of alcoholism.* Carbondale, IL: Southern Illinois University Press.

Ruskin, P. E., Silver-Aylaian, M., Kling, M. A., Reed, S. A., Bradham, D. D., Hebel, J. R., Barrett, D., Knowles, F. III, & Hauser, P. (2004). Treatment outcomes in depression: Comparison of remote treatment through telepsychiatry to in-person treatment. *American Journal of Psychiatry, 161,* 1471–1476.

Rutter, P. (1989a). *Sex in the forbidden zone: When men in power—therapists, doctors, clergy, teachers, and others—betray women's trust.* New York: Tarcher.

Rutter, P. (1989b, October). Sex in the forbidden zone. *Psychology Today,* pp. 34–40.

Ryder, R., & Hepworth, J. (1990). AAMFT ethical code: "Dual relationships." *Journal of Marital and Family Therapy, 16,* 127–132.

Safran, J. D., & Muran, J. C. (Eds.). (1998). *The therapeutic alliance in brief psychotherapy.* Washington, DC: American Psychological Association Books.

Safran, J. D., & Muran, J. C. (2003). *Negotiating the therapeutic alliance: A relational treatment guide.* New York: Guilford Press.

Safran, J. D., & Segal, Z. V. (1996). *Interpersonal process in cognitive therapy* (2nd ed.). Northvale, NJ: Aronson.

St. Paul Fire & Marine Insurance Co. v. Love, 447 N.W.2d 5 (Minn. Ct. App. 1989); 459 N.W.2d 698 (Minn. 1990).

Samuel, S. E., & Gorton, G. E. (1998). National survey of psychology internship directors regarding education for prevention of psychologist–patient sexual exploitation. *Professional Psychology: Research and Practice, 29,* 86–90.

Samuel, S. E., & Gorton, G. E. (2001). Sexual exploitation: An extreme of professional deception. *American Journal of Forensic Psychiatry, 22,* 63–81.

Saul, L. J. (1962). Erotic transference. *Psychoanalytic Quarterly, 31,* 54–61.

Schachter, J. (1990). Post-termination patient–analyst contact: I. Analysts' attitudes and experience; II. Impact on patients. *International Journal of Psycho-Analysis, 71,* 475–486.

Schachter, J. (1992). Concepts of termination and post-termination patient–analyst contact. *International Journal of Psycho-Analysis, 73,* 137–154.

Schank, J. A., & Skovholt, T. M. (1997). Dual-relationship dilemmas of rural and small-community psychologists. *Professional Psychology: Research and Practice, 28,* 44–49.

Schetky, D. H. (1994, November-December). Boundaries: When the therapist intrudes upon the patient's space. *AACAP News,* pp. 18–19.

Schoener, G. R. (1989a). Administrative safeguards. In G. R. Schoener, J. H. Milgrom, J. C. Gonsiorek, E. T. Luepker, & R. M. Conroe (Eds.), *Psychotherapists' sexual involvement with clients: Intervention and prevention* (pp. 453–467). Minneapolis, MN: Walk-In Counseling Center.

Schoener, G. R. (1989b). A look at the literature. In G. R. Schoener, J. H. Milgrom, J. C. Gonsiorek, E. T. Luepker, & R. M. Conroe (Eds.), *Psychotherapists' sexual involvement with clients: Intervention and prevention* (pp. 11–50). Minneapolis, MN: Walk-In Counseling Center.

Schoener, G. R. (1992). Psychotherapist–patient sexual contact after termination of treatment (letter). *American Journal of Psychiatry, 149,* 981.

Schoener, G. R. (1995a). Assessment of professionals who have engaged in boundary violations. *Psychiatric Annals, 25,* 95–99.

Schoener, G. R. (1995b). Employer/supervisor liability and risk management: An administrator's view. In J. C. Gonsiorek (Ed.), *Breach of trust: Sexual exploitation by health care professionals and clergy* (pp. 300–316). Thousand Oaks, CA: Sage.

Schoener, G. R. (1999). Preventive and remedial boundary training for helping professionals and clergy: Successful approaches and useful tools. *Journal of Sex Education and Therapy, 24,* 209–217.

Schoener, G. R., & Gonsiorek, J. C. (1989). Assessment and development of rehabilitation plans for the therapist. In G. R. Schoener, J. H. Milgrom, J. C. Gonsiorek, E. T. Luepker, & R. M. Conroe (Eds.), *Psychotherapists' sexual involvement with clients: Intervention and prevention* (pp. 401–420). Minneapolis, MN: Walk-In Counseling Center.

Schoener, G. R., Milgrom, J. H., Gonsiorek, J. C., Luepker, E. T., & Conroe, R. M. (Eds.). (1989). *Psychotherapists' sexual involvement with clients: Intervention and prevention.* Minneapolis, MN: Walk-In Counseling Center.

Schultz-Ross, R. A., Goldman, M. J., & Gutheil, T. G. (1992). The dissolution of the dyad in psychiatry: Implications for the understanding of patient–therapist sexual misconduct. *American Journal of Psychotherapy, 46,* 506–514.

Scott, C. D., & Hawk, J. (Eds.). (1986). *Heal thyself: The health of health-care professionals.* New York: Brunner/Mazel.

Searight, H. R., & Campbell, D. C. (1993). Physician–patient sexual contact: Ethical and legal issues and clinical guidelines. *Journal of Family Practice, 36,* 647–653.

Sederer, L. I., & Libby, M. (1995). False allegations of sexual misconduct: Clinical and institutional considerations. *Psychiatric Services, 46,* 160–163.

Sell, J. M., Gottlieb, M. C., & Schoenfeld, L. (1986). Ethical considerations of social/romantic relationships with present and former clients. *Professional Psychology: Research and Practice, 17,* 504–508.

Shackelford, J. F. (1989). Affairs in the consulting room: A review of the literature on therapist–patient sexual intimacy. *Journal of Psychology and Christianity, 8*(4), 26–43.

Shepard, M. (1971). *The love treatment: Sexual intimacy between patients and psychotherapists.* New York: Wyden.

Shopland, S. N., & VandeCreek, L. (1991). Sex with ex-clients: Theoretical rationales for prohibition. *Ethics and Behavior, 1,* 35–44.

Shor, J., & Sanville, J. (1974). Erotic provocations and dalliances in psychotherapeutic practice: Some clinical cues for preventing and repairing therapist–patient collusions. *Clinical Social Work Journal, 2,* 83–95.

Shuman, D. W., Greenberg, S. A., Heilbrun, K., & Foote, W. E. (1998). An immodest proposal: Should treating mental health professionals be barred from testifying about their patients? *Behavioral Sciences and the Law, 16,* 509–523.

Siegel, L. (2004, December 13). The attraction of repulsion. *The New Republic,* pp. 40–47.

Simmons v. U.S., 805 F.2d 1363 (9th Cir. 1986).

Simon, G. E., Ludman, E. J., Tutty, S., Operskalski, B., & Von Korff, M. (2004). Telephone psychotherapy and telephone care management for primary care patients starting antidepressant treatment: A randomized controlled trial. *Journal of the American Medical Association, 292,* 935–942.

Simon, R. I. (1991a). The practice of psychotherapy: Legal liabilities of an "impossible" profession. In R. I. Simon (Ed.), *American Psychiatric Press Review of Clinical Psychiatry and the Law* (Vol. 2, pp. 3–91). Washington, DC: American Psychiatric Press.

Simon, R. I. (1991b). Psychological injury caused by boundary violation precursors to therapist-patient sex. *Psychiatric Annals, 21,* 614–619.

Simon, R. I. (1992). Treatment boundary violations: Clinical, ethical, and legal considerations. *Bulletin of the American Academy of Psychiatry and Law, 20,* 269–288.

Simon, R. I. (1994). Transference in therapist–patient sex: The illusion of patient improvement and consent: Part 1. *Psychiatric Annals, 24,* 509–515.

Simon, R. I. (1995). The natural history of therapist sexual misconduct: Identification and prevention. *Psychiatric Annals, 25,* 90–94.

Simon, R. I. (1999). Therapist–patient sex: From boundary violations to sexual misconduct. *Psychiatric Clinics of North America, 22,* 31–47.

Simon, R. I. (2001). Commentary: Treatment boundaries—flexible guidelines, not rigid standards. *Journal of the American Academy of Psychiatry and the Law, 29,* 287–289.

Simon, R. I., & Williams, I. C. (1999). Maintaining treatment boundaries in small communities and rural areas. *Psychiatric Services, 50,* 1440–1446.

Singer, E. (1977). The fiction of analytic anonymity. In K. A. Frank (Ed.), *The Human dimension in psychoanalytic practice* (pp. 181–192). NY: Grune & Stratton.

Slovenko, R. (1991). Undue familiarity or undue damages? *Psychiatric Annals, 21,* 598–610.

Smith, B., & Gutheil, T. G. (1993). Unusual patient case report: A patient's false claim of therapist sexual misconduct. *Hospital and Community Psychiatry, 44,* 793–794.

Smith, D., & Fitzpatrick, M. (1995). Patient–therapist boundary issues: An integrative review of theory and research. *Professional Psychology: Research and Practice, 26,* 499–506.

Smith, E. W. L. (1985). *The body in psychotherapy.* Jefferson, NC: MacFarland.

Smith, J. T., & Bisbing, S. B. (1988). *Sexual exploitation by health care and other professionals* (2nd ed.). Potomac, MD: Legal Medicine Press.

Smith, S. (1977). The golden fantasy: A regressive reaction to separation anxiety. *International Journal of Psychoanalysis, 58,* 311–324.

Smolar, A. I. (2002). Reflections on gifts in the therapeutic setting: The gift from patient to therapist. *American Journal of Psychotherapy, 56,* 27–45.

Smolar, A. I. (2003). When we give more: Reflections on intangible gifts from therapist to patient. *American Journal of Psychotherapy, 57,* 300–323.

Smolar, A. I., & Akhtar, S. (2002). Why no sex? *American Journal of Psychotherapy, 56,* 260–261.

Snyder, S. (1986). Pseudologia fantastica in the borderline patient. *American Journal of Psychiatry, 143,* 1287–1289.

Sonne, J. L. (2005). Nonsexual multiple relationships: A practical decision-making model for clinicians. Available at *http://kspope.com/site/multiple-relationships.php* (accessed on August 15, 2007).

Sonne, J. L., Borys, D. S., Haviland, M. G., & Ermshar, A. (1998, March). Subsequent therapists' reports on the effects of nonsexual multiple relationships on psychotherapy patients: An exploratory study. Paper presented at the annual convention of the California Psychological Association, Pasadena, CA.

Sonne, J. L., Meyer, C. B., Borys, D., & Marshall, V. (1985). Clients' reactions to sexual intimacy in therapy. *American Journal of Orthopsychiatry, 55,* 183–189.

Sonnenberg, S. M. (1992). Psychotherapist–patient sexual contact after termination of treatment (letter). *American Journal of Psychiatry, 149,* 983–984.

Spindler, A. C. (1992). Psychotherapist–patient sexual contact after termination of treatment (letter). *American Journal of Psychiatry, 149,* 984–985.

Spruiell, V. (1983). The rules and frames of the psychoanalytic situation. *Psychoanalytic Quarterly, 52,* 1–33.

Stake, J. E., & Oliver, J. (1991). Sexual contact and touching between therapist and client: A survey of psychologists' attitudes and behavior. *Professional Psychology: Research and Practice, 22,* 297–307.

Stark, M. (1995). The therapist as recipient of the patient's relentless entitlement. In M. B. Sussman (Ed.), *A perilous calling: The hazards of psychotherapy practice* (pp. 188–199). New York: Wiley.

Stone, A. A. (1983). Sexual misconduct by psychiatrists: The ethical and clinical dilemma of confidentiality. *American Journal of Psychiatry, 140,* 195–197.

Stone, A. A., & MacCourt, D. C. (1999). Insurance coverage for undue familiarity: Law, policy, and economic reality. In J. D. Bloom, C. C. Nadelson, & M. T. Notman (Eds.), *Physician sexual misconduct* (pp. 37–88). Washington, DC: American Psychiatric Press.

Stone, M. H. (1975). Management of unethical behavior in a psychiatric hospital staff. *American Journal of Psychotherapy, 29,* 391–401.

Stone, M. H. (1976). Boundary violations between therapist and patient. *Psychiatric Annals, 6,* 670–677.

Storring, V. (Producer). (1991). *My doctor, my lover* (Videotape). Boston: Frontline Production.

Strasburger, L. H. (1999). "There oughta be a law": Criminalization of psychotherapist–patient sex as a social policy dilemma. In J. D. Bloom, C. C. Nadelson, & M. T. Notman (Eds.), *Physician sexual misconduct* (pp. 19–36). Washington, DC: American Psychiatric Press.

Strasburger, L. H., Gutheil, T. G., & Brodsky, A. (1997). On wearing two hats: Role conflict in serving as both psychotherapist and expert witness. *American Journal of Psychiatry, 154,* 488–456.

Strasburger, L. H., Jorgenson, L., & Randles, R. (1991). Criminalization of psychotherapist–patient sex. *American Journal of Psychiatry, 148,* 859–863.

Strasburger, L. H., Jorgenson, L., & Sutherland, P. (1992). The prevention of psychotherapist sexual misconduct: Avoiding the slippery slope. *American Journal of Psychotherapy, 46,* 544–555.

Strean, H. S. (1991). Extra-analytic contact can disrupt an analysis. *Psychodynamic Letter, 1* (3), 1–4.

Strean, H. S. (1993). *Therapists who have sex with their patients: Treatment and recovery.* New York: Brunner/Mazel.

Stricker, G., & Fisher, M. (Eds.). (1990). *Self-disclosure in the therapeutic relationship.* New York: Plenum.

Sussman, M. B. (1992). *A curious calling: Unconscious motivations for practicing psychotherapy.* Northvale, NJ: Aronson.

Sussman, M. B. (Ed.). (1995a). *A perilous calling: The hazards of psychotherapy practice.* New York: Wiley.

Sussman, M. B. (1995b). Intimations of mortality. In M. B. Sussman (Ed.), *A perilous calling: The hazards of psychotherapy practice* (pp. 15–25). New York: Wiley.

Szekacs, J. (1985). Impaired spatial structures. *International Journal of Psychoanalysis, 66,* 193–199.

Talan, K. H. (1989). Gifts in psychoanalysis: Theoretical and technical issues. *Psychoanalytic Study of the Child, 44,* 149–163.

Tansey, M. J., & Burke, W. F. (1989). *Understanding countertransference: From projective identification to empathy.* Hillsdale, NJ: Analytic Press.

Tauber, E. S. (1954). Exploring the therapeutic use of countertransference data. *Psychiatry, 17,* 331–336.

Taylor, B. J., & Wagner, N. N. (1976). Sex between therapists and clients: A review and analysis. *Professional Psychology, 7,* 593–601.

Thompson, T. L. (1989, October). Bias and conflict of interest alleged in handling of malpractice suit. *Psychiatric Times,* pp. 1, 26.

Twemlow, S. W. (1995a). The psychoanalytical foundations of a dialectical approach to the victim/victimizer relationship. *Journal of the American Academy of Psychoanalysis, 23,* 543–558.

Twemlow, S. W. (1995b). Traumatic object relations configurations seen in victim/victimizer relationships. *Journal of the American Academy of Psychoanalysis, 23,* 559–575.

Twemlow, S. W. (1997). Exploitation of patients: Themes in the psychopathology of their therapists. *American Journal of Psychotherapy, 51,* 357–375.

Twemlow, S. W., & Gabbard, G. O. (1989). The lovesick therapist. In G. O. Gabbard (Ed.)., *Sexual exploitation in professional relationships* (pp. 71–87). Washington, DC: American Psychiatric Press.

Tyler, J. M., & Sabella, R. A. (2003). *Using technology to improve counseling practice: A primer for the 21st century.* Alexandria, VA: American Counseling Association.

Van der Kolk, B. A. (1989). The compulsion to repeat the trauma: Reenactment, revictimization, and masochism. *Psychiatric Clinics of North America, 12,* 389–411.

Vasquez, M. J. T. (1991). Sexual intimacies with clients after termination: Should a prohibition be explicit? *Ethics and Behavior, 1,* 45–61.

Viederman, M. (1991). The real person of the analyst and his role in the process of psychoanalytic cure. *Journal of the American Psychoanalytic Association, 39,* 451–489.

Wachtel, P. L. (2007). *Relational theory and the practice of psychotherapy.* New York: Guilford Press.

Waldinger, R. J. (1994). Boundary crossings and boundary violations: Thoughts on navigating a slippery slope. *Harvard Review of Psychiatry, 2,* 225–227.

Waldinger, R. J., & Gunderson, J. G. (1987). *Effective psychotherapy with borderline patients.* Washington, DC: American Psychiatric Press.

Walen, S., DiGiuiseppe, R., & Dryden, W. (1992). *A practitioner's guide to rational-emotive therapy.* New York: Oxford University Press.

Walker, E., & Young, T. D. (1986). *A killing cure.* New York: Henry Holt.

Walker, R., & Clark, J. J. (1999). Heading off boundary problems: Clinical supervision as risk management. *Psychiatric Services, 50,* 1435–1439.

Weiner, M. F. (1983). *Therapist disclosure: The use of self in psychotherapy* (2nd ed.). Baltimore, MD: University Park Press.

Weiner, M. F. (2002). Reexamining therapist self-disclosure (letter). *Psychiatric Services, 53,* 769.

Welfel, E. R. (2002). *Ethics in counseling and psychotherapy: Standards, research, and emerging issues* (2nd ed.). Pacific Grove, CA: Brooks/Cole.

Welt, S. R., & Herron, W. G. (1990). *Narcissism and the psychotherapist.* New York: Guilford Press.

Wettstein, R. (2001). Ethics and forensic psychiatry. In Ethics Committee of the American Psychiatric Association (Eds.), *Ethics primer of the American Psychiatric Association* (pp. 65–73). Washington, DC: American Psychiatric Publishing.

Williams, M. H. (1992). Exploitation and inference: Mapping the damage from therapist–patient sexual involvement. *American Psychologist, 47,* 412–421.

Williams, M. H. (1995). How useful are clinical reports concerning the consequences of therapist–patient sex? *American Journal of Psychotherapy, 49,* 237–243.

Williams, M. H. (1997). Boundary violations: Do some contended standards of care fail to encompass commonplace procedures of humanistic, behavioral, and eclectic psychotherapies? *Psychotherapy, 34,* 238–249.

Williams, M. H. (2000). Victimized by "victims": A taxonomy of antecedents of false complaints against psychotherapists. *Professional Psychology: Research and Practice, 31,* 75–81.

Willison, B. G., & Masson, R. L. (1986). The role of touch in therapy: An adjunct to communication. *Journal of Counseling and Development, 64,* 497–500.

Winnicott, D. W. (1949). Hate in the countertransference. *International Journal of Psychoanalysis, 30,* 69–74.

Winnicott, D. W. (1965). *The maturational processes and the facilitating environment: Studies in the theory of emotional development.* New York: International Universities Press.

Wohlberg, J. W. (1990, February 10). *The psychology of therapist sexual misconduct.* Presented at panel discussion, "Psychological Aspects of Therapist Sexual Abuse," Boston Psychoanalytic Society and Institute, Boston.

Wohlberg, J. W. (1997). Sexual abuse in the therapeutic setting: What do victims really want? *Psychoanalytic Inquiry, 17,* 329–348.

Wohlberg, J. W., McCraith, D. B., & Thomas, D. R. (1999). Sexual misconduct and the victim/survivor: A look from the inside out. In J. D. Bloom, C. C. Nadelson, & M. T. Notman (Eds.), *Physician sexual misconduct* (pp. 181–204). Washington, DC: American Psychiatric Press.

Wohlberg, J. W., & Reid, E. A. (1996). Helen Bramson: Treatment after sexual abuse by a mental health practitioner. *Bulletin of the Menninger Clinic, 60,* 52–61.

Woody, R. H. (1998). Bartering for psychological services. *Professional Psychology: Research and Practice, 29,* 174–178.

Yenney, S. L., & American Psychological Association Practice Directorate. (1994). *Business strategies for a caring profession: A practitioner's guidebook.* Washington, DC: American Psychological Association Books.

Younggren, J. N. (2002). Ethical decision-making and dual relationships. Available at *http://kspope.com/dual/younggren.php* (accessed on May 13, 2007).

Younggren, J. N., & Gottlieb, M. C. (2004). Managing risk when contemplating multiple relationships. *Professional Psychology: Research and Practice, 35,* 255–260.

Zagha v. Kroplick, Los Angeles County (CA) Superior Court, Case No. LC 042770 (2000).

Zelen, S. L. (1985). Sexualization of therapeutic relationships: The dual vulnerability of patient and therapist. *Psychotherapy, 22,* 178–185.

Zipkin v. Freeman, 436 S.W.2d 753 (Mo. 1968).

Index